# ALFALFA TO IVY

# ALFALFA TO IVY

## *Memoir of a Harvard Medical School Dean*

Joseph B. Martin

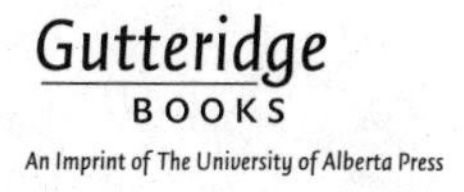

Published by

The University of Alberta Press
Ring House 2
Edmonton, Alberta, Canada T6G 2E1
www.uap.ualberta.ca



Library and Archives Canada Cataloguing in Publication

Martin, Joseph B., 1938–
Alfalfa to ivy : memoir of a Harvard Medical School
dean / Joseph B. Martin.
Includes bibliographical references and index.
Issued also in electronic format.
ISBN 978-1-55195-701-2 (bound).--ISBN 978-1-55195-700-5 (pbk.)

1. Martin, Joseph B., 1938-. 2. Neurobiologists--Massachusetts--Boston--Biography. 3. Deans (Education)--Massachusetts--Boston--Biography. 4. Harvard Medical School--Employees--Biography. 5. Mennonites--Alberta--Duchess--Biography. I. Title.

QP353.4.M37A3 2011 616.80092 C2011-905838-3

First edition, first printing, 2011.
Printed and bound in Canada by Houghton Boston Printers, Saskatoon, Saskatchewan.
Copyediting and Proofreading by Meaghan Craven.
Maps by Wendy Johnson.
Indexing by Noeline Bridge.



The University of Alberta Press is committed to protecting our natural environment. As part of our efforts, this book is printed on Enviro Paper: it contains 100% post-consumer recycled fibres and is acid- and chlorine-free.

The University of Alberta Press gratefully acknowledges the support received for its publishing program from The Canada Council for the Arts. The University of Alberta Press also gratefully acknowledges the financial support of the Government of Canada through the Canada Book Fund (CBF) and the Government of Alberta through the Alberta Multimedia Development Fund (AMDF) for its publishing activities.

Canada

Canada Council for the Arts
Conseil des Arts du Canada

Government of Alberta

*To Rachel Ann, my partner,*
*whose equipoise guides and sustains.*

# CONTENTS

# FOREWORD

*Professor David Hubel*
*Harvard Medical School*

WHEN JOE MARTIN ASKED ME to read over the manuscript of this book I was surprised and flattered. And, when I got back to him a week later to tell him how much I enjoyed reading the material, I was amazed that he asked if I would write a foreword to it.

My background, of hands-on research with only one brief foray into administration, could not have differed more from Joe's long and successful career of leadership in both medical administration and research. After some reflection, however, I can see the striking similarities between our career trajectories. We were both born in Canada of parents who were US citizens; and so we both grew up as dual citizens, with consequent advantages and disadvantages of both citizenships—not the least being subject to military service in both countries. Both of us went to school in Canada—from elementary school through college and medical school. Elementary schools and high schools were small; we walked to our schools, which never closed because of bad weather. Our schools were run and financed by provinces rather than immediate municipalities, so schools in poor neighborhoods did not suffer the way they do in the United

States. After medical school we both did protracted residencies in neurology and in research, at starvation wages or no wages at all. We both did stints at the Montreal Neurological Institute (MNI) and the Montreal General Hospital ("MGH North"), and we both ended up, finally, at Harvard. Today we are both semi-retired members of the Harvard Medical School Department of Neurobiology. There the similarities end. Joe's career rose to top-level administration positions, with brief, highly successful lapses into research, which resulted in his major role in tracking down the gene locus for the defect responsible for Huntington's Chorea. And my dogged and long career in research on the visual cortex was interrupted, if only for some months, by a not-too-successful lapse in administration.

Along the path to Harvard, however, we both worked on farms—milked cows, hitched up horses, fed pigs, chased roosters.

In coming to Harvard, in 1958, from Walter Reed and Johns Hopkins, I found the change depressing. The informality and friendliness of Hopkins contrasted with the pomposity and stiffness of Harvard Medical School. (Torsten Wiesel and I were welcomed by being demoted from the assistant professorships we enjoyed at Hopkins to an obscure position called "associate," to make the point that Harvard had high standards.) But of the leadership of HMS over the years I have had nothing but praise. I experienced the tenures of four deans. George Berry, grouchy and determined, ran the school with the sole help of a financial genius, Henry Meadow. Bob Ebert was kind and flexible, so unable to say "no" that I at times felt sorry for him. (Without Bob, our Department of Neurobiology would never have come about.) Dan Tosteson, always friendly and supportive, reformed the teaching at HMS completely. Finally, Joe Martin!

For me, our paths crossed in an important way twice in Joe's ten-year term as dean. The chairmanship of my department, neurobiology, fell vacant when Gerry Fischbach left in 1998. Joe Martin, who had just arrived as dean, wanted to recruit Carla Shatz as Gerry's successor. Carla had been my first graduate student in the 1960s, and I looked forward enthusiastically to her coming. But there was a hitch: Carla needed more space than was available, and the extra adjacent space she would need was occupied by my office and lab. Moving to a different floor in a different building promised to be a huge pain, and I was determined to stay put. Persuading me to move fell to Joe, and I can still hear him saying, "Put yourself in my place." In the course of our discussions, Joe's reasonableness and gentlemanly attitude won me over. I gave up, and Carla came. I ended up far better off, with better quarters in a new building, and the school even agreed to make operable what once were sealed windows so that I could enjoy fresh summer breezes.

My other major encounter with Joe occurred when I retired as University Professor. I was determined to keep on with research and needed to keep some funds amassed over the years through various awards. Minor HMS administrators wanted to grab those funds to support the ever-growing list of medical school deans, but a five-minute meeting with Joe quickly settled that difficulty, and I kept the funds.

I was fascinated to read the long story of Joe's administrative successes and travails, especially as I, too, had travails, though on a far smaller scale and a decade or so earlier, both at the Montreal Neurological Institute and at Harvard. I know, or knew, many of the *dramatis personae* at both places who are mentioned in this book. Having been at the MNI, at the bottom of the hierarchy, and at Harvard during a half-century at levels from bottom to close to the top, I know of no better story than Joe's telling of the deep satisfactions and the frequent deep frustrations of administrative leadership.

At the MNI, I was an assistant resident on the neurology service and well remember how neurologists were made to feel like poor cousins of the surgeons. Wilder Penfield, known as "the Chief," was a strong, outwardly kind leader who had the status of a demigod. In Montreal the relationship between McGill University and the hospitals (the Montreal Neurological Institute, the Royal Victoria Hospital and the Montreal General Hospital) must have been complex, but there can hardly be an institution with more complex and baffling relationships than the ones between Harvard Medical School and its associated hospitals. The extent to which Joe was able to navigate these waters tells us much about his patience, his serene disposition and his common sense.

Joe had adventures, tangles and great successes at every step in his amazing journey: at the Montreal Neurological Institute, at the Massachusetts General Hospital, at the University of California at San Francisco as dean of the medical school and then chancellor, and finally back at Harvard Medical School. Bench research, as both Joe and I can attest, can be full of frustrations and successes, and I find it fascinating to be reminded that the same is true of top-level leadership.

PROFESSOR DAVID HUBEL is Professor Emeritus of Neurobiology, Harvard Medical School, and Nobel Laureate in Physiology or Medicine in 1981 for work with Torsten Wiesel on elucidating the function of the visual system.

# ACKNOWLEDGMENTS

THE DEEP GRATITUDE I WANT TO EXPRESS to all the colleagues, friends and family members who contributed to this manuscript transcends the customary ritualistic gesture of ordinary acknowledgments. Almost every page of what follows has been touched by their ideas, suggestions and scrutiny, reflecting the role each has played in my life's journey. Not only did discussions with friends and colleagues here in Boston, and with others across the North American continent, encourage me to tell my story but these conversations, replete with recollections and insights, have also enriched my narrative.

In the first two chapters I've relied on written and oral family histories. I am grateful to Gerald Brunk, whose knowledge of Mennonite history guided the accuracy of my account in the first chapter. In reconstructing early family life and circumstances in Duchess, *Tapping the Bow* by R. Groos and L.N. Kramer proved most helpful in providing a valuable account of the impact of irrigation in the region; contributions from Dick Martin and his wife June were also especially helpful, as were conversations with J. Robert Ramer and with Sam Martin and his wife Beulah. The story of Sam Martin, on which I expand in the second chapter, is also found in several online publications and in audio format (see chapter two n.2). I am especially grateful to Darvin Martin for reading and commenting on the first few chapters of the manuscript and for providing a sage guided tour of the ancestral homesteads in Lancaster, Pennsylvania. For the chapters that describe my academic journey from Montreal to my final return to Boston, I am grateful to many colleagues who took the time to read parts or all of the sections. For material dealing with my years in Montreal, the perspectives and unique insights that Garth Bray, Don Baxter and Don Lawrence generously offered were immeasurably enriching, as were Rich Murphy's comments on the later history of the Montreal Neurological Institute. Equally enriching was the forthcoming publication entitled *Neurology at the Montreal General Hospital* by Garth Bray and Don Baxter, as well as Preston Robb's 1989 publication, *The Development of Neurology at McGill.*

Kay Bander, whose support and direction I was fortunate enough to enjoy at the MGH during the 1980s, scrutinized the material describing my years at the MGH, as well as the entire manuscript, criticizing and encouraging me with many helpful suggestions. Three profoundly helpful meetings with Susan Leeman also clarified many issues relating to my years at the MGH, for which I remain grateful. For the history of the MGH, the 1983 publication *The Massachusetts General Hospital 1955–1980* edited by Benjamin Castleman, MD, David C. Crockett and S.B. Sutton was a very useful resource. Of great value also were the suggestions made by Howard Goodman and Ed Kaplan regarding the Hoechst agreement with the MGH.

The chapter on Huntington's disease benefited from perspectives of several colleagues who were willing to read the chapter and comment on it. In particular, I am grateful to Rudy Tanzi, Kurt Isselbacher, Lou Semonovich, Alex Rich, Phil Leder, Adrian Ivinson, Steve Hauser, Verne Caviness, Chris Gates and Mike Brownstein, who also read many other sections of the manuscript. I was assisted by Verne in shaping this chapter's conclusion. Discussion with Jim Gusella helped clarify important dates and events. The chapter that recounts my life at UCSF could not be what it is if it weren't for Steve Hauser, Bruce

Spaulding and Holly Smith. Their combined wisdom, advice and analyses were invaluable in structuring one of the most challenging periods of my career.

For the chapters that relate to my deanship at Harvard Medical School (HMS), I relied on the input of many colleagues to whom I extend my gratitude: Paul Russell, David Nathan, and Barbara McNeil for their unique perspectives; Jules Dienstag, who gave generously of his knowledge and who also read other chapters of the manuscript; Dan Federman, whose full knowledge of the New Pathway I have welcomed, as I have his willingness to read and comment on the entire manuscript; Margaret Dale, Joyce Brinton and Christopher T. Walsh, who advised me on the material related to conflict of interest, as did Hamilton Moses, who was also kind enough to read and comment on this and other chapters. I have also benefited from the 2001 publication *Conflict of Interest in Medical Research, Education, and Practice*, edited by Bernard Lo and Marilyn J. Field and from Jeffrey Toobin's 2008 book entitled *The Nine: Inside the Sacred World of the Supreme Court*. For aspects of the history of Harvard Medical School, two of Nora Nercessian's publications were useful resources: *A Legacy So Enduring*, outlining the transformation of the Administration Building since its construction to the year 2000, and *Against All Odds*, recounting the predicament and lives of graduates of Harvard Medical School of African descent at HMS before affirmative action. I gained information about the founding of the Alberta Heritage Foundation for Medical Research from Robert Lampard's *Alberta's Medical History*.

My gratitude is also extended to colleagues and friends who agreed to read the full manuscript from various perspectives: Stacey Smith, who read and commented on several chapters; Tim Johnson, Fred Lovejoy, Joseph Smucker, Lorraine Caristo, Don Gibbons, Verne Caviness and Robert Neal, all of whom read the full manuscript and made insightful suggestions. I shared the entirety of chapters eight through eleven with my friend and colleague Larry Summers.

Looking back, a few individuals stand out among the many who influenced my career decisions. Each exemplified what I hoped to become. Lionel McLeod urged me to seek an academic career; Joseph Foley introduced me to the Big Leagues; Seymour

Reichlin provided my grounding in scientific scholarship; and Donald Baxter gave me my first job, with the assurance that I would have time and resources to do my own work.

A number of outstanding mentors and colleagues helped me along the way. Albert Aguayo, Garth Bray, Charles A. Sanders, Haile T. Debas, Lloyd Hollingsworth (Holly) Smith and Eugene Braunwald each entered my academic life at critical points. Larry Summers was the best boss I ever had.

Throughout the time it took to write this book, my mother has been there to listen to my descriptions and add to the family history. My father did not live long enough to see the completed work, but he has been a major contributor—albeit posthumously—through his rich and detailed oral and written accounts of many aspects of life in Alberta.

The project would never have been realized without the kind wisdom and guidance provided by Nora Nercessian, who, over the course of a year commented on the content and organization of the text. Her deep knowledge of the communities at HMS and Harvard University, based on her experiences of nearly twenty-five years at Harvard, gave me new perspectives on the school, its students and alumni, and the school's relationship with affiliated hospitals and the university. I am grateful to Patricia Cleary for her expert copy editing of the entire manuscript. Vanessa Osgood provided outstanding editorial control of the process.

I am grateful to University of Alberta President Indira Samarasekera, who when I contacted her in June 2010, encouraged me to work with University of Alberta Press (UAP) to publish my memoir. UAP had always been my first choice and the response I received from Publisher Linda Cameron encouraged me to proceed. My thanks to Alan Brownoff, Cathie Crooks, and Mary Lou Roy, each of whom diligently worked to produce the best possible outcome. Of great benefit to me was the skillful advice and editorial assistance of Meaghan Craven, who confirmed my organizational outline and provided astute guidance for generating a coherent story.

Last, but not least, I am grateful to Rachel, who kept me focused, who read my drafts, who understood the message I wanted to share with my readers and helped me say what I wanted to say. She has stood by me, throughout this writing as throughout my life's journey, and has been the inspiration that has driven me forward. She has been the anchor of my life through easy times and foul weather; she has listened, probed, pushed and urged patience when impulsive acts were my foil.

Finally, I cannot conclude without a note of gratitude to our four children.

Our years in Belmont, Massachusetts, were formative for our four children. Each was born in a different city, but all graduated from Belmont High School, although our oldest son Bradley only lived there two years before leaving for college.

Brad chose to attend Cornell University in Ithaca, New York, graduating with a degree in chemical engineering. After obtaining an MBA from Boston University, he was hired by Analog Devices, a Massachusetts-based semiconductor company. He married Karen Lenington, who grew up and attended school in Lincoln, Massachusetts. Karen attended the University of Massachusetts and Bentley College gaining a degree in marketing/management. She then completed an MBA degree at Bentley College. They have two children, Josh and Courtney.

Melanie attended Brown University and the Stanford University School of Medicine. An interest in primary care led her to a primary care / internal medicine residency program at Santa Clara Valley Medical Center in San Jose, California. Melanie met Jeff Fowler at Stanford, where he earned a PHD in chemical engineering. Jeff works at Syngenta, an agrochemical company based in Greensboro, North Carolina, where Melanie and Jeff have lived for the past twelve years. Melanie directs a clinic for underinsured and Medicaid patients in High Point, North Carolina. They have two children, Gareth and Charlotte.

Doug attended McGill University in Montreal and the University of Pennsylvania School of Medicine. After residency in internal medicine at the Brigham and Women's Hospital in Boston, he joined McKinsey & Company and then Leerink Swann in Boston, where he works as a medical consultant to pharmaceutical and biotechnology companies.

Doug married Elizabeth Goodz, who he met in Montreal. Their marriage ended in divorce after ten years. We are blessed with their two sons, Cole and Dylan.

Neil attended my alma mater, the University of Rochester. After graduating with a joint degree in psychology and business he obtained a certificate in graphic design from Clark University and worked as a graphic designer for a mutual fund company. He is currently associate creative director at MMB, an advertising company in Boston. Neil married Clare Conroy, a nurse, and they have two children, Luke and Lila.

Rachel and I feel fortunate to be grandparents. "If we'd known they would be so much fun we would have had them first!" And from Joan McIntosh, "They say genes skip generations. Maybe that's why grandparents find their grandchildren so likeable."

# ABBREVIATIONS

AAMC—Association of American Medical Colleges
ACOs—accountable care organizations
AD—Alzheimer's disease
AHFMR—Alberta Heritage Foundation for Medical Research
ALS—amyotrophic lateral sclerosis (Louis Gehrig's disease)
AMA—American Medical Association
BALSA—Bay Area Life Sciences Alliance
BI—Broad Institute
BIDMC—Beth Israel Deaconess Medical Center
(formerly BIH—Beth Israel Hospital)
BML—Boston Medical Library
BWH—Brigham and Women's Hospital
CAG—community advisory group
CEQA—*California Environmental Quality Act*
CIRM—California Institute for Regenerative Medicine
CME—continuing medical education
CML—chronic myelogenous leukemia
CO—conscientious objector
COI—conflict of interest
CPR—Canadian Pacific Railway
CRO—clinical research organization
CT—computerized tomography
CTSC—(Harvard) Clinical and Translational Science Center
DFCI—Dana-Farber Cancer Institute
DF/HCC—Dana-Farber/Harvard Cancer Center
DNA—deoxyribonucleic acid
EIR—environmental impact report
EMC—Eastern Mennonite College
FAS—Faculty of Arts and Sciences
FDA—Food and Drug Administration

FMGs—foreign medical graduates
FTE—full-time equivalent
GCRCs—General Clinical Research Centers
GH—growth hormone
GHRH—growth-hormone-releasing hormone
HCA—Hospital Corporation of America
HCRI—Harvard Clinical Research Institute
HD—Huntington's disease
HHMI—Howard Hughes Medical Institute
HIID—Harvard International Institute of Development
HILS—Harvard Integrated Life Sciences
HIM—Harvard Institute of Medicine
HMC—Harvard Medical Center
HMI—Harvard Medical International
HMS—Harvard Medical School
HNDC—Harvard NeuroDiscovery Center (formerly HCNR—Harvard Center for Neurodegeneration and Repair)
HPIM—*Harrison's Principles of Internal Medicine*
HST—Health Sciences and Technology
INSERM—Institut national de la santé et de la recherche médicale
IOM—Institute of Medicine
IP—intellectual property
JCSW—Joint Committee on the Status of Women
LCME—Liaison Committee on Medical Education
LDDN—(HNDC) Laboratory for Drug Discovery in Neurodegeneration
LGBT—Lesbian, Gay, Bisexual and Transgender
LHRH—luteinizing-hormone-releasing hormone
LOD—log of the (probability) odds
LRDP—long-range development plan
MCC—Mennonite Central Committee
MCH—Montreal Children's Hospital
MCOB—Mennonite Congregation of Boston
MDS—Mennonite Disaster Service
MGH North—Montreal General Hospital
MGH South—Massachusetts General Hospital
MIT—Massachusetts Institute of Technology

MNH—Montreal Neurological Hospital
MNI—Montreal Neurological Institute
MOU—memorandum of understanding
MRI—magnetic resonance imaging
MWRA—Massachusetts Water Resources Authority
NCI—National Cancer Institute
NEDH—New England Deaconess Hospital
NERCE—New England Regional Center of Excellence
NIA—National Institute on Aging
NIH—National Institutes of Health
NINDS—National Institute of Neurological Disease and Stroke
NSF—National Science Foundation
OTL—Office of Technology Licensing
PCE—principal clinical experience
PEPFAR—President Bush's Emergency Aid Package for African HIV (Human Immunodeficiency Virus)-AIDS (Acquired Immune Deficiency Syndrome) Research
PET scanning—positron emission tomography scanning
PIBS—program in biological sciences
PSA—prostate-specific antigen
RFLPS—restriction fragment length polymorphisms
RFP—request for proposal
RVH—Royal Victoria Hospital
SFGH—San Francisco General Hospital
SFVAMC—San Francisco Veteran's Administration Hospital
SNPS—single necleotide polymorphisms
SOD1—superoxide dismutase type 1
SPORE—Specialized Program of Research Excellence
TMEC—Daniel C. Tosteson Medical Education Center
TRH—thyrotropin-releasing hormone
TSH—thyroid stimulating hormone
UC—University of California
UCSF—University of California, San Francisco
UPSCE—University Planning Committee on Science and Engineering
USDA—United States Department of Agriculture
Z-DNA—reverse helix, left-handed DNA

## ONE

# *The Journey from Bern to Duchess*

MY GRANDFATHER, SAMUEL MARTIN, migrated from Pennsylvania to the prairies of Alberta, Canada, after World War I. The town he chose for his family was Duchess, a tiny outpost along the newly formed Canadian Pacific Railway (CPR), one hundred miles southeast of Calgary. I grew up along a two-lane gravel highway near Duchess that served as the main route from neighboring Saskatchewan westward to Calgary, and on to Edmonton, the provincial capital. During World War II, it was a principal route for US troops and armored vehicles headed to or from Alaska, for which it was dubbed the "Alaska Highway."

Poignant in my recollections of the World War II era was the arrest and imprisonment of my uncle, Sam, my father's younger brother, who was denied exemption as a conscientious objector. As I stood along the road at age seven, marveling at the huge tanks and artillery carriers that lumbered by, I wondered what war was about and why some had to go while others escaped, and still others found imprisonment on our own soil. I soon learned that my family had a long-standing familiarity with persecution.

My curiosity grew into an understanding and appreciation of the underpinnings of human nature and the motivations that draw people together and then drive us apart. I wanted to be an active participant in what was happening in the world.

From these early roots I found my way to medical school with a plan to become a missionary. Along the way, I got sidetracked.

This is my story.

## In the Canton of Bern

The historical roots of my family can be traced to Switzerland and the canton of Bern. The city of Bern, founded in 1191, joined the Old Swiss Confederacy in 1353. Its influence in Central Europe grew, and, by the seventeenth century, Bern was the largest city north of the Alps, where it would play a major role during the Thirty Years' War (1618–48). It was during this time that the name Martin (also spelled Marti, Marten and Martyn) appeared in local genealogies and church and court records, as well as in documents from the neighboring Rhineland region of Germany.[1]

By 1669, when Christian Martin was born, Bern had become a center of peasant uprising and discontent, where persecution was common for political and religious dissent. The founding member of North American Martins of Swiss–German descent, Christian was born into an Anabaptist family.[2] There was endless oppression of the Anabaptist (Mennonite) sect throughout German-speaking Europe. Farmlands were possessed, active participants imprisoned and death sentences commonly metered out. As a result, my forbearers fled the region in the early eighteenth century, landing in Philadelphia and migrating to Lancaster County, Pennsylvania.[3]

The Anabaptists had emerged as a religious group less than a decade after Martin Luther had posted his ninety-five theses on the doors of the castle church in Wittenberg in 1517, calling for reform in the Catholic Church. That act and its aftermath would end the religious unity imposed by institutionalized medieval Christianity in Europe, including the Old Swiss Confederacy, forging the way for diverse and often more radical interpretations of reform.

The Anabaptists, one of the most radical of the new Christian groups, formed in 1525. The group consisted of young students, patricians and artisans led by Conrad Grebel, George Blaurock and Felix Manz, who had broken away from Ulrich Zwingli, the leader of the Swiss Reform Church. They protested that Zwingli's church was neither quick enough nor comprehensive enough in restoring "biblical Christianity." When dialogue and public debates with Zwingli failed, the young group, in a bold act on January 21, 1525, baptized Felix Manz at his home. The next day, the others were baptized by the well in the village of Zollikon on Lake Zurich. The unprecedented act of the "Swiss Brethren," as they were later called, signaled a final break from established religious authority, defying the state and Church—Catholic and Protestant alike—which would derisively label them "Anabaptists," a term derived from the Greek and literally meaning "re-baptizer" or "again baptizer." Zollikon became the first important stronghold of Anabaptism, and from there, the movement soon spread to the other cantons of the confederacy as well as to Germany, Austria and Holland.

"Believer's baptism," the notion that baptism should be administered only to adults as a voluntary act and as a sign of personal commitment to Christ, became one of the chief principles that defined the Anabaptists. In that, as in other beliefs held by Anabaptists, the authorities saw a rejection of Church hierarchy and the authority of civic bodies in religious matters. The result was a relentless campaign of persecution that targeted all Anabaptists on charges of sedition, heresy and anarchy, punishable by drowning, burning at the stake and other forms of torture. Between 1527 and 1533, at least 679 Anabaptists were executed in Switzerland and southern Germany; by the end of the sixteenth century the number of martyred Anabaptists had risen to 2,000, with thousands more imprisoned and exiled.

The first victim of the persecution, Felix Manz, was drowned in the Limmat River in Zurich in 1527, one year after the death penalty had been imposed on the Anabaptists. George Blaurock, another member of the group, was exiled from Zurich and two years later burnt at the stake in Tyrol. The persecution of Anabaptists was especially intense after 1535, following the attempt by a small revolutionary Anabaptist faction to establish forcefully the "Kingdom of God" on Earth in the German city of Münster in 1534, only to be overthrown the next year by the bishop's armies. Such events, including the May 1530 failed attempt to take over the city of Amsterdam, proved devastating to Anabaptists, and led authorities to conclude that religious dissent had escalated into political revolution.

The challenge of reorganizing the Anabaptist communities was taken up in 1536 by Menno Simons, a Dutch reformer and former Catholic priest, who would emerge as one of the most important—and more moderate—leaders of Anabaptism. The Anabaptist group under his leadership emerged as a distinct entity that came to be known first in Holland, and later in the Old Swiss Confederacy and the Rhine region, as Menists or Mennonites. Using his formidable talents in theological discourse and his organizational skills, Simons was able to direct the Anabaptists toward pacifism and an ideal of Christianity removed from any involvement in the political structures of society, with an emphasis on nonviolence and peacemaking. Earlier Anabaptist leaders had voiced the themes of nonviolence and peacemaking, but Simons transformed them into the hallmarks of Anabaptism. From Holland, Simons's movement expanded to other regions of Switzerland, Germany and eventually to America.

Despite their pacifism and nonresistance, the persecution of Mennonites continued in Switzerland into the early eighteenth century. Rather than engage in violence, the majority survived by fleeing to safer environments or by going into hiding. The experiences from decades of persecution were recorded in numerous martyrologies, including *Martyrs Mirror*, which marked its 350th anniversary in 2010, having been first published in 1660.[4] Next to the Bible, *Martyrs Mirror* held the most prominent place in Mennonite homes, including mine, where it was a fixture on the table next to my father's favorite chair. In graphic detail, the pages of *Martyrs Mirror* contained accounts and wood block illustrations of the thousands of men and women who had been persecuted and tortured, and whose memories, through this book, remain alive for generations to come.

## Christian Martin: Imprisonment and Escape to Bockschaft

Christian Martin Sr. was born at a time when the persecution of Anabaptists was common and when the thirteen cantons of the Old Swiss Confederacy were divided into hostile camps. Conflicts on economic and religious issues led to the Thirty Years' War (1618–48) in neighboring Germany. Subsequent peasant uprisings in Germany and the confederacy ended in economic ruin, with large numbers of the population killed by war and plague. The peasant revolt of 1653 was suppressed when the leaders were executed, many more exiled, and the communities involved in the rebellion heavily fined.

Christian Martin would not be spared the fate of other Anabaptists. He had married Ells (short for Elizabeth, b. 1672) sometime in the late seventeenth century. They would have four sons—Christian Jr. (b. 1694), Jacob (b. 1696), David (b. 1698) and Hans Heinrich (b. 1701)—and a daughter, Veronica (b. 1707). In 1720 he was arrested, his family possessions were seized, and he was sent to prison, most likely in the Trachselwald Castle in Bern, where the leader of the Swiss peasant rebellion had been imprisoned in 1653. The length of his prison sentence is not known, but the oral tradition in our family maintains that, while in prison, he told his sons who had come to visit him to leave Bern without him and seek safe haven, with the promise that he would follow them when he was free. Evidently his sons followed his advice and left Bern for the Rhine region known as the Palatinate. According to a few existing documents, my ancestor Hans Heinrich and his family went to Bockschaft, near Biegelhof in southern Germany, where they were tenant farmers from 1727 to 1731 (see Map 1).

Christian Martin Sr. escaped from prison in Bern some time after and made his way to Bockschaft with Ells, bringing two unknown young children with them. Bockschaft was a farming community situated midway between Heidelberg and Stuttgart, in an area east of the Rhine and close to the Neckar River that flows through Heidelberg to the Rhine. According to Bockschaft's November 1731 census, Christian Martin, his wife and the two children stayed there for some time, where he was listed as a member of the Mennonite community.

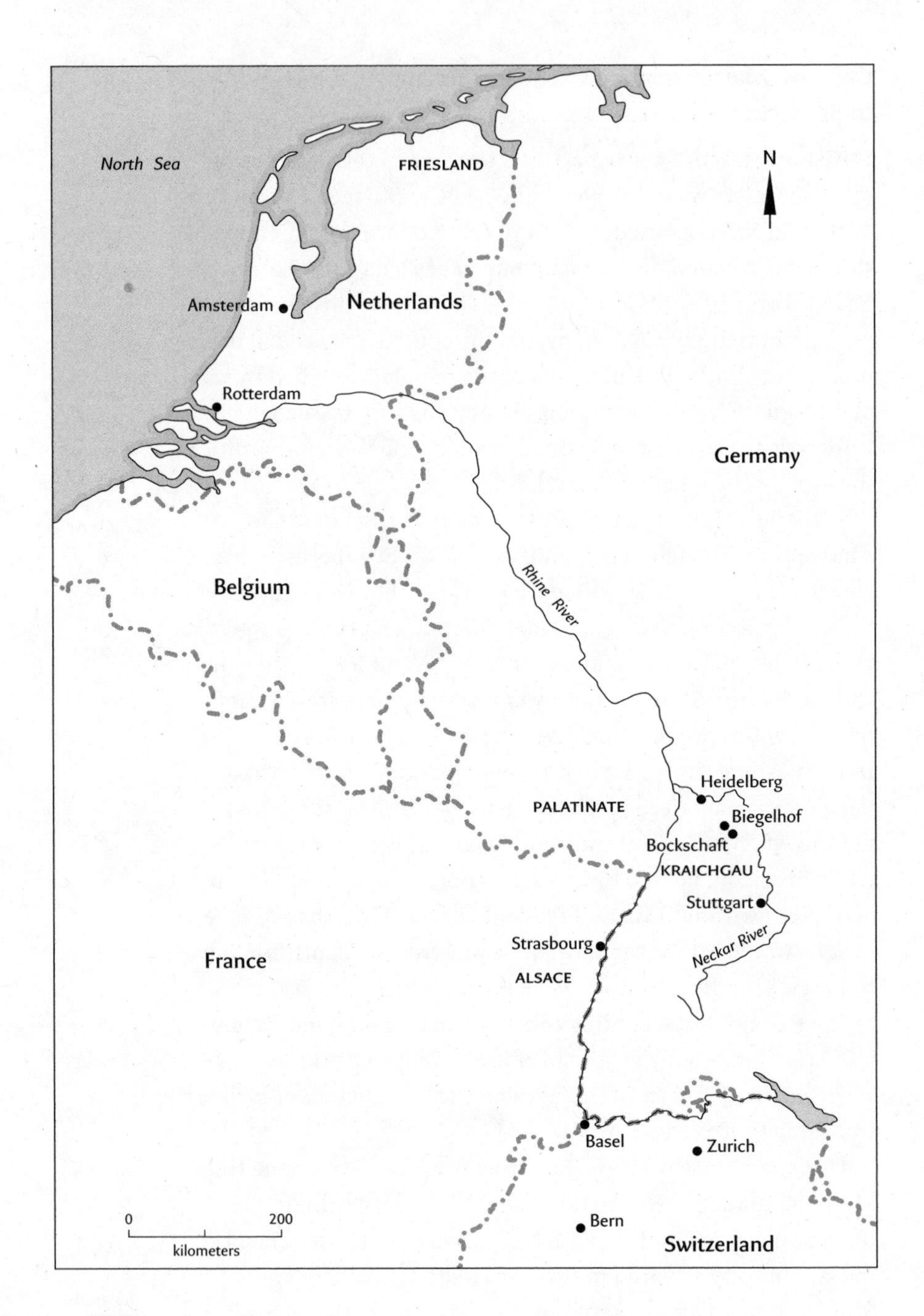
North Sea
FRIESLAND
N
Amsterdam
Netherlands
Rotterdam
Germany
Belgium
Rhine River
Heidelberg
PALATINATE
Biegelhof
Bockschaft
KRAICHGAU
Stuttgart
Strasbourg
Neckar River
France
ALSACE
Basel
Zurich
0
200
kilometers
Bern
Switzerland

The escape route from Bern Christian used had been a well-trodden path during the large migrations of mostly destitute Swiss Mennonites to the Palatinate in 1671 and 1709. Among those who had escaped north in 1671 were my wife Rachel's ancestors, the Wengers. The Palatinate was especially attractive to Anabaptists after 1684, when the Palatinate elector granted refuge and limited religious liberty to expelled Swiss Mennonites, hoping to rebuild his farmlands—wasted during the Thirty Years' War—through Mennonite labor. The Wengers and the Martins, like the other Mennonites who streamed into the Palatinate, were farmers and were barred from many professions and occupations. According to the terms of the elector, the migrants were free to hold the Mennonite faith but were forbidden to build their own churches or hold meetings in public buildings. They were not allowed to meet in groups larger than twenty members; they were not to advocate political revolt; and they were required to pay an annual tax. Later, they would be denied the right to live in cities and could marry only with the consent of the elector.[5]

< Map 1: Switzerland and the Palatinate, home of the author's ancestors.

These restrictions, along with the rising burden of taxation and the impending danger of war, would compel many Mennonites and other groups to search for a better and freer place to live and worship. That safe haven had been promised in William Penn's promotional tracts describing the advantages of Pennsylvania in the New World. Penn had visited Germany in the later part of the seventeenth century and met with the Mennonite communities along the Rhine. His promotional writings were subsequently translated into German and widely distributed in the towns and villages of the Rhine valley, particularly in the Palatinate region on the Upper Rhine, and were largely responsible for the two large migrations—of 1714 and 1717—of Swiss and German Mennonites to Pennsylvania by way of Rotterdam in Holland. He offered fertile land for settlement in Pennsylvania, north of Philadelphia, the first Mennonite settlement being located in Germantown in 1683.

## Rotterdam

To get to Rotterdam, migrants from the Palatinate region traveled down the Rhine River, through a number of locks, in small flat-bottomed boats known as scows. The trip took four to six weeks. By February 1722 the first of the Martins to begin the journey to the New World was Christian Jr. Five years later, in 1727, he was followed by his brothers, Jacob and David. Hans Heinrich and his wife, Anna, left Germany in 1731. Hans Heinrich had lost his buildings and crops to a fire in the winter of 1730–31 and had soon after asked for letters of recommendation from a minister of the Biegelhof Anabaptist congregation and from his landlord's agent. According to the minister, Hans Heinrich and his family had received good feedback from his brothers in Pennsylvania and were "undertaking to go to Pennsylvania with other good friends...."

The last to leave were Christian Sr. and Ells Martin, arriving in Rotterdam sometime in 1732 and sailing for America not long after. There, like thousands of others, they were processed by the Dutch Mennonite Commission for Foreign Needs (DMCFN). According to the commission's records at the Mennonite Archives in Amsterdam, Christian Martin had only one hundred guilders to cover the Atlantic voyage, but he had assured the commission, "The rest is promised from his friends from 'Bensilvania' so then no other sharing is needed."[6]

The DMCFN, as well as the Anabaptist community in Holland, provided invaluable assistance to refugees seeking passage to the New World. By the late seventeenth and early eighteenth centuries, Mennonites had enjoyed tolerance in Holland and had come into positions of authority, assuming financial and civic responsibilities. According to some reports, famous landscape artists Christian and Jacob van Ruisdael were among the Mennonites in Holland, and the great painter Rembrandt Harmenszoon van Rijn is speculated to have been closely associated with the Mennonite community; there is evidence to suggest that his wife was a Mennonite.

## "Bensilvania"

Estimates of the number of Germans arriving in Pennsylvania during this period vary, but based on ship passenger lists, most agree that between 10,000 and 15,000 made port by 1727. By 1750 the number had grown to 70,000–80,000, of whom about 2,500 were Mennonites, having traveled for months in overcrowded ships, with scant provisions of food and water, and high mortality rates.[7]

Christian Jr. and his wife, Maria Magdalena, had arrived in the New World before passenger lists were collected, probably in early 1722. Their departure was recorded by a Lutheran pastor in the Kraichgau town of Berwangen in 1722: "Christian Martin, an Anabaptist, who earlier was Lutheran but who again backslid, moved from Bockschaft to Pensylvanien with his wife Maria Magdalena...."[8]

In the next group was Jacob and David with their families. They boarded the ship *Molly* in Rotterdam and arrived in Philadelphia on September 30, 1727. Neither David nor Jacob had needed assistance from the DMCFN and paid their own way across the Atlantic. In the passenger list, David's name is spelled David Mardtin, while his brother's name appears as Jacob Marttin. About three hundred passengers (including, men, women and children over sixteen years) disembarked from the *Molly*. David's wife was not among them since she died en route to Pennsylvania and was buried at sea.

Onboard the good ship *Molly* were also twenty-nine-year-old Christian Wenger and his wife, Eva Graybiel, twenty-two years old, listed in the minutes of the provincial council as being from Rothenbach in the Swiss canton of Bern.[9] If and how well the Wengers and Martins knew each other is not clear. But 233 years later, their eighth-generation offspring, Rachel Ann Wenger, would become my wife on June 18, 1960, in Columbiana, Ohio.

The third group of Martins to arrive was Hans Heinrich, our family's progenitor, with his wife, Anna, their five children and Hans Heinrich's sister, Veronica, having boarded the *Britannia* in Rotterdam and having disembarked in Philadelphia on September 21, 1731. On the *Britannia*'s passenger list his name appears as Hans Hendrik Martin.

Before the passengers left the *Britannia* it was discovered that the captain had no license to transport the passengers to Philadelphia. The issue was resolved by having the passengers, including Hans Hendrik Martin, take the oath of allegiance and declare their good intentions to settle down and live in peace. The court document reads in part:

*At the Courtho. of Philadia., Sepr. 21st, 1731....*

*A list was presented of the Names of One hundred & six Palatines, who with their Families, making in all Two hundred & sixty nine Persons, were imported here in the ship Britannia, of London, Michael Franklyn, Mr., from Rotterdam, but last from Cowes, as by Clearance from that Port. The Master being Examined said he had no particular License for their Transportation. They were then called in, & having declared that their Intentions were to settle & live Peaceably in this Province, the several persons whose Names are subjoyned, did repeat and sign the Declaration inserted in the Minute of the 21st of Septr., 1727, & likewise took & subscribed the Declaration of Fidelity & Abjuration.*[10]

The document ends with a listing of 106 men's names. Women and children were not required to take the oath.

The last to arrive were Christian Sr. and Ells, on the *Pink Plaisance*, which they boarded in Rotterdam. They arrived in Philadelphia on September 21, 1732, and joined the family in Lancaster, Pennsylvania. According to the ship's passenger list, they were accompanied by two children, Fronik Martin and Martin Marte, and another relative Fravin Martin, age sixteen. It is not known if they were grandchildren of Christian and Ells.

## Laying Roots in the New Land

Christian Martin was sixty-three years old when he first set foot in Philadelphia. The stories I heard about him, this patriarch of our family, were quick to point out that here was no ordinary man. He was, we were told, larger than life. According to one story, he had simply appeared, unannounced, in the barnyard of son David at Weaverland, a valley in Lancaster County, Pennsylvania. He had brought along the scythe he had used in Europe, and during haying season, despite his age, he could cut

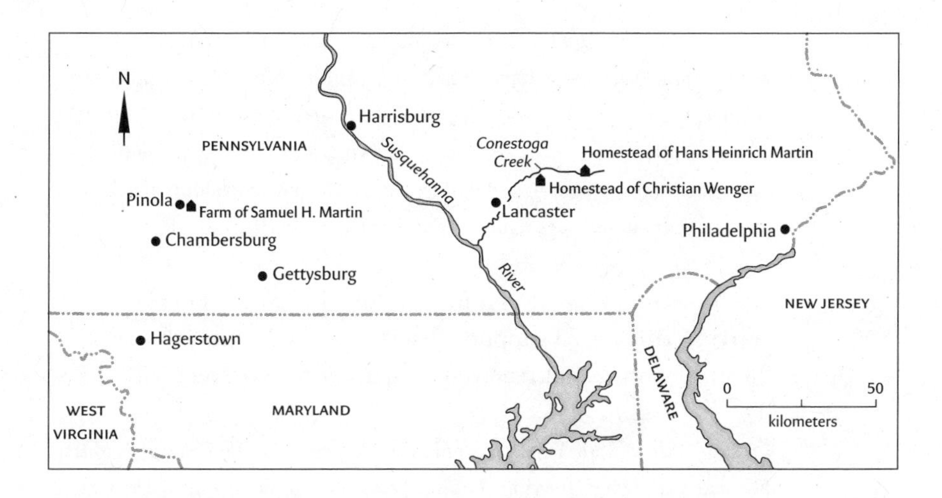


Map 2: Weaverland, Lancaster County, Pensylvania.

hay faster than any of his sons, who were then in the prime of their lives. In his mid-sixties, the story went, the swaths he cut were so heavy that those who raked behind him preferred to follow someone who was not as strong or as fast.

All of Christian's sons settled in Weaverland.[11] Located about seventy-five miles west of Philadelphia, Lancaster County became the heartland of individual farms—both Mennonite and Amish—and remains so to this day.[12] Christian Jr., who was ordained to the ministry after arriving in Philadelphia, settled on a tract along the upper reaches of Mill Creek, near the location of Summit Valley Elementary School in New Holland, Pennsylvania. By the 1740s he had resettled in Conestoga Manor, on a tract just west of present-day Millersville, Pennsylvania. David and Jacob settled in the Weaverland valley, near Christian Jr.'s first tract. Hans Heinrich settled east of Weaverland along Conestoga Creek, which led to his acquiring the nickname "Creek Henry" because his homestead was divided by the creek. He would later develop a mill at this site (see Map 2).

A glimpse of Christian Martin and his sons nearly twenty years after their arrival in Pennsylvania comes from a report by George Hantsch, a Moravian minister, who had been scouting the Lancaster Mennonites to explore support for a unified Christian faith for all Pennsylvania Germans. He visited the Martins on two occasions in 1748 to get their support. The first visit was on June 27, 1748, at the house of Christian Jr.

*We...went to Christian Marti's in Manor Land, also a preacher. There we were warmly welcomed but we stayed only a short while. He is a dear man and deeply sensitive. He was concerned for his soul. We testified to him about the sinners friend: the one who so eagerly draws them to himself if only they will recognize their misery and wretchedness. His wife and children also were eager to hear our message. Our time with them was well spent.*

The second visit was on July 12, this time at the home of David Martin, still to gain support. It seems, however, that this time the minister was not received with unanimous good will:

*Tuesday, July 12, 1748, Visited David Martin, also his brother Heinrich Marti who was with him at the time, but lived two miles from this place. With him also was their father, still living, an old man of 79 years. Our visit with these folk went quite well. They could tolerate us and understand us. Especially were the old man and his son David loving toward us. But Heinrich was only out for a good disputation.*[13]

## "Principles and Conscience"

The Martins and Wengers and many others of the Mennonite faith had come to the United States for the opportunity of a dignified life with religious freedom and good soil. They had left behind many of their possessions, but not their hymn books, their copies of *Martyrs Mirror* or their Bibles, in which their family histories were detailed. Christian Martin, "the old man," was able to see the "Promised Land" only when he was in his mid-sixties.

In 1782, during the heat of the Revolutionary War, the values Christian had passed on to his sons were to be tested yet again. In that year, six farmers from Earl Township were convicted of "basely and treacherously" assisting English prisoners of war to escape by providing them with meat, drink and lodging. Among them were Christian Martin Jr. and Henry (Hans Heinrich) Martin. They were convicted in October 1782 and received the substantial fine of fifty pounds. Henry petitioned the governor of Pennsylvania to reduce the fine. In this he was supported by Peter Miller, head of Ephrata Cloister, a pious religious group located in the nearby town of Ephrata, who appealed to the governor to reduce a fine that would ruin them, arguing that their actions were based on their "Principles and Conscience" since Mennonites would help anybody in need. The Pennsylvania Supreme Executive Council acceded, and the fine was reduced by two-thirds.

### The Descendants of Christian and Ells Martin

Christian Martin died around 1748, near the age of eighty; Ells had died before him that same year. According to family tradition, Christian Martin, who lived with his son, David, in Weaverland, asked David one morning to stay around the house because he felt a change was about to occur. Later that day he felt tired and was helped to his bed. He never woke up from his sleep. Christian and Ells had at least thirty-four grandchildren, and by 1757 the name Martin would become the most common name among Earl Township taxpayers. Descendents of Christian and Ells Martin would find their way to New York, Ohio, Maryland, Virginia and Indiana, as well as to Ontario and Alberta in Canada. Estimates indicate that, today, close to a half million descendants from this family are spread throughout North America. The majority no longer have any religious ties to the Mennonite churches of North America.

For five generations (more than 175 years) the patriarchal descendants of Hans Heinrich Martin (1701–84), my family's progenitor, lived within a hundred miles of the original Weaverland homestead in Lancaster, Pennsylvania. The patriarchal line included: Heinrich Jr. (1742–1819); Jacob (1781–1865); John (1818–1900); and Joseph H. (1861–1935). Each of the men married other descendants of the German (Pennsylvania Dutch) migrations of the seventeenth and eighteenth centuries, among them the Zimmerman and Horst families.

Records about the occupations of early Martin descendants are scant, but, as far as it is known, they were farmers. Many Martin descendants served in the ministry of the Mennonite Church, including the post of bishop (Joseph H.), but none attended college. Births, deaths and marriages were recorded in family Bibles and are available in court and county documents, but there are no detailed records of family events in the form of diaries or other writings. For the most part, the early Martins

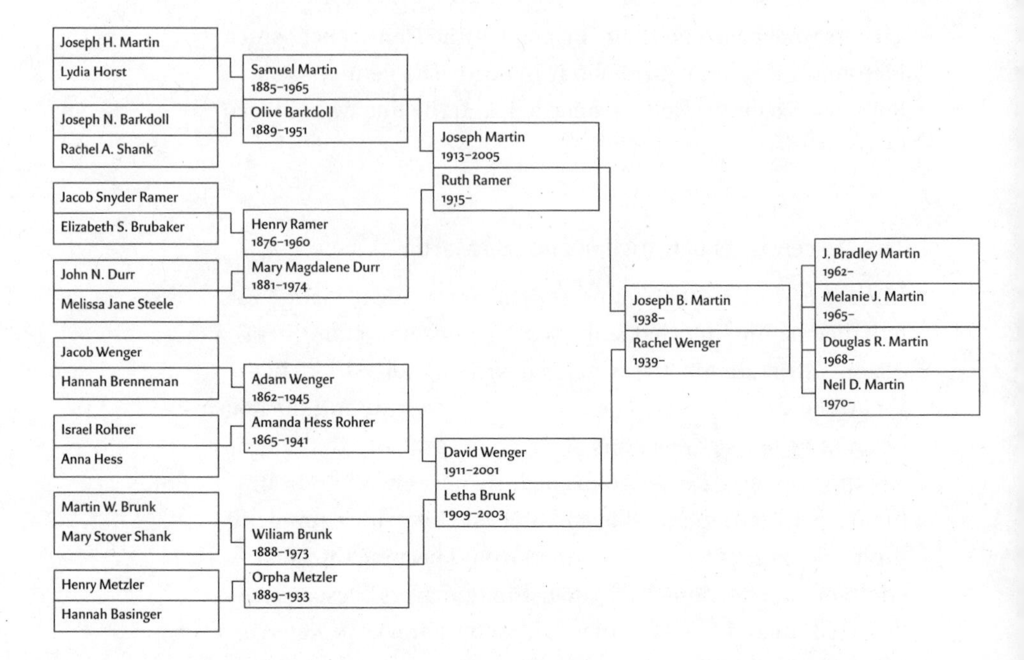


Martin family genealogy.

maintained conservative cultural habits and had large families. Ten to fifteen children were common in one family. The men tended to outlive the women.

In Pennsylvania, the preferred language was a Low German Pennsylvania Dutch dialect. My family, like many other settlers, maintained their customs and language and kept the dialect as one of their languages even into the mid-twentieth century. I still remember how my maternal grandparents, the Ramers, would put it to use when they didn't want us children to understand what they were saying, which, of course, only served to pique our curiosity even more.

My grandfather, Samuel H. Martin, who was born in Pinola, Pennsylvania, in 1885 proved to be an agent of change. He broke the mold! Soon after he married Grandmother Olive Barkdoll, the two crossed the Maryland line to live in Maugansville, Maryland, near Hagerstown, where my father was born in 1913. But the family soon returned to the Pinola area, not far from Gettysburg. From there, out of restlessness and the desire for new adventures, he would later migrate westward to Canada with his growing family (see Maps 2 and 3). The selection of Duchess was predicated on joining an already-growing

Mennonite settlement, which included the arrival nine years earlier of my mother's Uncle Sam and Aunt Hettie and, later in 1917, her own family, my grandparents Henry and Mary Ramer (anglicized from the German Römer).

## Alberta: "An Emptiness...Almost Frighteningly Total"

In 1883, only sixteen years after the Dominion of Canada was established as a confederation, Canadian Pacific Railway (CPR) workers completed the CPR through the western reaches of the Canadian Prairie provinces. In Alberta, which had officially become part of the dominion in 1905, the line stretched from the Saskatchewan border through Medicine Hat on to Calgary, and continued west to the Canadian Rockies (Banff and Lake Louise) across the Continental Divide to British Columbia.

It was a remarkable feat for the young country. The pace at which the railway extended through what is now southern Alberta was in itself remarkable, with the crews laying over six miles of railroad in a single day near the town of Brooks, only a few miles from my childhood home in Duchess, Alberta.[14] To complete a project of such a massive scale, 12,000 men, 5,000 horses, and 300 dogsled teams were put to use. The rugged terrain posed formidable challenges and dangers. The hard labor involved in clearing and grading the roadbed for the railway and in blasting tunnels through the rock in the foothills and the mountains cost the lives of many of the immigrant workers, the majority of whom were from Europe and China and worked under poor conditions with low pay.

The principal towns along the railroad in Alberta included Medicine Hat (near the border with Saskatchewan), Tilley, Brooks, Bassano, Cluny and Gleichen (the two centers of the Blackfoot Nation), continuing on to Strathmore to reach Calgary; the railroad's path through this string of towns covered a distance of about 250 miles. This stretch of southeastern Alberta consisted of treeless virgin prairie with tall grass, sagebrush and cactus. Surveyed in the 1880s by the Palliser Expedition, the area was recorded as being inhospitable to agriculture. Called the Palliser Triangle after Captain John Palliser, leader of the expedition, the area's apex is near Calgary and its base extends along the Alberta and Saskatchewan borders with the US. The prairies were populated with buffalo, antelope, badgers, gophers, coyotes, a few wolves, grasshoppers and rattlesnakes. Recounting his experience as a young boy living in Saskatchewan a few miles from the Alberta border in the early twentieth century, Wallace Stegner's *Wolf Willow* captures the character of the land:

*The rest of that country is notable primarily for its weather, which is violent and prolonged; its emptiness, which is almost frighteningly total; and its wind, which blows all the time in a way to stiffen your hair and rattle the eyes in your head.*[15]

The CPR was the initiative of a consortium of businessmen from eastern Canada and was to be financed, at least in part, by the sale of land to settlers along a twenty-four-mile swath on each side of the railway. Despite the Palliser Expedition's assessment of the area as unfertile, estimates in the early twentieth century indicated that the soil quality of the prairies was of good to high quality, but the annual rainfall averaging twelve to thirteen inches per year would not be sufficient to grow grain and alfalfa. To attract homesteaders, the CPR needed to provide more productive lands. A feasibility study indicated that a substantial area of up to one million acres in size could be supplied with water by damming the Bow River near the town of Bassano—a railway station along the Medicine Hat–Calgary line, and my birthplace. The gradual slope of the land from the Bow River eastward to the Red Deer River allowed irrigation water to flow west to east. The irrigated area was eventually named the Eastern Irrigation District.[16]

Construction on the dam began in 1910 and was completed four years later. Concomitant with the construction of the dam, the CPR built another rail line from the border of Saskatchewan to Bassano, designating it the Royal line. Stations were built at intervals of ten to fifteen miles along the line in Empress, Patricia, Millicent, Duchess, Rosemary and Countess. Some of these names harkened back to a distant, perhaps romantic, world. Bassano, for instance, was named after a beautiful village in northern Italy near Venice, which I had the pleasure to visit a few years ago. My hometown, Duchess, was named for the wife of the Duke of Sutherland, a wealthy British tycoon who invested in a large property near the town of Brooks, just a few miles away. Yet these towns were hardly more than stations. They were equipped with grain storage facilities and elevators for loading grain onto trains and, of course, marked the areas that were to be populated by future settlements.

With the completion of the railway and the damming of the Bow at Bassano, the CPR began to market the region to potential homesteaders in the eastern part of the country, as well as in England, Europe and the United States. But with the onset of World War I in 1914, many potential European settlers instead found themselves in the trenches of that dreadful conflagration. To compensate for this, the CPR more aggressively campaigned in the United States, particularly in Nebraska, Kansas, Colorado and Pennsylvania. It was at this time that a Mr. Harrison from Canada opened an office in Harrisburg, Pennsylvania, and it was through his notification that Sam Ramer, my mother's uncle, visited—and in 1915 purchased at approximately $50 per acre—a quarter section of land (160 acres) near the railroad station house of Duchess.

Duchess is located about ten miles north of Brooks, the railway station that served as the arrival point for easterners. When Sam Ramer arrived there were a few settlers and ranchers in the Brooks area, but his land was the first in close proximity to Duchess. During the first winter, the family lived in the station house while their standardized farmhouse was being constructed by CPR contract. Next to arrive, in the summer of 1917, were my maternal grandparents—Henry B. Ramer and his wife Mary Magdalene (Durr)—and their four children, to a homestead in Duchess near Sam Ramer's home.

My grandmother's family, the Durrs, included prominent leaders of the western Pennsylvania Mennonite Church, most notably Bishop John Durr, my grandmother's father, widely acknowledged for his leadership and oratorical abilities. When Henry, Mary Magdalene, and their children arrived in Duchess, my mother Ruth, two years old at the time, was the youngest of the children. Her three older siblings were Clarence, David and John. At fifteen, John would accidentally be killed by a shotgun blast while hunting for geese, instilling in my mother a lifelong fear of guns and of hunting.

Prairie life was rough. Cows provided milk, from which came butter and cheese; wheat and oats were ground into flour; pigs and cattle were sacrificed for meat; and chickens and geese provided eggs and meat. Vegetables grew in abundance, but the methods to preserve them for the long winters required special jars and equipment not easily available in those days. Then, in the second year of his settlement in Alberta, Henry Ramer, an ordained minister, became exceedingly and unexpectedly busy. The worldwide flu epidemic did not spare the prairies. Hundreds of settlers were afflicted and many died. During the winter of 1918–19, Henry visited community after community providing solace to families whose loved ones had died, conducting the funeral services in their homes and schoolhouses.

> Map 3: Eastern Irrigation District and the Duchess area in Alberta.

The new settlers had to learn the technology of irrigation. Each of the canals crossing the region gained its source at the main canal, which carried water from the dam at Bassano. Sequential tributaries brought water to individual farms, where smaller dams collected the water to be sent out across the farmland. Smaller irrigation ditches made by horse and plow allowed the running water to follow the contours of the land. The water in these smaller distribution ditches was contained by dirt-filled dams or by spreading a stretch of canvas from bank to bank attached to a wooden strut. The canvas was held in place by a few shovels of dirt at the bottom of the ditch, and the pooled water was released through small breaches on either side of the irrigation ditch. This was known as gravity, or flood, irrigation.

The crops of the first few years of settlement were abundant and the rainfall ample enough to provide lush pasture for the cows on the native prairie grass. But irrigation farming was extremely labor intensive. A strong motivated man might irrigate four to six acres a day, rising at 4 or 5 a.m. and working until the gathering darkness prevented him from identifying the best location for the last "set" of the canvas dam across the irrigation ditch. Every acre had to be irrigated twice during the late spring and summer. Rainfall was intermittent and hardly ever sufficient to call a halt to the irrigator's toil.

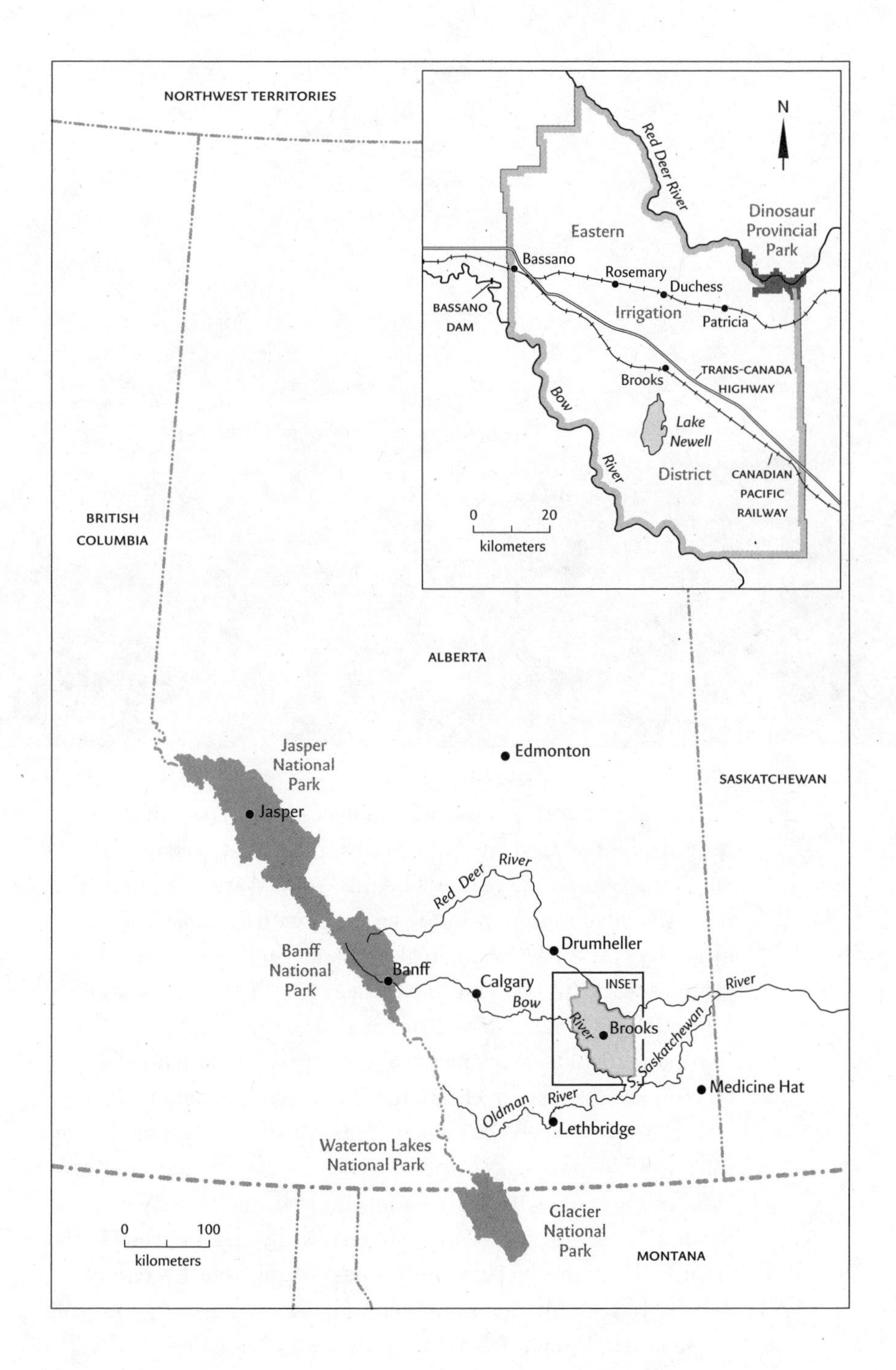
NORTHWEST TERRITORIES
N
Red Deer River
Dinosaur
Provincial
Park
Eastern
Bassano
Rosemary
Duchess
BASSANO
DAM
Irrigation
Patricia
Brooks
TRANS-CANADA
HIGHWAY
Bow
Lake
Newell
River
District
CANADIAN
PACIFIC
RAILWAY
0
20
kilometers
BRITISH
COLUMBIA
ALBERTA
Jasper
National
Park
Edmonton
SASKATCHEWAN
Jasper
Red Deer River
Drumheller
Banff
National
Park
Banff
Calgary
INSET
River
Bow
River
Brooks
Saskatchewan
S.
Medicine Hat
Oldman River
Lethbridge
Waterton Lakes
National Park
Glacier
National
Park
0
100
kilometers
MONTANA

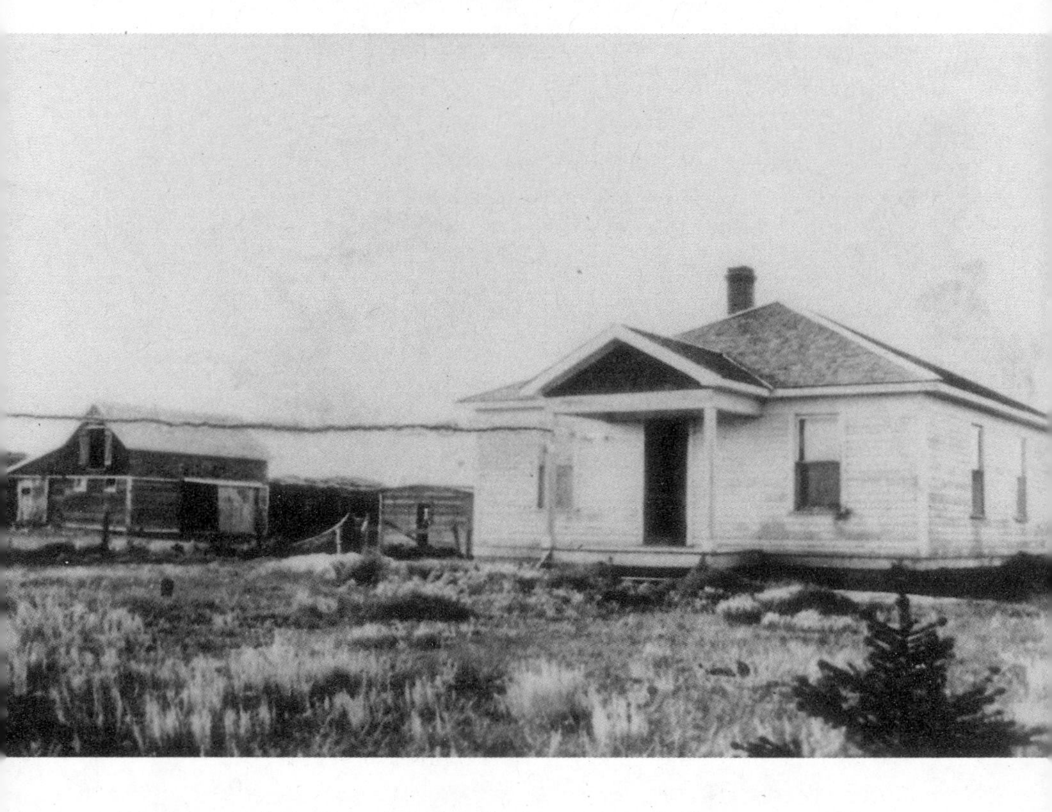

The CPR-constructed Martin homestead, circa 1924.

The influx of settlers to this region of Alberta, part of the carefully marketed strategy for settling the West, was remarkably successful in the years following World War I. Promises of rich soil and abundant rainfall, together with aggressive and ultimately false advertising regarding new methods of farming, proved successful in attracting farmers from England, Ireland, Germany and Poland, as well as the US.

Among them were my paternal grandparents, Sam and Olive Martin, and their seven children, ranging in age from one to eleven. They boarded the train in Pennsylvania on March 28, 1924, headed for Brooks, Alberta. With them were Sam's brother, Dan, and his wife with their young children, and Sam's younger brother, Jason, an eighteen-year-old whose behavior in the Pinola community had been sufficiently questionable that his parents decided to send him along to keep him in line.

My father, Joseph B. Martin, the second of Sam and Olive's seven children alive at the time, was ten years old. His siblings were Ethel, two years his elder, and younger sisters and brothers Fred, Lulu, John, Ruth and Sam. They traveled from Pinola to Harrisburg, Pennsylvania, on to Buffalo, New York and Toronto, where they transferred to the cross-country CPR to traverse Ontario, Manitoba and Saskatchewan before finally arriving in Brooks, Alberta.

During the journey, some in the group came down with whooping cough, keeping the others awake at night. A few of the older boys escaped to the forward cars and acted as though they didn't belong to the plain Mennonite group. They saw their first Royal Canadian Mounted Police (RCMP) in their bright red coats, riding breeches, special hats and shiny high-top boots, and they overheard them commenting on all the kids in the Martin group, saying that there must be an incubator back there.

Although Sam and Olive relocated to Alberta in 1924, this was not the first time that Sam had visited Alberta. In 1903, at the age of seventeen, he had left school after completing the minimal requirement—seventh grade—and ventured forth from Pennsylvania to the western states, working as an itinerant laborer in Ohio, Illinois and Kansas. He then worked for a time as a logger in British Columbia and as a farmhand in Carmangay, Alberta, before settling in Corning, California, a small farm community seventy miles north of Sacramento. Altogether, he had roamed the western regions of the United States and Canada for more than three years. In Corning, he purchased a forty-acre farm and for four years grew garden vegetables, taking them by train to markets in Sacramento and San Francisco. After suffering several bouts of malaria, he abruptly returned to Pennsylvania, where he married Olive Honora Barkdoll, my grandmother. At his return, he was just past his twenty-fifth birthday.

This time, the move to the West, with a large family, to a climactically unfamiliar and unfriendly land, was final. Wanderlust and dissatisfaction with farming conditions in southeastern Pennsylvania, contrasted with the promising expanses of grain farms Grandpa Martin had seen as a teenager, were factors that led to the family's move. An additional factor was the encouragement of the emerging Mennonite community in Duchess, Alberta, where several families, including my mother's, had already settled and reported favorable crop conditions and excellent, fertile, prairie soil.

My father remembered the train ride to Alberta well. One of his aunts had prepared a trunk full of food and other items for the ride, but by the time they had reached the western parts of Ontario, the food had become putrid. "It was disposed of," my father would say, "by throwing it from the train somewhere west of Winnipeg." The train ride from Toronto lasted three nights and four days. They were met at the train station in Brooks by Henry Ramer, my mother's father, and John Brubaker, the two settlers who had already braved the Alberta prairie for nearly a decade. Henry and John took the Martins to Duchess in a Model T Ford, where they stayed with local families until their farmhouse was ready for occupancy a few weeks later. My mother recalls that my uncle, Sam, eighteen months old, and his sister, Ruth, three years old, stayed with them for several months in the spring of 1924.

Olive had been four months pregnant when they arrived at the station in Brooks. Jim would be born at home soon after they moved into their CPR-constructed home, which had earlier been occupied by my grandfather Ramer's brother, Ammon, a settler who by then had relocated to the United States. It was a square single-floor structure with a combined kitchen and eating area, a front room for entertaining guests and two bedrooms. Interior bathroom facilities would not be available for many years. The house was set back from the dirt road by about seventy-five feet to provide space for a grass lawn kept green by periodic watering from the irrigation ditch. The front door opened onto the roadside but was rarely used. All the traffic to the homestead came into the barnyard, and the entrance to the house was located there. The barn housed a few cows for milk, a pig or two, lots of chickens, and later, a stable for horses.

In this remote region of the prairies stray cats and skunks were common. Children who accidentally confronted a skunk in the springtime suffered for days. The treatment for skunk odor was never entirely successful, and it was not unusual at school to have a classmate bring along the scent for the day.

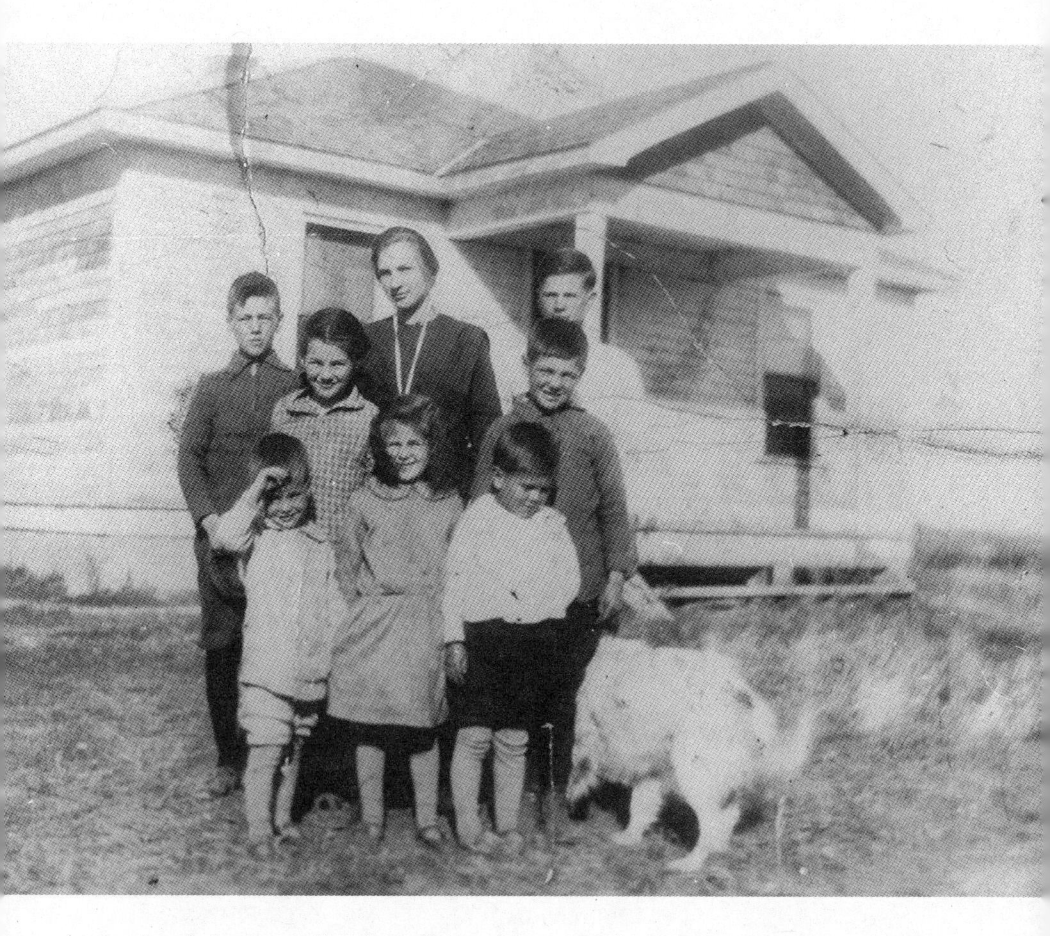

The Martin children outside the family homestead. Ethel, the oldest, wears a church-endorsed head covering and a cape dress. Joseph, the author's father, is in the back row on the right.

My father's recollection of school was mostly negative. He was not a good student. He skipped school when he could, preferring to be outside doing farm work to sitting at attention in a classroom. After attending classes sporadically during his teenage years, he was delighted at age fifteen to leave school permanently. He would never admit to any regrets for having left when he did. His younger brother, Uncle Fred, who would later be a business partner, stayed on and finished high school.

## TWO

# *Emerging as a Family in the New Land*

IN THE MID-1920S CROPS WERE BOUNTIFUL, rainfall abundant and the promise of agricultural success from the prairie soil high. Wheat sold for a dollar a bushel, and the yield was up to forty to sixty bushels to the acre. Alfalfa grew well. It provided a substantive diet for the livestock in the winter and also fortified the soil by introducing nitrogen back into the ground. I would learn about alfalfa's qualities years later in Howard Goodman's laboratory at the Massachusetts General Hospital, which had a research interest in plants. I learned there that the nodules on the roots of the alfalfa plant contain highly specific saprophytic bacteria that cause "nitrogen fixation," a process that replenishes the environment with natural fertilizer in the soil around the plant's root. When I once asked my father about this, he smiled and noted that it was customary to pull the alfalfa plants to view the nodules, which, when abundant, meant that the soil fertility would be restored. He knew nothing about the science, but he did know about the mysteries of successful farming.

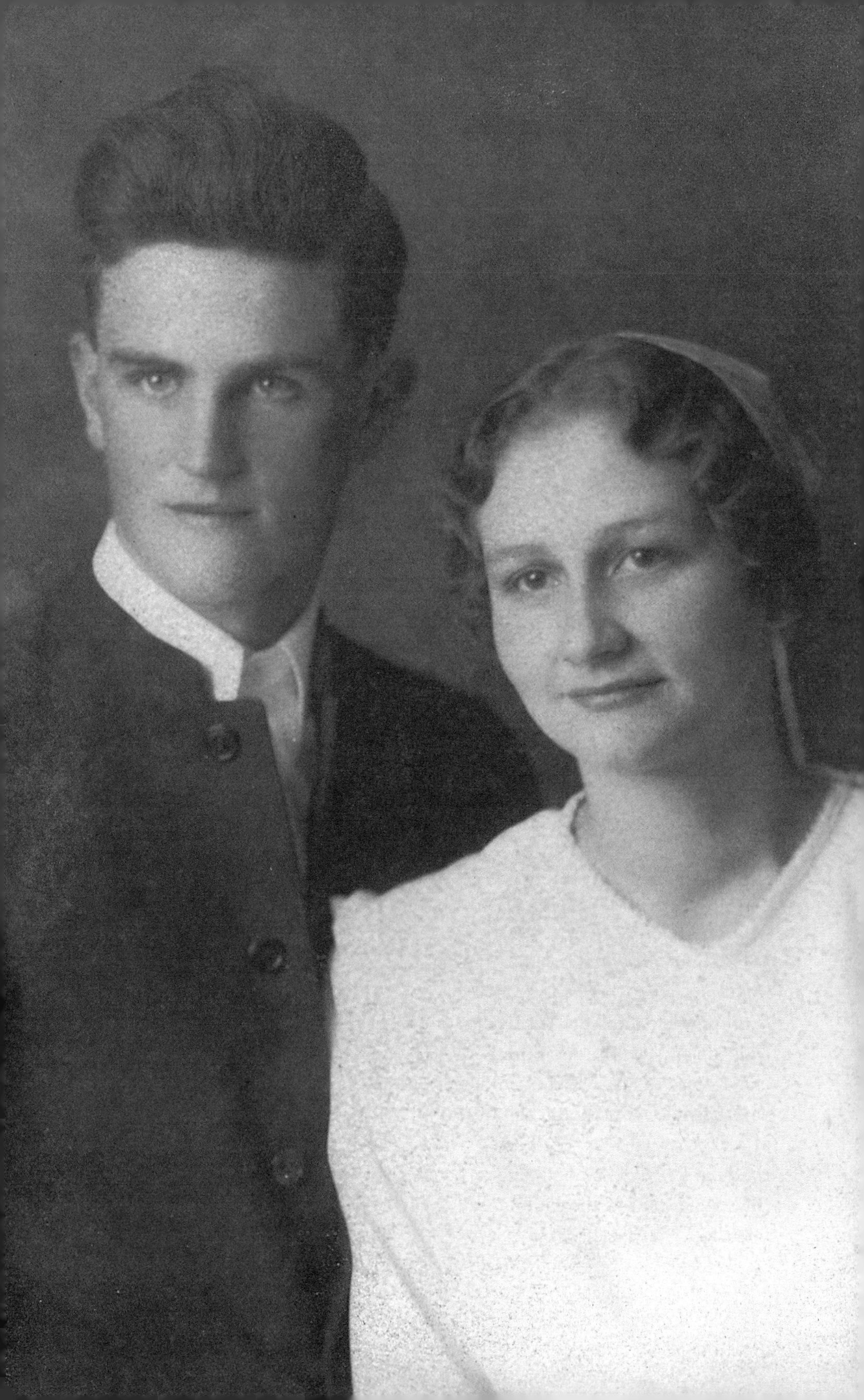

Sam and Olive Martin's family grew from seven to ten children with the arrival of three more sons—Jim, Paul and Richard. With seven healthy young boys, Grandpa purchased more land and tripled the farming effort. He put the boys to work as soon as they were able to do chores and, with their help, harvested the first crops in Alberta in 1925 and 1926. The growing family needed new accommodations. During the first summer and winter after their arrival, the boys slept in a granary near the barn. The next summer, Grandpa Sam purchased a two-roomed teacher's house located near town and moved it to the farm next to the house to provide what would be known as the "shack." It was connected to the house by a short narrow walkway. Neither insulated nor heated, the shack became the sleeping quarters for the boys. They used animal hides for comforters to survive the cold nights of winter. One can only imagine the scene each winter morning as the lads ran the short distance from their warm beds to the house in their underwear.

< The author's parents on their wedding day, 1936.

My father was the eldest son. In 1927, when he was thirteen, he left eighth grade to help support the family. He was assigned his own team of horses and a wagon at harvest time to gather wheat bundles from the stooks, pyramids of grain sheaves in the field. He had to deliver a wagonload in turn, with five or six other drivers, to the threshing machine. The threshing machine was powered by an idling tractor via a belt. I remember as a youth standing and marveling at the long leather belt, twenty-five feet or more in length and six to eight inches wide, swirling with a half-rotation around the two pulleys between tractor and machine. It went at a remarkable speed, and I was amazed that it didn't come off the pulleys. Dad insisted with great pride that he never missed his turn delivering a load to the threshing machine. At age fifteen, my father became the senior farm manager alongside his father and assumed full duties organizing irrigation, building the ditches that traversed the fields, and spending long hours, seven days a week, in watering the entire 160-acre patch.

It was then that he first came to know my mother, two years younger, who busied herself helping with the meals the hungry threshers gorged on during harvest and preparing food for canning to survive the long dreary winters. My father spent the years between 1928, as his key role evolved at the Martin homestead, until his marriage to my mother in 1936, when he was twenty-two, in various local farm-related jobs, saving every penny to eventually acquire a farm of his own. In addition to working full time for his father, he made himself available to the neighbors, including the Ramer homesteaders, whose farm was adjacent to the Martin's.

My mother insists it was a long time before she took any notice of my father and before she agreed to date and marry him. My mother's family had lived in a city, Altoona, Pennsylvania, where the customs of table and household etiquette were noticeably different from those of rural Pennsylvania. In Grandma and Grandpa Ramer's home, the table was set with linen and English china, and the house was kept spotlessly clean. The Martins, by comparison, either didn't know or didn't care about such niceties. Long after my parents had married, my mother persisted in feeling that the Martins considered her to be elitist, overly interested in "nice things," and too aware of the manners of others. She was, however, acknowledged by everyone to be a superb cook and seamstress. In the days when suits purchased at the local store required "making over" into "plain suits" to meet the Mennonite tradition of eschewing fashion, she was the best at alterations and the most popular. She could create the high tight collar, à la Nehru, getting them to look right and straight.

IN EARLY 1937, AFTER THEY MARRIED and Dad finished the harvest, the couple set out in a Model A Ford coupe for a deferred honeymoon trip to California. They arrived in the San Francisco Bay area just after the opening of the San Francisco–Oakland Bay Bridge. Years later, while shopping on Haight Street in San Francisco, I stumbled upon a vintage photo of the bridge showing vehicles crossing over, one of which might well have been the one they drove. I sent it to my parents on their sixtieth wedding anniversary in 1996.

The young couple was open to the idea of resettling in California if employment opportunities had been available, but that seemed unlikely, and they returned home to live in an addition to the rear of Grandma and Grandpa Ramer's house, which had two bedrooms, a kitchen and a living room but no

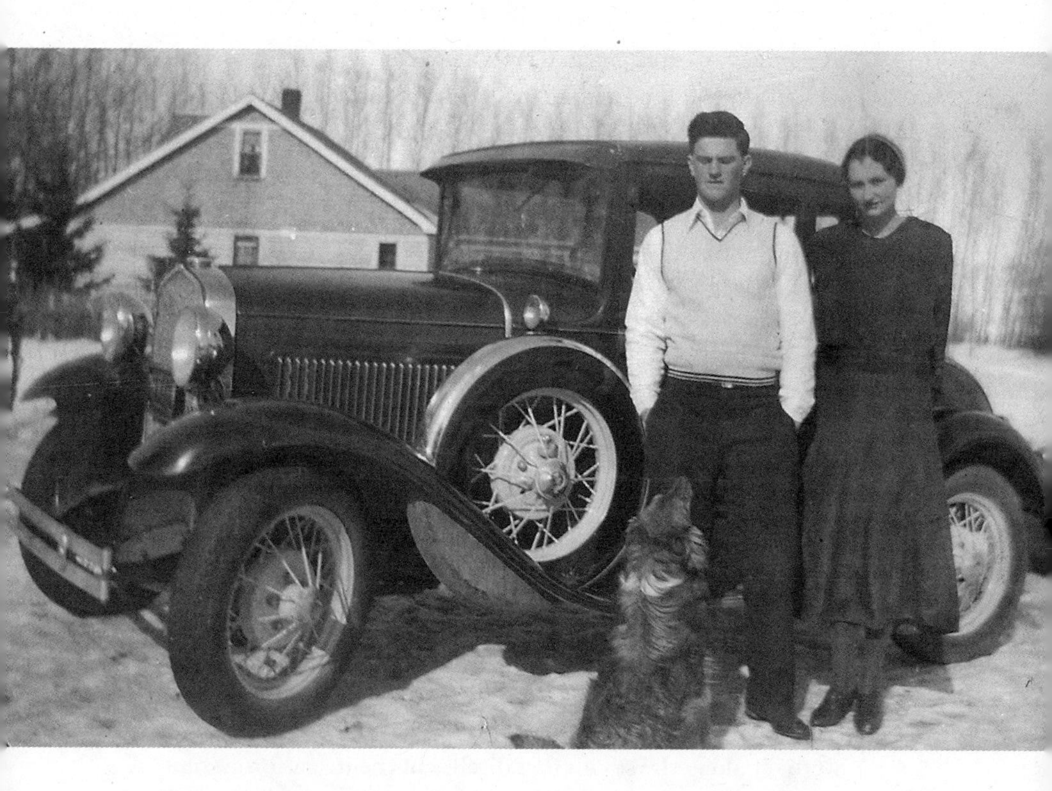

The author's parents prepare for a trip to California in their Model A Ford coupe, 1937.

bathroom. They lived there for five years, until I was three years old and my brother Dale had arrived. Eventually, my father grew to resent working for others at a wage of $25–30 a month, and he arranged to purchase a quarter section of land (160 acres). We moved there in the spring of 1942 and had a "hired girl" that summer and fall so my mother could spend the days helping with the farm work, driving the tractor, milking cows, and raising pigs and poultry for our meals.

## The Depression and the Dirty Thirties Strike Alberta

The optimism of the mid-1920s faded in 1929 when wheat prices plummeted and the country entered the Great Depression. The worldwide crash in grain prices made it increasingly difficult for the homesteaders in the US and Canada to meet mortgage payments on the land and, in the case of irrigated regions, the water assessment tax critical to support the irrigation infrastructure. The price of wheat declined to a few cents a bushel, and the mortgages on farmland and late tax payments led to a succession of bankruptcies and abandoned farms in the Duchess district. Grandfather Martin's brother, Dan, left Alberta for the US, relocating to Wisconsin. His farm sale yielded enough to pay most of his debts and transportation out of the country in a Model T. Grandfather's other brother, Jason, also left for Wisconsin.

Emigration became common. Disillusioned by unfulfilled promises of riches, families forsook the land to return east or to migrate south to Kansas and Nebraska. Grandma Ramer told me that the Martins and the Ramers were too poor to move back to their origins in Pennsylvania. Irrigation provided adequate food for survival, and readjustments on mortgage obligations permitted survival without total bankruptcy; still, it was necessary to find other means of financial and nutritional support. My father was forced into trapping and hunting, not only for the revenues from the pelts of coyotes, muskrats, weasels and mink but also for the food provided by the antelope, deer, elk and moose that abundantly inhabited the foothills and mountains to the west.

A coyote pelt fetched $1 as did a weasel or muskrat. Traplines were set along the canals and ditches of the irrigation system and near the water's edge of the few lakes that were formed for irrigation reservoirs. A typical day took my father a distance of twenty to fifty miles on his horse along the traplines to secure a half dozen or so animals from two hundred or more traps. As the years advanced, however, the animals became scarce and the efficiency of the enterprise marginal. By then, my father had become an accomplished marksman. He would later acquire a sporting goods license and import rifles, ammunition, gunpowder and telescopes from the US.

## Early Memories of Life in Duchess

I arrived on the scene October 20, 1938, born in the hospital at Bassano. My earliest memories are about farm life. Some childhood memories survive as fragments, but they are vivid nevertheless. Among my first recollections at age four or five are of my father building a barn and delivering milk by car to the growing village of Duchess, which had a population approaching one hundred. I recall finding my way to the outhouse summer and winter. We had no indoor plumbing and no electricity. It was exciting to help my father deliver milk door-to-door early in the morning. And I remember learning to drive a tractor when I was five years old, taking it to my cousin's house when I started school in 1944 so I could walk with them the additional mile.

I remember making my first allowance at age seven or eight by preparing the bullets for my father, which would be placed into the end of the brass cartridge to make ammunition. I filled hollow copper jackets with pieces of lead cut from a spool of coiled lead; the lead segments were carefully placed into the copper jackets and crimped into a bullet shape by a specially designed mold I operated by hand. When completed, the sharpened end of a bullet had a short piece of lead protruding from the copper sleeve. To prepare loaded ammunition, my father filled the brass cartridge with gunpowder, inserted a "primer" into the end of the cartridge to explode the gunpowder and inserted "my" bullets tightly into the firing end. The ammunition was now ready for use in the bolt action of the rifle. Telescope sights mounted on the top of the rifle allowed accuracy of two to three inches at one hundred yards, and it was not uncommon to "take" a coyote at 250 to three hundred yards and a large game animal at up to three or four hundred yards.

In 1945, when I was seven, we moved from the dairy farm to a newly built house on the main highway linking Duchess to Brooks, less than a quarter mile from Grandmother Ramer's home and across the road from Uncle Clarence, my mother's brother.[1] The acre of land was part of the original Ramer homestead, which Dad purchased from his father-in-law. My father had sold the farm and joined his brother, Fred, in the car and farm machinery business, which was called the Duchess Garage. Uncle Fred, who had contracted to sell John Deere tractors and machinery, was short on cash, and my father, of whom neighbors said still had the first nickel he ever made, provided new capital by selling the farm. My father moved from being a dairy farmer to a successful automobile (Chrysler and Plymouth cars and Fargo trucks, a brand sold by Chrysler in Canada) and farm implement (John Deere) dealer at the Duchess Garage.

One of the great blessings of the move to our new house was its close proximity to Grandma and Grandpa Ramer. I could walk across the field and arrive unannounced any time of the day and get a welcome and a glass of milk or a cookie, or better yet, a dish of homemade ice cream. On Saturday nights, I could stay over. I would climb the steep stairs to the second-floor room familiar to me from the time we lived with them. One winter, I spent days lying there, delirious from measles, with a temperature that rose to 105°F.

On one occasion, late at night after I had been sent to bed, I quietly crept into my parents' room and took a $20 bill from my father's wallet. In the morning, I retrieved it from under my pillow and, putting it into a front pocket, set off to tell Grandma about my fortune. She asked where I got it, and I said that my daddy had given it to me. A call to my mother straightened things out all too quickly. My punishment was straightforward. I had to surrender the money immediately with the warning that another effort like that would get me into serious trouble.

Sunday mornings I helped gather eggs in the barn and watched Grandma cook oatmeal in a double boiler. Sometimes we had "pap," a mixture of flour and milk cooked into custard and served with brown sugar and more milk. It came out flat onto the plate, and I suspect it was the sweetness from the sugar that made it so special. On Sunday afternoons the Martin and Ramer grandchildren convened in Grandma Ramer's large front yard and played tree base, prisoner's base and kick-the-can. We spent hours running and playing. The trees planted out behind the farmhouse provided an ideal venue for playing "cowboys and Indians." Contests were a regular part of the fun. Who could throw the farthest, pee the highest or run the fastest played out in many of our best times together. I was competitive and was surprisingly able to keep up with the older cousins without great difficulty. At least that's how I remember it.

When we had lived on the farm, the walk to Grandma Ramer's place went past Grandma Martin's house. Somehow it was never so welcome to stop there. I don't remember any laughter or happiness in the house of my Martin grandparents, and I rarely visited them, except with my parents. Grandma Martin was about five foot five, slightly overweight, shy and tired. She had a facial tic that led to frequent irregular squinting, and I remember wondering whether it was due to nervousness

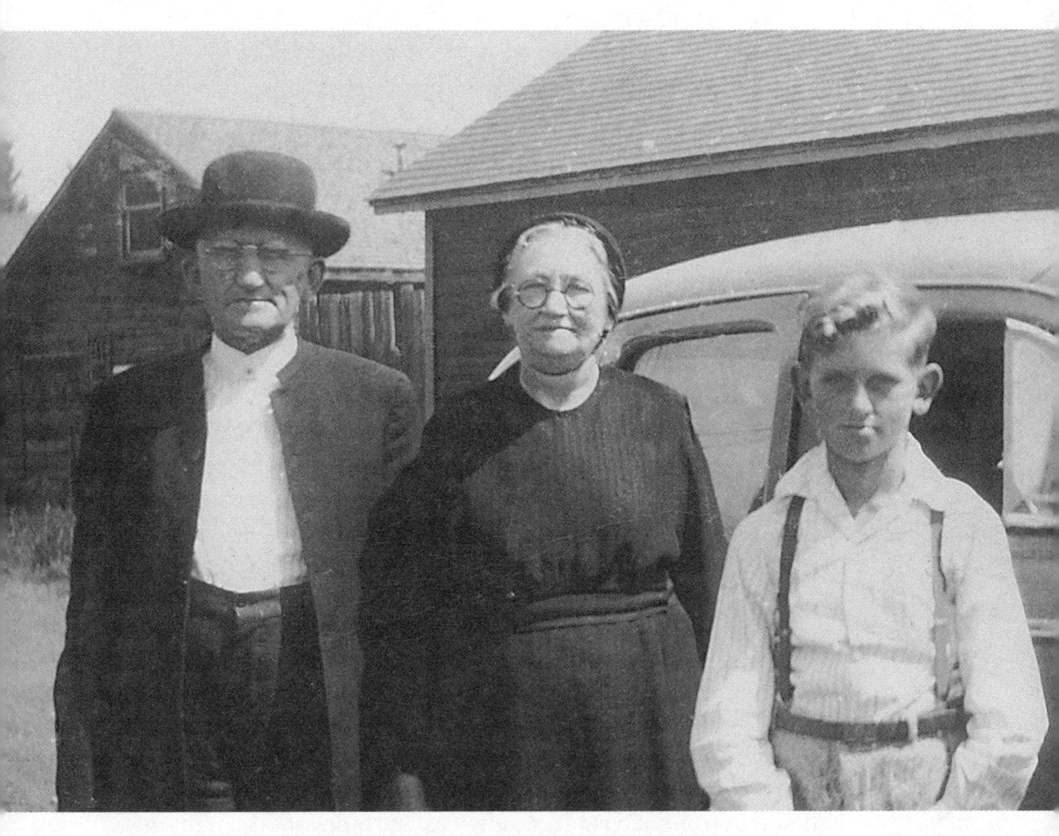

The author, age nine, poses with Grandma and Grandpa Ramer, on the day of his baptism.

or something more serious. In the fall of 1950, Grandpa took Grandma to visit relatives in Pennsylvania, returning to Alberta for the Christmas holidays. After that, Grandma grew frail with respiratory complaints and was hospitalized. She died in January 1951. Her death certificate listed tuberculosis as a cause.

Grandpa was hard to approach and seemed uninterested in children's activities. He was stern and short tempered but widely respected in the community for his work ethic and integrity. He always paid his bills on time and did not encourage borrowing money. After Grandma died, his interests in farming waned, and the boys took over the property. He moved to Duchess to live in one of the original CPR-constructed homes, which stands occupied today. He took over the management of Slatter's Meat Shop, a longtime fixture on the desultory east side of the main street in Duchess. Located next to the Purcell General Store, which also held the post office in a rear corner, Slatter's was owned by George Slatter, who was recuperating from an illness

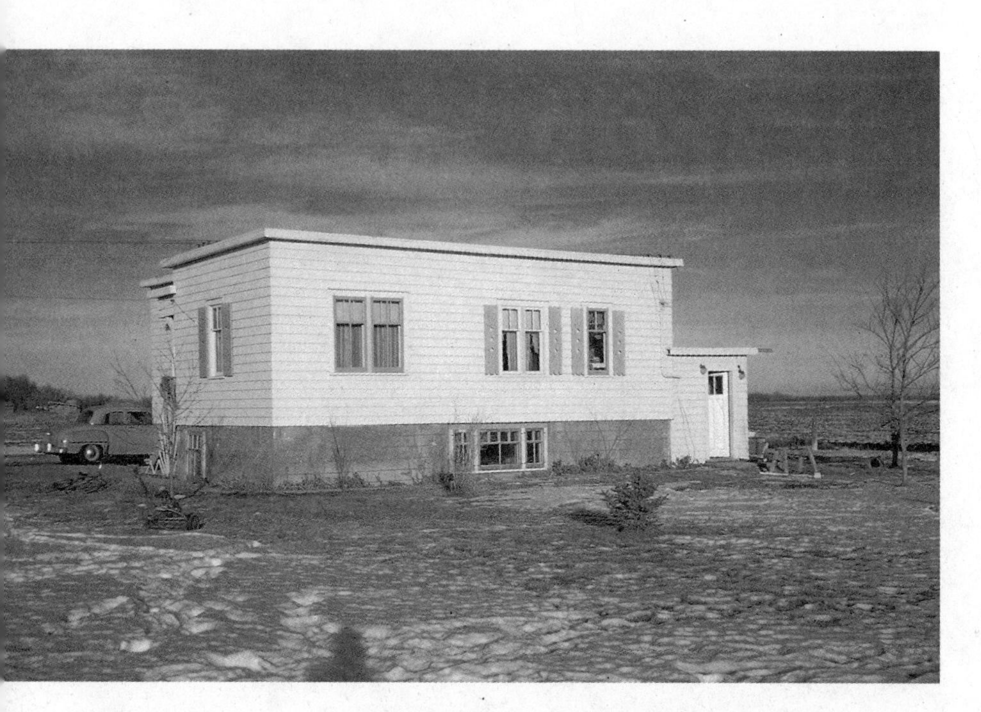

The Martin house, off the gravel road known locally as the "Alaska Highway."

after serving in World War II. On the west side of the street was the Duchess Hotel, the lumber yard and the pool hall. The local telephone system, the "Central," was located next to the pool hall and in front of a small residence. One block south on main street, near the residential quarter, stood Doctor Porter's chiropractic office in a vacated bank building.

I grew closer to Grandpa Martin in the last decade of his life, beginning when I spent a couple of summers helping him on weekends, listening to the stories he loved to tell. He had mellowed out quite a bit by this time, and I grew quite attached to him. After my fiancé Rachel arrived on the scene in 1959, we visited him to learn of an interesting coincidence that carried him back on memory lane to his teenage westward travels. He was telling us about the time he had spent in Rachel's community in eastern Ohio, working at odd jobs, when he had fallen in love with a young lady, Melissa Weaver, who Rachel knew as an older woman. We could see a beam on Grandpa's face as he told us about his first love. He told us he stopped by to seek her out on his return from his western sojourn seven years after first meeting her. But she apparently had evinced no interest in

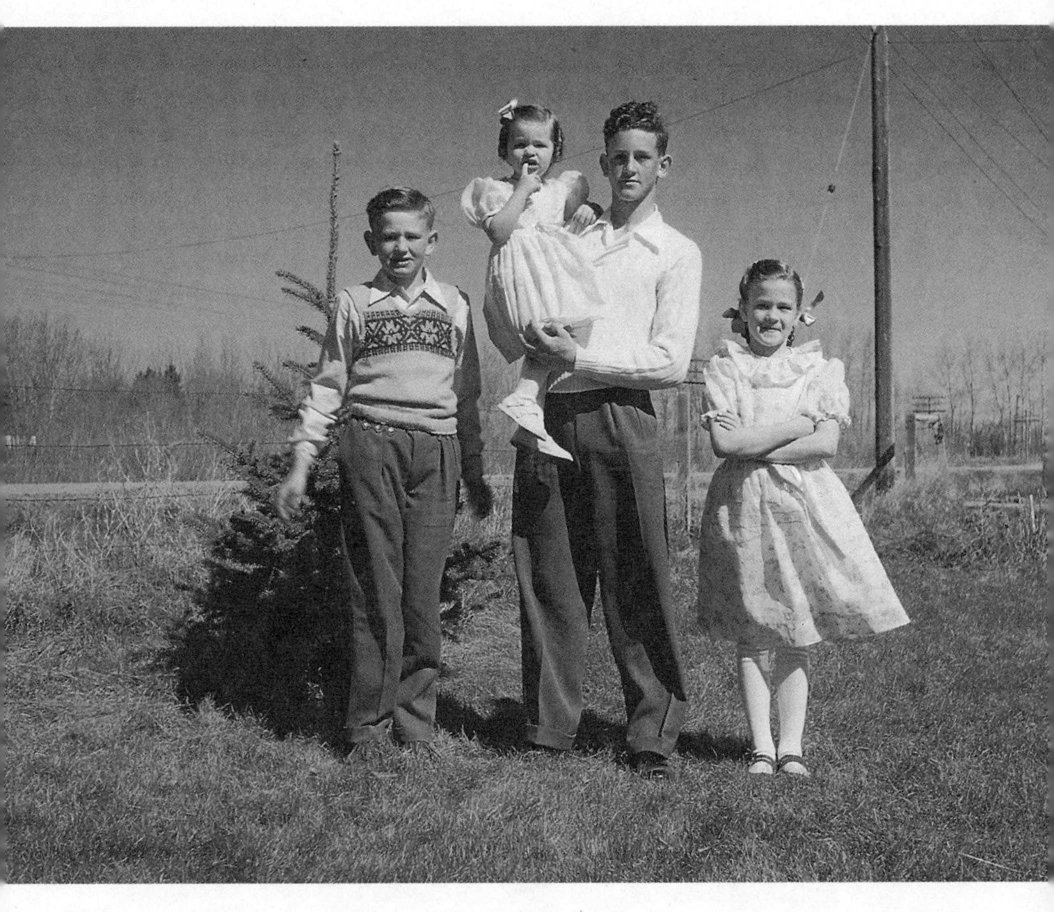

The author with brother Dale (left) and sisters Marian and Linda (in arms) in the farmhouse yard, 1953.

reciprocating his attention, and Grandpa had returned to Pinola to marry Grandma.

My parents took us often to the United States, their native land. These trips, to venues like Great Falls, Montana, or Glacier National Park were customarily heralded on our arrival, after passing customs and immigration, with my father's recitation of the famous 1805 poem *The Lay of the Last Minstrel* by Sir Walter Raleigh Scott:

*Breathes there a man with soul so dead,*
*Who never to himself has said,*
*'This is my own, my native land!'*
*Whose heart hath ne'er within him burn'd*
*As home his footsteps he hath turn'd*
*From wandering on a foreign strand?*

Neither of my parents ever fully accepted their Canadian implantation, and neither ever made the gesture to inquire about Canadian citizenship. For me, this meant dual citizenship, which would come in handy when I moved to Boston in 1978.

Perhaps the biggest adventure of my childhood was our trip in August 1948 to New York to "see the Empire State Building." Dad and Mom, my brother Dale, then six, my sister Marian, three, and I, aged nine, set out in a 1948 Plymouth four-door sedan to travel the 2,200 miles across the American plains, through Illinois, Indiana, Ohio and Pennsylvania, where we visited an endless number of relatives, both close and distant, before the big day when we traveled from Lancaster, Pennsylvania, to New York City. We were awed by the sheer enormity of the big-city skyscrapers, and the memories provided "bragging rights" for years to come.

The trip to New York in the summer of 1948 opened my eyes to a world I had never imagined—I rode my cousin's bicycle on a paved road and saw traffic congestion in the big cities. And my parents showed us the small hilly farms and dense populations in Pennsylvania, so unlike the sparsely populated prairie sites. My plans for my adult years loomed large. Combining my beliefs with my new desire to travel, I decided I wanted more than ever to be a missionary doctor, and I told everyone that was what I planned to be.

## Church Life

For a young Mennonite boy growing up in a farming community, social life consisted almost entirely of church activities. I regularly attended church twice on Sundays, sang hymns for the ill at the hospital in Brooks with a youth group on Sunday afternoons and, more often than not, attended prayer meetings on Thursday nights. I was a pious young man.

For forty years my father led the congregational singing on Sunday mornings. He would rise from his seat in the second row, tap the tuning fork on the first bench to get the pitch and launch *a cappella* singing. He stood erect in the center aisle below the raised platform where the central pulpit stood, and those of us who could carry a tune were given an opportunity to sing parts, from an early age. His was a clear, crisp, tenor voice. My father never looked up as he led the congregation in singing. Not once in all the years I watched him did he acknowledge the congregation. He looked embarrassed, and I was embarrassed for him. What was he thinking?

Men and women were separated in the church. The male elders of the congregation, including ministers, deacons and bishops, sat in the front right pews in the "amen" corner. The other men, including the boys, sat on the right side of the auditorium, and the women and girls were on the left. Sermons were delivered by my grandfather, Henry Ramer, or Uncle Clarence. We petitioned serious prayers in a kneeling position, the congregation rising, turning and facing the rear of the church. The women wore white devotional "coverings" on their heads after they were baptized, and the more conservative men wore "plain" coats, many of which my mother had remodeled from regular suits.

Church was serious business and misbehavior was not tolerated. One of the few spankings I got occurred after church one Sunday evening for not showing the requisite degree of deference, sitting midway up in the church pews and turning around to grimace at my friends in the rear of the church. I knew from my father's stony silence in the car going home that I was in deep trouble. When we arrived, I was taken behind the garage, placed over his knee—he never bothered to sit down—and walloped fifteen to twenty times. It hurt my feelings as much as it hurt my posterior, and I saw to it that it never happened again.

Misbehavior of a more serious type was confessed in church during annual revival meetings, conducted by a God-fearing visiting dignitary, who brought awe and respect. That was a time when we boys, growing up in a bewildering world of sexual exploration, were especially vulnerable to guilt and remorse.

## Uncle Sam Goes to Jail

Of memories I have of family members, the one about my Uncle Sam's arrest on April 19, 1944, and his imprisonment, which became legendary in our community, left an indelible mark.

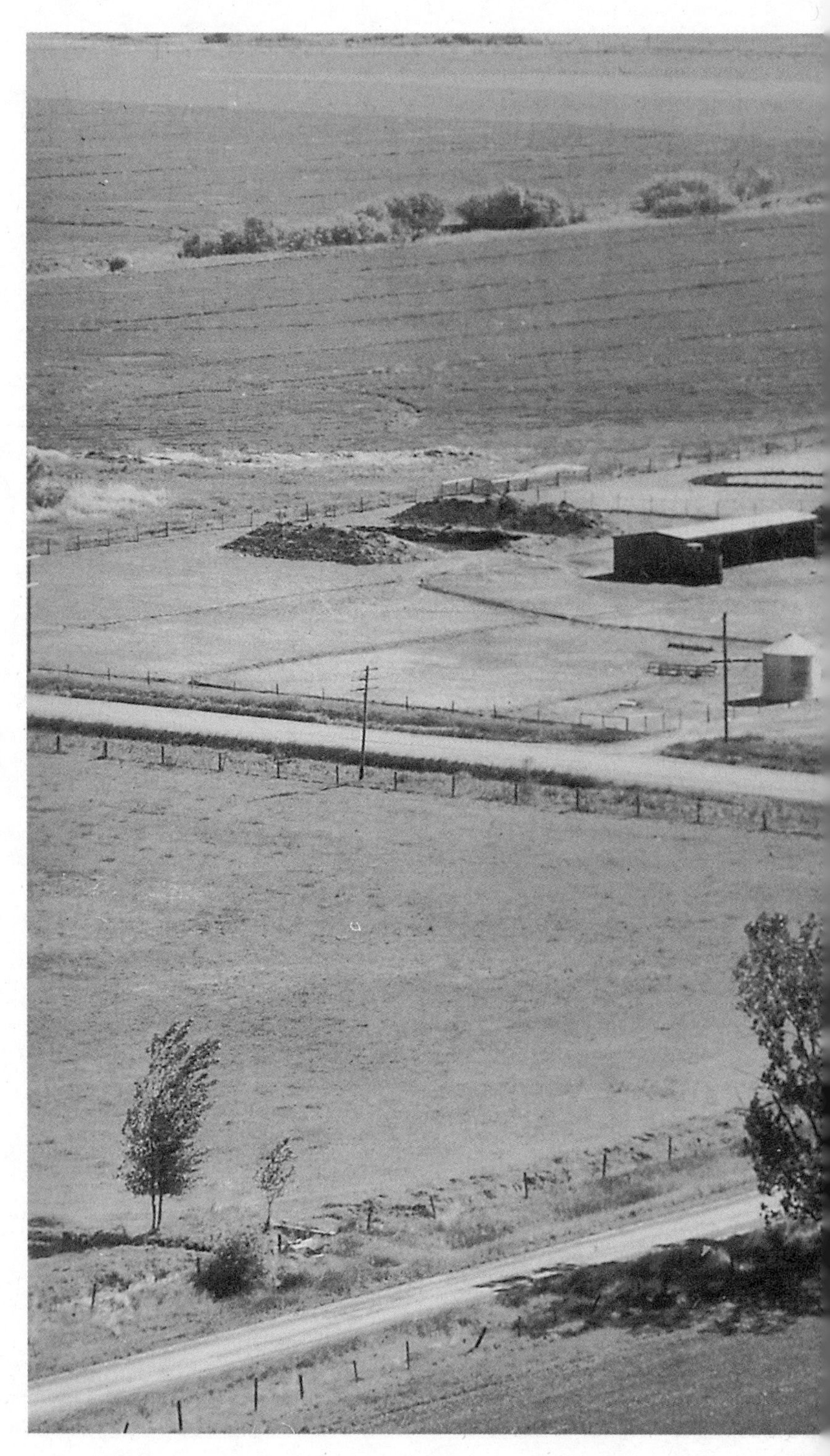

Aerial view of the author's home and intersecting roads, circa 1956. The horizontal road is the gravel "Alaska Highway." The road leading upward passed the Martin homestead one-half mile away. Irrigation ditches beyond the house traverse a part of the Ramer homestead inherited by the author's mother.

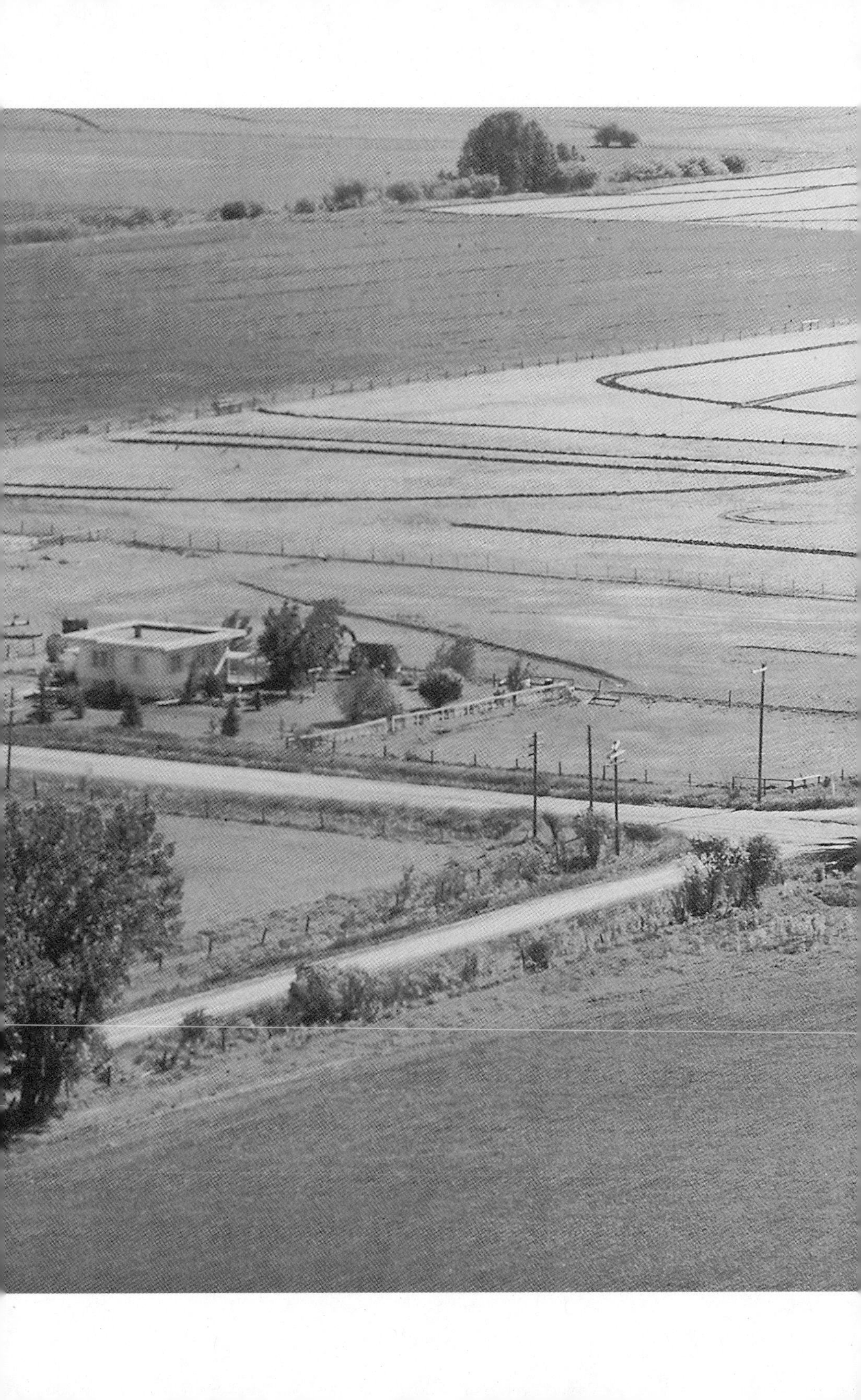

Uncle Sam was born in the US and was eighteen months old when the family moved to Duchess. He had been baptized into the Mennonite Church and attended regularly.

The Mennonite Church in Duchess had taken a strong stand against military involvement in the early part of World War II, and getting deferrals as conscientious objectors (COs) had not been difficult for its members. My father, who was twenty-six years old at the beginning of the war, was drafted by both countries. His appearance before Canadian authorities was limited to an interrogation with an army official and his request for exemption was granted on two counts: his religious convictions as a CO and his occupation as a farmer on his own property. A few months later, he received a letter of inquiry from the US and was granted a similar exemption. Uncle Jim, two years younger than Uncle Sam, was granted CO status and served two years in alternative service in a government-sponsored logging camp.

Uncle Sam's turn to state his case came when he was twenty-one. At first, it seemed that Sam's problems in claiming an exemption arose from a series of inadvertent events. It was thought that the judges and officers reviewing his case wanted to make an example of Sam to others who thought military conscription could be easily avoided. Other Mennonites had enlisted under pressure, after all. Another factor leading to the judges' refusal of deferment was that Sam had recently decided to leave farming to work as a mechanic in Fred's auto shop.

On December 28, 1942, Sam received a call to report for military training. He responded by applying for military exemption as a CO, following the path his other brothers had taken. In late February, he appeared before the Military Mobilization Board in Edmonton. During an interview with the judge, he stated he attended church regularly and had no prior arrest except for a speeding ticket. His request for exemption was rejected; he was offered alternative service with Canada' merchant navy, which he refused. He was given a one-year postponement, a delay in military prosecution.

In early 1944, as the period of postponement was ending, Uncle Sam requested another extension; the request was denied, and a notice to report for military service was issued and Sam was arrested. His first court appearance was before the Royal

Canadian Mounted Police in Brooks on the charge of failing to report for military training after being instructed to do so. His reply to the court was unambiguous and succinct: "Sir, I will not be a soldier. I am a conscientious objector. Three times I have been told to join the military, but my answer is unchanged. The Scriptures, as I understand them, tell me not to kill."

Sam's refusal to accept induction resulted in trials and imprisonment that lasted over the next eighteen months. On April 19, 1944, he was arrested again by the RCMP for failing to report for induction into the army, handcuffed and led across the familiar streets of Brooks to the train station where RCMP officers escorted him to Calgary. He remained shackled during the train ride, and, after arrival at the RCMP barracks, he was photographed, fingerprinted and body-searched. A few days later, the RCMP transported him by train in a cohort of thirty prisoners to the provincial jail in Lethbridge, Alberta. On arrival, his head was shaved, treatment for lice administered, prison clothes assigned, and a thirty-day jail term began.

At the time Lethbridge was a small town one hundred miles southwest of Duchess on the route we often took from our place to the Alberta–Montana border crossing. My parents visited Sam in the months—as the original one-month term was extended—that followed. Sometimes I went along, waiting anxiously in the car with my brother, Dale, until they returned. The visits were short. I had a mixed understanding of the goings-on around me. I knew bad people went to jail, and I knew that Uncle Sam was not bad. So why was he in jail? At five years of age, I was confused.

During the spring of 1944, Sam was permitted to spend time outside in the Alberta sunshine doing farm work. Grandpa Martin and Uncle Clarence, by then a well-known Mennonite minister, importuned the Mobilization Board in Edmonton to secure his release. They were joined by the Conference of Historic Peace Churches in Kitchener, Ontario, in raising concerns about the proceedings. But the authorities refused any further consideration of Sam's sentence.

On May 13, 1944, with four days off his thirty-day sentence for good behavior, he was handed over to the military police and taken back to the Mewata Armory in Calgary to be inducted into the army. Built during World War I, the armory looked like a medieval fortress from the outside, complete with towers and turrets and crenellated rooflines. Its name was borrowed from Cree, an Algonquian language spoken in a variety of dialects by Aboriginal peoples from the Northwest Territories down to Alberta and across Canada to Labrador; ironically, *Mewata* means,"Oh, Be Joyful."

Uncle Sam was subjected to physical examinations and intelligence tests, and the favorable results led to a recommendation of appointment as a junior officer. A uniform was issued, and he was ordered to appear at installation ceremonies. Again, Sam refused. So, on May 24, he was charged with disobeying a lawful command and given a second sentence of twenty-eight days in a military prison, where he was placed into confinement with soldiers found guilty of desertion and disobedience.

The treatment Uncle Sam received at Currie Barracks, a military outpost in Calgary, was denigrating and cruel. After persistent refusal to wear a military uniform, Uncle Sam was stripped, given only underwear, and placed in a small cell. To emphasize the army's view of the seriousness of his failure to enlist, the four-week sentence included a severe curtailment in diet, with two days of bread and water followed by two days of a normal diet.

The military leaders at the Mewata Armory demanded another appearance from Sam on June 23, 1944. Again, Uncle Sam refused to take up the mantle of military service. With his continued refusal to don a military uniform, the army issued a third sentence of twenty-eight days, this time with twenty-one days of bread and water and solitary confinement, where from 10 p.m. to 6 a.m. he was given three blankets to use while sleeping on a hard shelf. He was allowed no visitors during the twenty-eight days of this sentence. Uncle Sam's optimism began to ebb, and he became despondent. He wondered what family and friends were doing to help. And he wondered if Beulah, whom he had started to date before the trouble began, would wait for him until he was free again. He wondered if he might die in prison, and, if he did, would he be missed by anyone?



One day, near the end of his period of isolation, a guard appeared and threw forty-five letters on the floor with the injunction, "You have fifteen minutes to read them." But the guard did not return right away, and he was able to read all of them. The demonstrations of love and support contained in the letters rallied Uncle Sam's spirit. During the last week of the twenty-one-day imposed fast of bread and water, he was finally given access to a normal diet again.

The family and church leaders were devastated. Sam sought assistance from the United States government since he had been born and remained a US citizen. An officer granted him an informal hearing but judged his health too precarious to be moved to the US. The appeals sought by family and church leaders had included the request for consideration of alternative service, as long as it was under civilian and not military management. But Sam's appeal was denied, seemingly because other Mennonites of German-Russian origin had been willing to serve in the medical corps.

A petition objecting to Sam's treatment was signed by 140 Duchess community members, who, although they did not share pacifist beliefs, felt his treatment uncivil and unfair. Two non-Mennonite ministers helped collect the names on the petition, which Uncle Clarence delivered to the commanding officer. Sam was also permitted to have a visit with Clarence, but only if their conversation could be monitored. Clarence requested permission to pray with Sam. The guard, embarrassed by the whole affair, moved away, and Clarence proceeded to tell Sam all the news from the family and the efforts underway to gain his release. Of greatest importance to Sam was Clarence's assurance that Beulah still cared for him.

While Uncle Sam was serving this latest in the string of sentences, another Mennonite appeared at the Currie Barracks. After similar treatment, this man relented and joined the army. "Am I being too adamant in refusing to wear a uniform?" Sam found himself asking. They took away his Bible because, he was told, it was warping his views. But Uncle Clarence complained about this when he heard of it, and the orderly officer returned the Bible. It was illegal to withhold the Scriptures from a defendant.

My puzzlement over Uncle Sam's jail sentence grew in the summer of 1944 when I watched as my parents welcomed Ralph

Sass, a German prisoner-of-war, to our home. Mr. Sass was assigned to farm labor for my dad. I knew we were still fighting the Germans. I could not understand why Uncle Sam languished under tight security in the Lethbridge jail while Mr. Sass was free to walk into town for a package of cigarettes. He seemed to be able to do as he pleased, although he was required to wear a special uniform with a red mark on the back of the shirt. Still, his life seemed altogether quite normal. And why was Uncle Jim permitted to go free logging trees in the mountains.

Later that summer, Uncle Sam was summoned to a hearing regarding a court-martial. Despite testimonial support from Uncle Clarence about Sam's character and sincerity, the military prosecutor recommended an additional sentence of ninety days at Currie Barracks. His fifth sentence was again in solitary confinement with a diet of bread and water.

A few days later, again refusing to wear a uniform, he was forced to march in the prison courtyard with other soldiers. Military activities were part of the daily routine in "rehabilitating" soldiers who had been sent to prison as a disciplinary measure. Having no other clothes, Uncle Sam marched from the barracks into the courtyard where he was left standing in his underwear, while the others marched to the sergeant's cadence, calling out "right-left, right-left." Just then, a voice came over the loudspeaker. "Sam Martin, you are sentenced to eighteen months in the Lethbridge Provincial Jail, with hard labor."

Returning to his cell, he discovered that a uniform had been delivered to him. He looked at it for a while; the temptation was strong. What was the fight about anyway? Why had he been singled out for humiliation from the thousands of Mennonites, Doukhobors, Jehovah's Witnesses, Quakers and other COs? How much longer could he bear it?

Before he was transferred back to Lethbridge, a doctor examined Sam and concluded that the authorities needed to do something about him. His health had become precarious. He had lived on bread and water for forty-nine days over the previous three months. My father remembered him as a skeleton.

Lethbridge seemed like a homecoming for Sam, but he was too weak to carry out his work assignment: hoeing weeds in the sugar beet field. As a result, he was put in charge of the horse cart that ferried food around the prison grounds. In October Sam was given a weekend pass to Duchess. He saw Beulah and his family and participated in the semi-annual communion service held each fall and spring at the Duchess Mennonite Church. He once again enjoyed his mother's cooking, and he and Beulah spent hours together sharing experiences that would eventually become a major part of their lives. On Sunday evening, my father and Beulah took him back to Calgary, as required. He was once again transferred to Lethbridge to complete the remainder of the eighteen-month sentence.

Fortunately, Sam's subsequent stay in the Lethbridge jail turned out to be a friendly one. By now Sam was well known and respected by the warden. He was assigned to regular duties, and somehow the hard labor stipulation was overlooked in the conveyance of orders. He was put in charge of the maintenance and repair of the twelve lawn mowers the jail used to maintain the property. He soon noticed that prisoners were sabotaging the mowers to get time off to rest. Sam urged rest breaks and the misbehavior abated. When the warden needed a mechanic to fix his car, Sam's experience in Fred's garage came in handy. The warden extended Uncle Sam's work to include repairing the farm machinery, hauling grain during the harvest on the prison farm, and Sam was the first prisoner at that jail permitted to drive the prison truck into town on local errands. The other prisoners seemed to respect him for his efforts, and, as far as Sam recalled years later, did not resent his new liberties.

During this period of thawed relations between Sam and prison authorities, a member of the prison community assigned as manager of the prison farm was found guilty of embezzling money. Sam and an older "convict" were put in charge of the farm. Sam was responsible for directing the prisoners' farm duties throughout the spring and summer of 1945. The warden congratulated the two: "Boys, we just want you to know that we are very pleased with the way you're running the farm. For the first time in its existence, this farm has made a profit."

By this time, events in the European theater of the war were drawing to a close. On April 27, 1945, Allied forces closed in on Milan; Mussolini was executed on April 28; and Hitler committed suicide on April 30. A day later, German forces in Italy

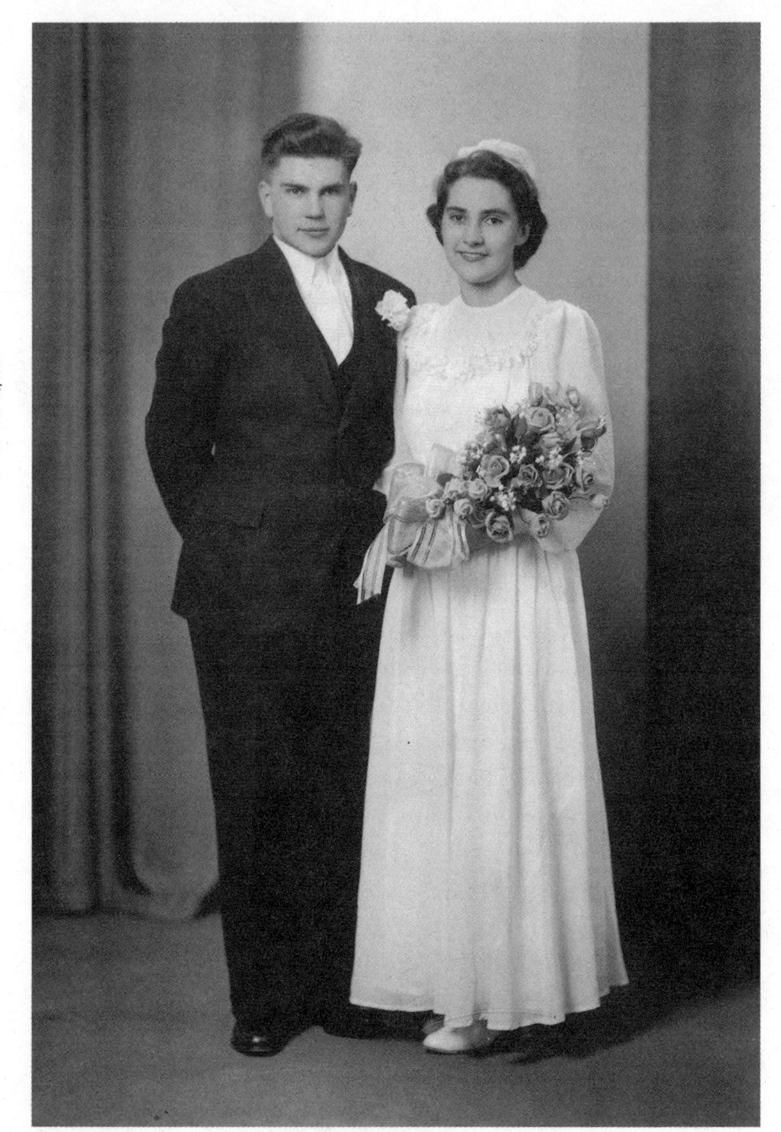

Wedding photograph of Uncle Sam and Aunt Beulah Martin.

surrendered, and between May 2 and May 4 the remainder of German forces throughout Germany surrendered. An unconditional surrender by the Axis powers occurred on May 7 and 8. But Japan continued on in its efforts in the Pacific theater. Atom bombs released on Hiroshima and Nagasaki in early August led to Japanese surrender.

Early in November 1945, after completing two-thirds of the eighteen-month sentence, Uncle Sam was summoned to the warden's office and informed that the remainder of his sentence had been "remitted." The many appeals to Edmonton and Ottawa appeared to have had their effect. As well, Canada's involvement in the war had ended in the summer of 1945. The Canadian military operation was being dismantled.

I recall standing by the highway watching military convoys lumber by on the gravel road, one of the main routes for US troops returning from Alaska, and thinking about Uncle Sam going to jail for not wanting to fight. I couldn't understand why the war had lasted for more than six years, and why a disagreement between a few countries had taken so long to resolve. And, at the age of seven, I couldn't conceptualize the human loss, but the tanks, trucks and machine guns that moved along the Alaska Highway within one hundred feet of my house as they were transported from Alaska back to the continental US made a deep impression on me.

Sam requested an "industrial leave" to assist in the work at his brother's garage. The commanding officer agreed, and he was released on November 8, 1945. His first call was to Beulah—from a hotel in Calgary. He asked her to come and get him. When she arrived, he proposed on the spot, and she agreed to marry him. In mid-April, 1946, nearly a year after the war had ended and two years after his initial confinement, Sam received a formal military discharge—an honorary discharge that carried the addendum, "twenty-three months non-effective service."

After being released from prison, Uncle Sam became the shop manager at the Duchess Garage, now run by Uncle Fred and my father. He was a capable mechanic, eventually assuming the role of foreman. There seemed no vehicular mechanical or electrical problem that he could not track down and solve. During my early teenage years, I worked in the front section of the business, pumping gas, finding machinery parts for customers and assisting with office paper work. I admired Sam enormously and often asked him to repeat stories of his time in jail, which he seemed very reluctant to talk about. I wondered whether the prison experience had affected him in ways that he found difficult to describe.

Reflecting on his experiences more than a half century later, Sam would encourage young people to "stand up for their convictions and to remember that such decisions are not made in isolation." He did not regret his decision:

> *If anything, I suppose I would have to say that my convictions are even stronger now than they were then...It's just that coming from where I came from... my background...it was impossible for me to take arms and destroy human lives or even to support a system that did...*[2]

> Grades five, six and seven, Duchess Elementary School, 1951. The author is in the back row, center, with the prominent ears. Teacher Jean Murray recommended the author's promotion from grade seven to grade nine, which permitted him to graduate from high school at age sixteen.

Sam and Beulah lived in Duchess for their entire married life.[3] On April 8, 2010, Uncle Sam had a fall, likely from a heart arrhythmia, and suffered a subdural hematoma, with death occurring within twelve hours. I was in Alberta visiting my mother, planning to see Sam and Beulah the very next day. He was a remarkable man and his passing was quick, as he would have wanted it.

My last memories of the war as a child came about two years after Uncle Sam returned home, when Uncle Clarence brought to our church a Jewish friend, Joseph Herscowitz, whom he had met on a trip to Chicago. Mr. Herscowitz told us all of the death of Jews in Europe, the transport from the cities to the gas chambers in the death camps. I felt again the incredulity of war and what humans are capable of doing to each other. I was determined more than ever to explore the horizons beyond the environs of my upbringing.

## School Days in Duchess

In the 1920s there was a one-room schoolhouse that served grades one through eight. The school I remember had three rooms for grades one to three, four and five, and six through eight, linked by a common hallway. Later, a fourth classroom was added and grades eight through ten were located there. I completed ten years in Duchess and was then bused to Rosemary, ten miles away, for the final two years of high school.

Farm schoolyards always had a barn located a few hundred feet away from the school to house the horses that some students rode to school, and the outhouses were near the barn. At our school, there was one outhouse for each sex, located at the perimeter of center field of the ball diamond. The memory

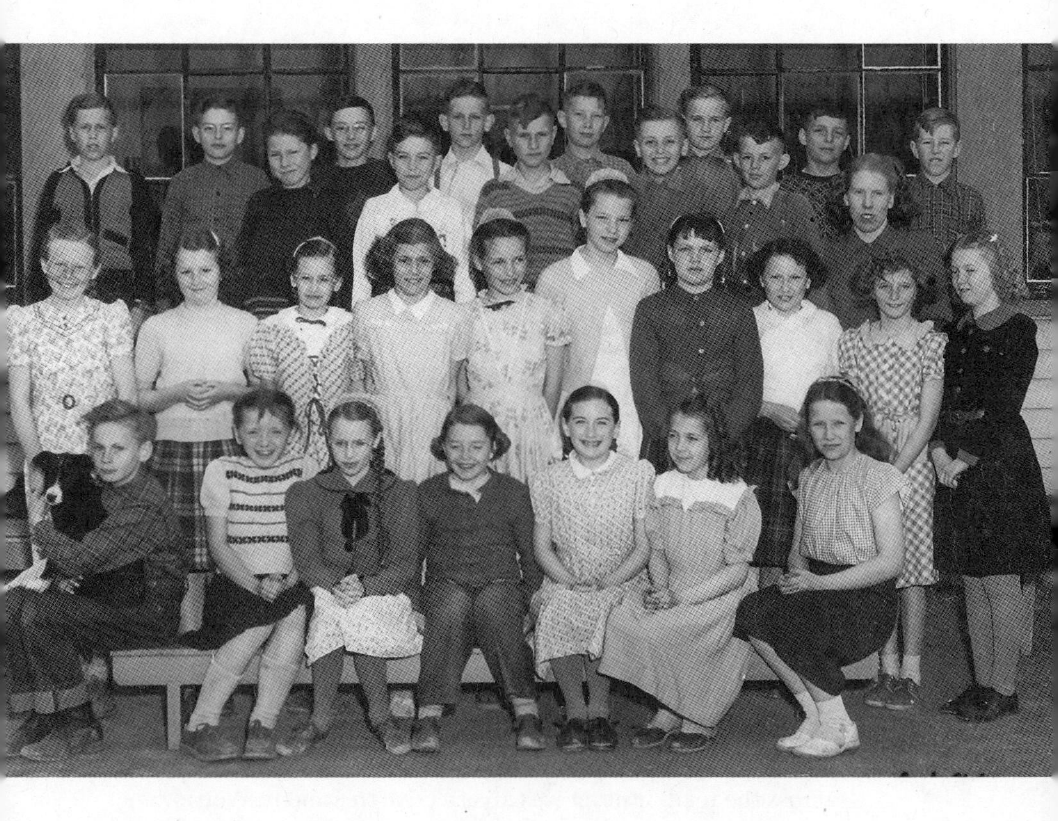

remains fresh of recovering a wayward baseball from the toilet when the door had been left open and, on at least one occasion, from the hole itself. Balls were valuable, and we only had one. Halloween invariably led to upending the school toilets, particularly those used by the principal and teachers. It was a great accomplishment to tip it over when it was occupied, especially if you got away with it afterward.

For a while, in grade school, I appointed myself the music teacher to a group of young Mennonite students. It didn't matter that I had had no instruction in music! I bought music books to first teach myself and then the younger kids at the Mennonite church across the street from the schoolyard, helping them master the four parts of singing that would later become useful as they sang *a cappella* in church.

School was always easy for me, and I don't remember ever taking homework with me after school. I loved geography, memorizing country capitals, rivers, mountains and famous landmarks. I read widely in history and immersed myself in the assignments in literature. Education in Alberta was by this time highly structured, and province-wide examinations were given at the end of grades nine and twelve. One of my favorite teachers, Jean Murray, arranged for my transfer from grade seven directly to grade nine. I had to hustle that year to pass the standardized province-wide exams.

## My Friend Spot

Spot was a two-year-old cocker spaniel, brown with white patches and dangling ears that flopped when he ran. He came from a neighbor's litter—free, if I promised to take good care of him. He waited for me in the driveway of our country home each day when I returned from school, rushing out to greet me, cautious not to go onto the road. Somehow he never got attached to chasing cars, a common pastime of rural hounds, such as my cousin Robert's collie, which lived across the road from our place. Chasing cars was dangerous for dogs. An irritable driver en route to town could time the sudden opening of the car door to strike a blow to the chasing animal, sending him sprawling across the road. It never was an effective treatment. Worse yet was the trick of tying a gunnysack to the wheel hub cover and driving toward the dog; the hound's teeth would catch in the mesh and it would twist and turn with the movement of the wheel, sometimes suffering fatal injuries. It is said that you can't teach an old dog new tricks. Equally difficult, I learned, is to unteach a young dog with bad habits.

Spot was not a house dog; he slept in a kennel near the rear door even during the bitter cold days of winter. There he waited patiently for food and water whenever the door opened.

Spot was a "bird dog." He chased anything that ran or flew nearby, almost never successfully but never seeming to give up. It was easy to take Spot hunting. I would take my favorite shotgun, a 14-gauge Browning over/under model from my father's rack, climb the chain-link fence I'd helped build between the house and the open farmland, and we'd set off, Spot flushing out ring-neck pheasants and I, usually inaccurately, trying to hit one. When successful, my mother would prepare the bird for a delicious meal for me and the family.

Spot loved to hunt birds, so how would he know that baby chicks were off limits? One spring afternoon, with temperatures soaring from chinook breezes blowing in over the mountains, Grandpa Ramer released a brood of chicks into a low fenced-in area outside the barn. It was a great find for Spot. When I returned from school that day, he dashed eagerly to meet me, tail wagging furiously, a chick in his mouth, proudly demonstrating his canine talents. On approaching the pen, I found the remains of his successful hunt—twenty-five to thirty chicks piled together neatly in one corner.

Dad was furious. "You'll never be able to trust that dog again," he said.

The next thing I knew, Spot was in the back of Dad's pickup truck heading to the open prairie, where a single shot heard from afar told me of Spot's demise. I was heartbroken, but these were the rules of prairie life. Spot was only three years old when he died. I never again had a dog as a pet.

The deep hurt (was it anger?) was assuaged somehow later that year when hunting for coyotes with my dad. Driving across the prairies west of Duchess near the Rocky Lake reservoir we came upon a coyote sleeping in the grass. Dad swerved the car to put me in line with the coyote as it ran away.

"This one is yours," he said.

I put my .22–250 rifle out the open window, took a bead on the coyote in the telescopic sight and followed it moving the rifle to keep pace with the animal aiming carefully for the heart just behind the shoulder. I pulled the trigger and the coyote collapsed. We drove to the site and, assured that the animal was dead, my father put out his hand with a friendly gesture, "Good job, now you are a man." I was very pleased, and the rift between us closed.

## The Call of the Wild

Nature's mysteries, its wilderness and its bounty were ever present in my everyday existence. Although we lived relatively close to the Canadian Rockies, which were about two hundred miles away, I pled unsuccessfully for the opportunity to learn to ski; we were too poor to purchase equipment and pay the fees for skiing.

In its place, my numerous cousins and I took up inexpensive avocations like Sunday-afternoon hikes in the Badlands, now part of Alberta's Dinosaur Provincial Park, on the banks of the Red Deer River, where we looked for fossil bones and animal remains.

Once or twice a year we visited and hiked in the Rocky Mountains of Banff and Jasper National Parks, nestled in the majesty of nature. Banff National Park, established in 1885, is the oldest of Canada's national parks. Located eighty miles west of Calgary, the park features 2,564 square miles (6,641 square kilometers) of valleys, mountains, glaciers and forests. Its natural phenomena were first "discovered" by transplanted Europeans in 1883 when three CPR workers stumbled across a cave containing hot springs on the eastern slopes of the Rocky Mountains. With close to 3,894 square miles (11,000 square kilometers) of mountain wilderness, Jasper is the largest national park in the Canadian Rockies. The two parks are home to many of North American's big game animals, including grizzly bears, moose, elk, and mountain sheep and goats.

As I grew older, my interactions with nature also involved my father; he began taking me along on his hunting adventures. The highlights occurred in late summer and early autumn with hunting trips on the eastern fringe of Banff National Park. These two-week escapades with my father, his guide and close friends involved remote campsites, finicky horses not accustomed to riders and long horseback treks deep into the mountains, where I often felt no man could ever possibly have gone before. He had already made sure I was properly educated in hunting and gave excellent instructions. Before setting off on large expeditions, I learned how to safely hold a loaded gun while walking through the fields with Spot in search of partridge or pheasant, and Dad urged me never to prop a loaded gun next to me while driving across the prairie.

Early morning was the best time to spot coyotes on the prairies. We traveled along the back roads at dawn, along the banks of the canals, or across the ranges of prairie where cattle grazed. Young coyotes were particularly vulnerable, born in the spring and striking out on their own in the fall. We used gophers for target practice. At 100 to 150 yards, a direct hit was a sure sign that the scope was properly aligned on the rifle barrel. Other target options were crows and magpies on fence posts, and occasionally a sparrow hawk, but never an eagle. We knew better than to shoot the American bird.

Big game hunting in the Canadian Rockies was best in late August and early September. Elk and moose were in full "heat" at that time of year, eager for reproductive action. At this time of year the males had fully developed antlers that gave them the equipment necessary not only for aggressive challenges to competitors but also to attract females. Under testosterone stimulation, the antlers grow over a few months from small stumps in the spring to formidable racks that would be larger each year the animal aged. The antlers fall off in the late fall when seasonal changes in circadian rhythms cause levels of the hormone to decline rapidly.

We also shot mountain sheep and occasionally a mountain goat. Bears could not be hunted in the regions outside the immediate boundaries of the park, but they were plentiful in parts of northern Alberta. By contrast to elk, deer, moose and mountain sheep, which were quite edible, bear meat made terrible steaks and hamburgers because of its gritty fatty texture. As a result, bears were shot mostly for their trophy value. The head and the skin of a bear looked impressive on the floor in the den or hung on the wall, head down. My father in his later years managed to ambush a full-sized grizzly bear, and for years to come the hide, carefully prepared by a taxidermist with head remaining attached, hung in the entry of my parents' house. It was to become a gift to my nephew, Jeff Shantz, who after being drafted by the Chicago Blackhawks began playing for the Calgary Flames. That was just fine with me, and I hope with other members of the family. My mother, certainly, was not troubled by its departure from her home. After my father died, all of the trophies ended up as gifts to friends or family. He had left me one of his favorite rifles, a caliber .22–250 with a beautiful laminated stock that he had carved. But it disappeared from his nearly empty gun cabinet a few years later. I have no idea who took it, but I'm not too concerned since I had no idea how it would be transported across the 49th parallel separating our two countries. "Gun control" works in peculiar ways in the US!

My experience in the art and science of hunting was unique in the setting of a pacifist Mennonite community, especially during World War II when some of our neighbors went off to war. Then there was my mother's aversion to shooting guns, associated with her brother's tragic accidental death. No question, the avocation had a particularly bloody tinge. Yet for me it was invigorating, and it was the time I spent alone with my father that made it so special.[4]

## My Life as a Trapper

The time I was able to spend with my father hunting, and the lessons I learned from him during our trips, resulted in him placing an interesting responsibility on my shoulders later in my youth. On October 20, 1952, as I turned fourteen years old, I looked forward to a new adventure. Each fall, in early November, the trapping season opened. I had learned the ropes from my father, who had depended on the income from catching and selling ermine (weasel), muskrat and mink furs during the Great Depression. Weasels, normally chocolate brown, turn snow white in early November as the days shorten and temperatures fall. Their bodies are about ten inches long, with an equally long tail ended in a black tip.

My father provided me with a 1950 Fargo truck, fitted with a flat five-foot-wide box with ten-inch-high sides and an open back. I drove along my trapline three times a week, following fence lines over the prairie or along the irrigation canals, where weasels liked to spend the winter.

To attract the weasels' interest, I stapled pieces of carcasses to fence posts about eighteen inches above the metal traps. The bait consisted mostly of prairie snowshoe hares, which could be shot during the night from our car as we drove country roads with a spotlight. Transfixed in the glare, the hare were easy marks for a rifle with a telescope sight.

A weasel caught a day or two before I found it was frozen solid, its extended limbs caught in the jaws of the trap as it struggled to get free. When I came upon recently captured animals, however, I knew I would be in for a ferocious fight. They would lunge at me as I swung my hatchet, aiming to strike them

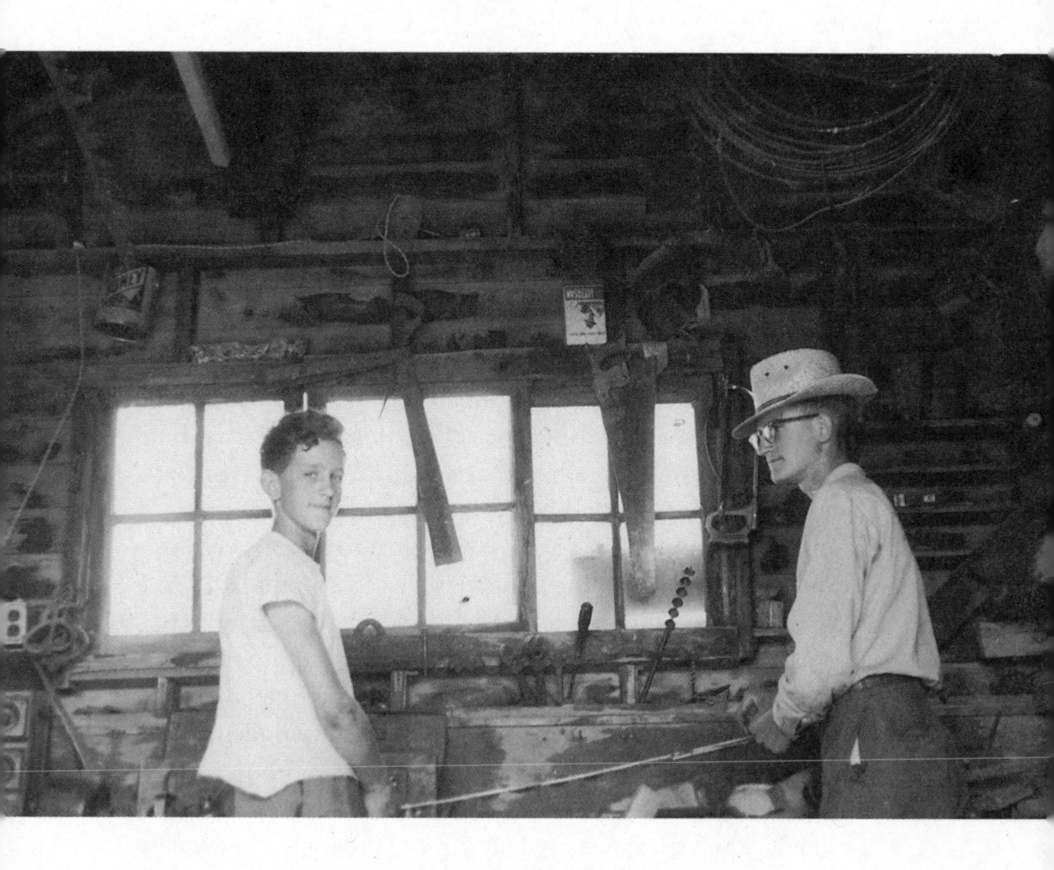

on the head. It was crucial not to damage the fur covering the body.

After completing the five-mile run in the truck, past traps placed every one hundred to two hundred yards, I skinned each animal I'd caught. I removed the hide from the body, beginning with the tail, carefully leaving it attached to the fur at the rear of the body. Then, I gently dissected each paw away from the hide and advanced forward, turning the hide inside out to maintain its integrity, careful not to sever a piece or cut a hole, which would greatly reduce its value. After dissecting the hide away from the four paws and cutting around the face, the skin and its fur was freed from the carcass and could be stretched inside out over a slat of wood about two inches wide and eighteen inches long. I hung each hide suspended vertically for a few days in the cold outdoors, until they dried to a firm texture.

My two months of trapping yielded a quite remarkable eighty-three weasel hides, about a dozen more than the number caught

The author with cousin Robert Ramer in the farm workshop, 1950.

by my father's friend, Jack Endersby, who was nine years older than me, and who I felt competed with me for my father's attention. At $3 a hide, I had enough money to buy my first 35mm camera, which heralded the beginning of a lifelong love of photography.

## It Could Have Ended For Me Then

My hunting trips ended when I left for university at age sixteen, but not before I nearly lost my life. It was the end of the summer in 1952. Bob Long, an experienced trapper and a big game hunter's guide in southern Alberta, as well as my father's friend of many years, took my father and me and three other friends on the first hunt of the year in late August to an area west of Sundre, Alberta, near the Banff National Park boundary. We set out the first morning on horseback to ride five to ten miles to the best hunting area. The horses had been brought into the corral a few days before, after running wild for the summer. They were an edgy lot and not quite sure they wanted to be ridden.

A short distance down the trail on the first morning, my cap blew off. I dismounted and, with my rifle strapped across my shoulder and back, retrieved my cap and proceeded to remount the nervous horse. I placed my left foot into the stirrup, grabbed for the horn of the saddle and made a lunge to mount. Just then, the spooked horse turned away from me. The saddle, which had not been tightly secured (horses can prevent the tightening of the cinch on the saddle by voluntary inflation of the lungs), swung in a circle around and under the horse, at which point my foot slipped fully into the stirrup. The horse ran down the trail toward my father who had dismounted to wait for me. My father saw what happened. The saddle and I were both under the horse, and the horse was lunging at full gallop toward him. I still remember keeping my grip on the horn of the saddle and drawing myself upward to keep my head off the ground. My father described vividly the image that flashed before his mind's eye, of traveling home with my corpse in the back of the pickup and trying to explain to my mother what had happened. By some miracle, the stirrup detached from the leg flap of the saddle and I was deposited at the side of the trail, unharmed. My rifle was

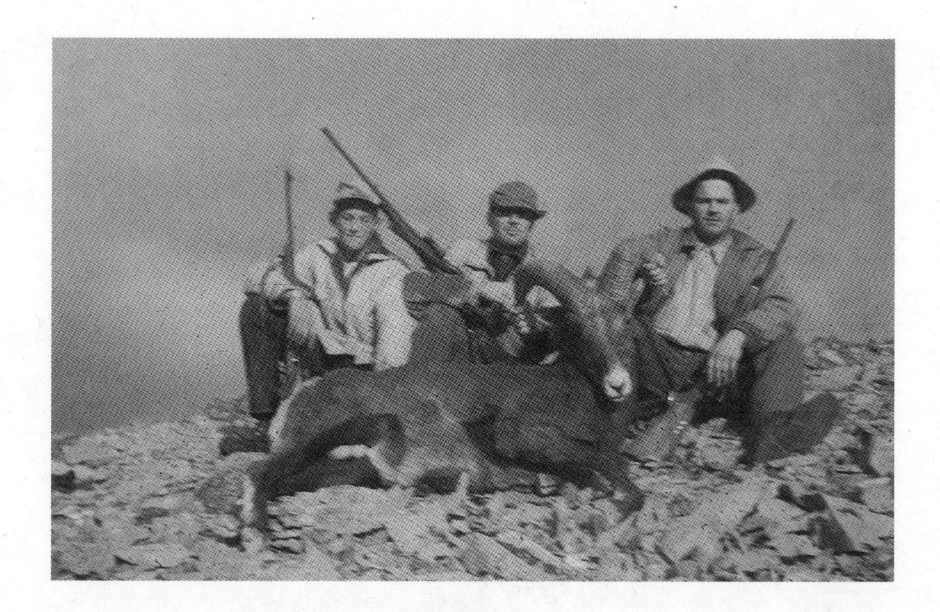

missing but a thorough search located it in the brush well off the trail with its sling broken, the stock having caught hold on the ground and flung it off to the side. My only residual predicament was a torn right pant leg from cuff to thigh. Bob Long pursued the horse for more than a mile. The saddle was torn to pieces as the horse stumbled over the fragments left hanging from its belly.

The author's father (right), rancher Gene Christianson, and the author on a successful hunt outside Banff National Park in the Rocky Mountains, 1953, (elevation 10,000 feet). The bighorn sheep head would soon adorn a wall in the author's father's den.

The call of the wild took only a momentary deflection. Bob returned to camp for another saddle, we exchanged horses and on we went with our hunting. Later, Bob commented on how he had noticed that the lacing on the leg strap that attached to that stirrup was broken, and that he had intended to repair it but had gotten heavy into the rum instead. I was glad Bob had become distracted! In the end, the hunt was successful; my father managed to shoot four deer over the next week, providing meat and a trophy to each of the other hunters. He used to insist that he had never shot a large game animal illegally, and I am inclined to believe him.

My father's hobby of guns and ammunition was quite out of the ordinary for a pacifist Mennonite. He became a charter member of the National Rifle Association and collected every volume of the association's monthly publication, *The National Rifleman*, from 1930 through 1990, all precisely and tediously

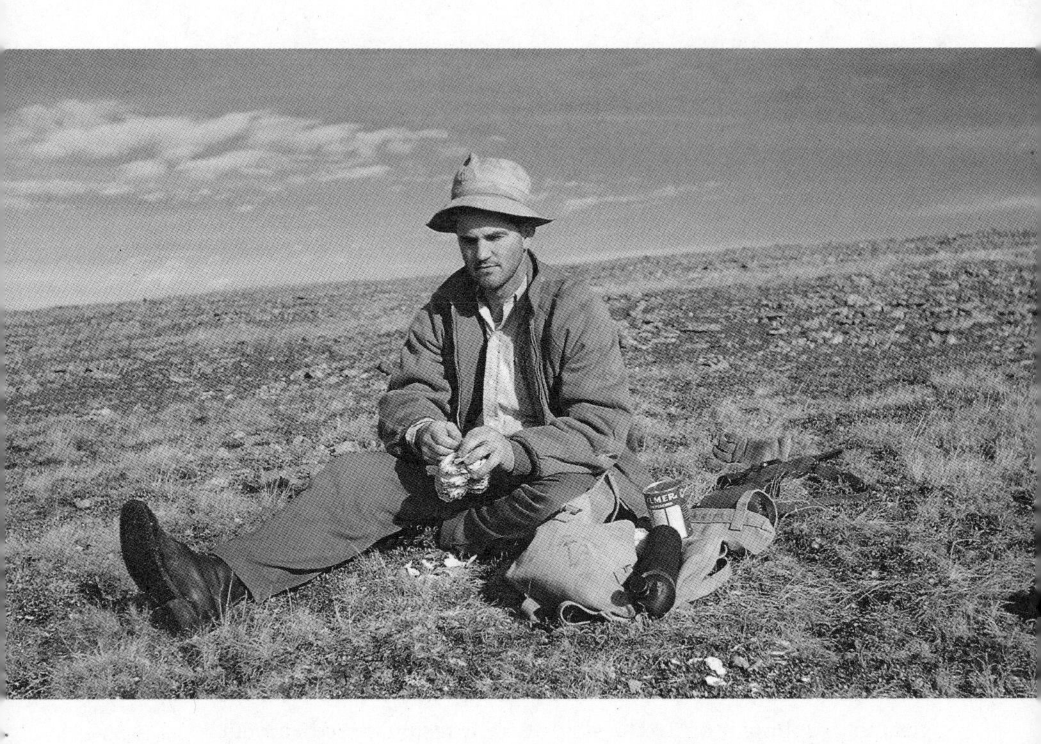

The author's father enjoying lunch on a hunting trip.

bound and organized on the shelves in his gunroom. I had not appreciated how deeply he felt about hunting until very recently when I discovered an extensive handwritten notebook he had been compiling about his adventures, meticulously recording every hunting experience he had ever had, beginning with the first big hunting trip he took in 1929, at the age of sixteen. He would not return to big game hunting—elk, deer, bear, mountain sheep and mountain goats—in the mountains again until 1938, the year I was born. After that year he would go hunting every fall along the foothills of the Rocky Mountains, staying there for a week or two at a time.

Although he took up hunting to provide for the family, it became a "hobby" for my father. At one point, his collection included more than eighty rifles and shotguns. In later years, his travels to the United States revolved around visits to gun shops to purchase copper jackets, gunpowder, telescopes and crudely shaped wooden "stocks" that he fashioned into handsome wooden supports to hold the embedded bolt action of the rifle. But, although he claimed never to have shot an animal illegally, not all of his ammunition importing was legal. In the days after World War II, there were ample supplies of bullets and gunpowder in the US, and my father's purchases far exceeded the limits Canadian authorities had imposed for bringing such items across the border. On one occasion, I watched my father take apart the upholstery lining the tire wells and inner parts of the doors to deposit his treasures, avoiding discovery. On another occasion, he had purchased a fifty-pound keg of gunpowder that would only fit upright in the trunk of the 1948 Plymouth sedan. Most border crossings were a mere formality, but to assure almost certain disinterest by the customs agent, my father waited until the lunch hour to cross the small border crossing a few miles north of Shelby, Montana. The lone agent asked about goods being brought across the border, and my father replied that he had some sporting goods, which, he always maintained, was an accurate accounting of the real nature of the items. The agent rose from his place behind the desk, saying he wanted to take a look. The opened trunk displayed the folly of my father's habits, and he was informed that there "was no way you can take that into Canada." My father insisted that it was for his own use, that he had a legitimate sporting goods license and that he believed there was no reason why it could not be taken into Canada, requesting that a higher-up be consulted. A telephone call and further insisting on my father's part led to a peaceful and entirely satisfactory conclusion. He drove off into Alberta with a ten-year supply of the explosive stuff. Stories like this became one of the family lodestones of triumph over adversity as posed by regulatory agencies. Storytelling became one of Dad's passions, and he was superb at rendering accounts of ordinary events into pearls of wisdom.

## The "Sweat Shop" and Myrtle Bast's Duchess Café

During most evenings of the week my father and Uncle Fred entertained local farmers and anyone else who might come their way. Uncle Fred, who since his early teenage years had been immersed in conversations with regular contacts around the world with his ham radio, would talk about conversations he had on the radio with his contacts, spurring on dialogue in the garage. The setting for this "salon" was the Duchess Garage, affectionately referred to as the "sweat shop" by my dad. The impression Uncle Fred and Dad gave to their families, who remained at home on these evenings, was that these events were sales "opportunities."

I joined in some evenings in my teens and remember energizing discussions on many topics. Religion and local politics were in general taboo, but national and business topics related to survival in a rural western Canadian farming economy were common. Discussions often revolved around the vagaries of the weather: cold icy winters and hail and drought in the summer; the prices of wheat, beef and pork; and the incessant failure of the citizens of eastern Canada to appreciate the contributions of the western provinces. It was explained to me that Alberta sent oil, minerals and foodstuffs at low transportation cost to the east, where they manufactured all types of goods—cars, trucks, machinery, radios and television sets, packaged cereals, other foodstuffs and perishables—then sent them back to us at great cost. Our political ineptness, in the view of Uncle Fred, kept us from significant intellectual deliberations and fair trade agreements with big government and the robber barons of Toronto and Ottawa. Perhaps it was this sentiment that led me to cheer for the Montreal Canadiens hockey team rather than the Toronto Maple Leafs. (The Detroit Red Wings were also a favorite in our family because they connected us to the automobile industry, to which we owed our livelihood.)

The other center where discussions took place was Myrtle Bast's Duchess Café, just down the street from the Duchess Garage, where a few of my uncles, along with the mechanics from the sweat shop, took their coffee breaks. Uncle Sam, who had a clever sense of humor, was usually the life of the party during coffee breaks at the café. A centerpiece of the action was the merciless teasing of the young waitresses, who seemed pleased with the attention.

While the men met and conversed at Myrtle Bast's café, the women of the Mennonite Church were a close-knit group who gathered regularly at the Sewing Circle where quilts were quilted and garments sewed for sale at the Mennonite Central Committee's annual fundraiser. My mother was an accomplished seamstress and my sister Marian took it up seriously,

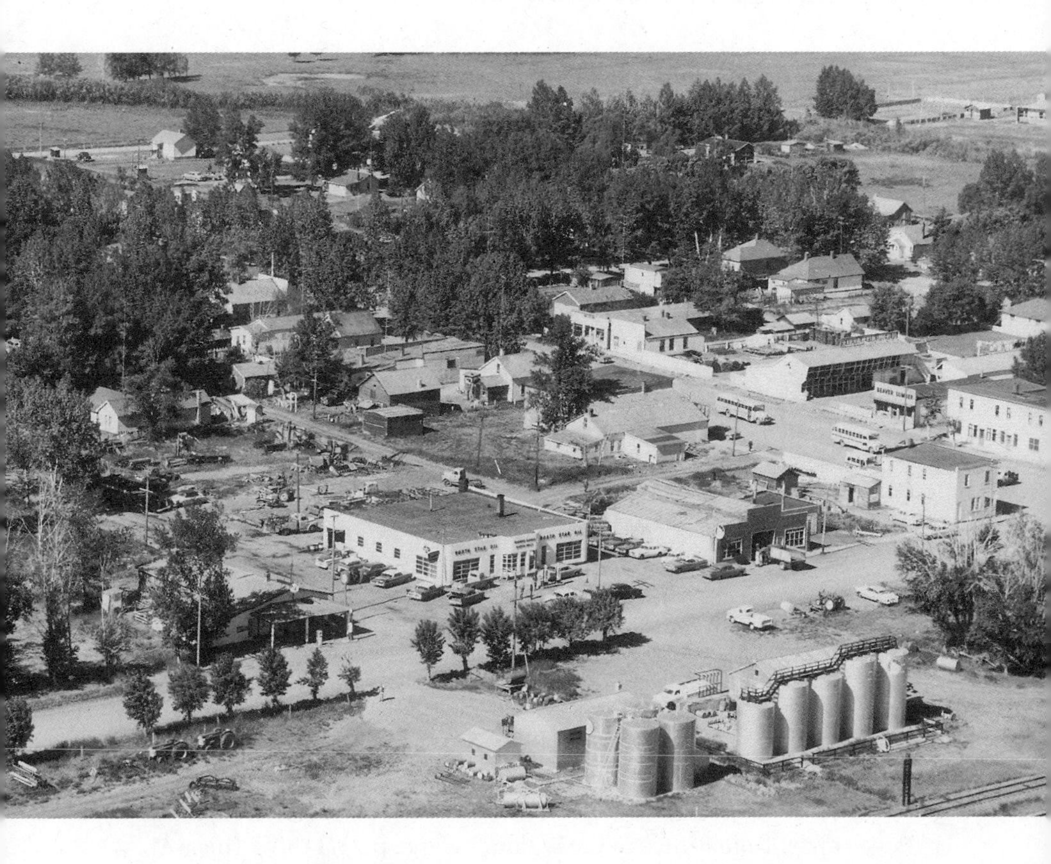

The village of Duchess, Alberta, circa 1952. The Duchess Garage is in the center foreground of the picture; Myrtle Bast's Duchess Café is on the lower right, at the corner of Main Street.

becoming an accomplished quilt designer and needlepoint craft expert, later creating objects that sold for hundreds of dollars.

## The End of an Era

Grandpa Martin died in 1964 at the age of seventy-nine, a few months short of his eightieth birthday. His ten children became pastors, homemakers and farmers, and some held dealerships in farm machinery, trucks and cars. My father lived a few months beyond ninety-one years. His health was affected at age sixty when he was diagnosed with prostate cancer, initially considered very serious. He responded to radiation treatment, however, and aside from the common side effects resulting from the treatment, he lived a healthy and full life. He was buried in 2005 next to a spruce tree in the Duchess cemetery.

As I think back to my days in Duchess, I realize that our experiences were unique in our community and set our family

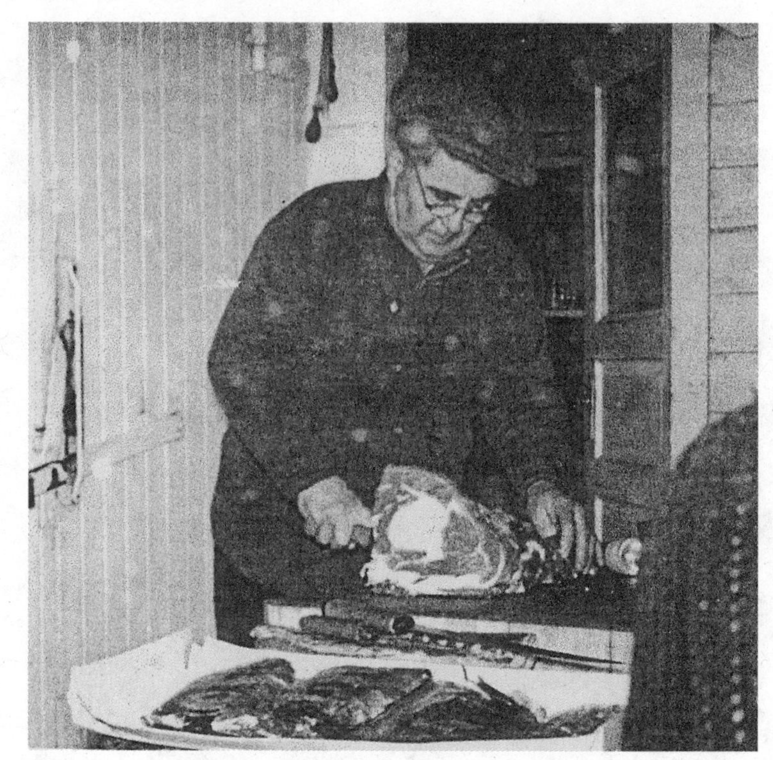

Grandpa Martin, 1958, cutting a beef roast in Slatter's Meat Shop, Duchess.

apart from others in the region. In large part, I think this was because of my father's restlessness, his seemingly relentless quest for adventure and knowledge of a world beyond the perimeters of a farm. That quest and his ability to adjust to situations drove him to achievements quite remarkable for an uneducated man. He used to read widely and could quote poetry from many sources. Intensely curious about world politics, particularly those affecting the United States, he received and read through several of the weekly newsmagazines—*Time*, *Newsweek*, and when it appeared, *US News & World Report*. He had changed careers from a dairy farmer to a successful automobile and farm implement dealer. I learned from him that much can be achieved if one really wants it badly enough.

I recall with great pride my dad's purchase of an entire Encyclopedia Britannica when I was twelve years old. He called the sales representative in Calgary, who appeared one day at the Duchess Garage armed with a sales pitch. Halfway through it, my dad stopped him with the warning, "If you go on much longer, you'll talk me out of it." They reached an agreement, a check was passed and, to this day, a familiar recollection is of Dad reaching for the encyclopedia to settle a dispute about history, politics or geography. His focus on facts probably accounts for my own predisposition toward reading history and biographies over novels.

In 2011 my mother, born in 1915, still was living in Duchess in the house that she and my father had built to their personal specifications in 1963. Nearby, in the village, live my two sisters, Marian and Linda, and their families. By 1980 my parents had begun migrating each winter to Florida to escape the cold dull days of an Alberta winter. They purchased a modest home in Sarasota on Florida's west coast, where we visited them.

My grandfather, Henry Ramer, died at home in 1960 at age eighty-four shortly after a period of congestive heart failure. Grandmother Mary Durr Ramer died a few months short of her ninety-third birthday, living alone in her own home until a few months before her death.

Looking back, by sheer numbers at least, ours had been the dominant Mennonite family in the area. My grandparents and parents had moved to the area early on and watched it grow from a group of homesteaders, with hardly anything to call their own, to a productive community. The whole family, including many first cousins who worked in the fields, drove tractors or did farm work during the holidays, lived within a radius of six miles. Although our family represented the primary social and cultural network of the area, no one ran for any political office; that remained outside the realm of permissibility. Running for political office or serving as a police officer was banned, like military service.

The first to leave Duchess and Alberta had been Uncle Dick, the youngest of Grandpa and Grandma Martin's progeny. He had finished high school in Brooks and left for college in Virginia in the early 1950s. In the decades that followed, many of my cousins would leave the world of Duchess to find their destinies in different parts of North America, entering the twentieth century in an inevitably sudden evolution. We currently range in age from Virginia, born in 1932, to Nanci, born in 1964 and two years younger than our son Bradley. From this generation of fifty-four cousins born in Alberta emerged college graduates (doctors, lawyers, teachers and nurses), accountants, successful farmers and businessmen.

As I finished my high-school classes in 1954, I prepared to do as Uncle Dick had done and enter the wide world beyond Duchess. I was still keen to become a missionary doctor, and I had been accepted into pre-med at the University of Alberta.

## THREE

# *Transitions*

I WAS SIXTEEN WHEN I ARRIVED in Edmonton to begin studies at the University of Alberta—and I was frightened. The world outside Duchess seemed overwhelming, the big city huge and forbidding. It was vibrant with sophistication I felt I lacked. I had made arrangements to stay with Leonard and Florence King, a young married Mennonite couple with three children; I was given room and board, including laundry, for a monthly stipend of $60.

University was very difficult at first. My pre-med class consisted mostly of kids from large cities who had attended comprehensive high schools populated by up to a thousand students. During high school, they had been offered preparatory courses for university admission. (Qualification for university admission was determined by province-wide standardized examinations taken in June, with the report cards mailed to the students in mid-August.) The contrast between these students and my own pre-university studies was as overwhelming as the city itself. My graduating high-school class had twenty-one students, and we had two teachers for the six obligatory courses. Mr. L.J.

Shields, the principal, a sincere man who was an elder in the sizable local Mormon community, had minimal administrative responsibilities so that he could teach chemistry, physics and mathematics. Fortunately, he had a background that prepared him for the assignment. The other teacher, Mrs. A. Pead, had arrived in the summer before my senior year from Belgium. She taught Canadian history, of which she knew nothing, English, which she spoke poorly, and French, which she had mastered as her first language. My final year in Rosemary High School also required diligent effort from me to pass the required exams with a satisfactory grade point average to guarantee placement at the University of Alberta. I studied at home for the most part, using university preparatory materials and old examinations to help me cover the expected breadth of knowledge, always enjoying the full support of my parents, neither of whom had graduated from high school.

For as long as I can remember, I had wanted to be a doctor. As I think back now, that interest was probably fueled by the missionaries who visited our church, sharing dramatic stories of the plight of patients they had seen in India and Africa. I wanted to be a missionary doctor, and that remained my intent until the last two years of medical school when my advisors encouraged me to "specialize." In high school, I was aware that admission to pre-medical courses at university required a GPA of 65 or above. The Canadian scheme of grading was different than that in the US. In high school and university, an A was any mark over 80; a B was between 65 and 80; and a C between 50 and 65. It was rare to get a mark above 90 in any subject. I managed to get an average of 76 and learned in late summer that I was one of the few Rosemary High School students accepted at the University of Alberta. Many of my fellow students from the high school also eventually qualified to enter university, and six or seven of them graduated as teachers, nurses and at least two others as doctors. My high-school graduation class had been a potpourri of religious and cultural backgrounds: Mormon, Japanese (we didn't know whether Shinto or Buddhist), Mennonite, Catholic and Lutheran. I guess atheists were not admitting it in those days.

University education in Alberta was supported in large part by tax subsidies to the provincial school. In my case, tuition in the first year of university, 1955–1956, was $200 for courses that ran from September through April. There were few vacations during the year, and it was expected that students who had come from farms would need to complete studies in the spring to help get the crop in.

During my first year physics and English were disaster courses. My first essay describing the character of the duke in Robert Browning's "My Last Duchess" earned a 40 per cent mark from Mrs. White, an American. I flunked the first physics test and felt that my dream of a romantic life in medicine was permanently shattered. In those trying times, I relied on and received the sustenance to continue my studies from my hosts, the Kings, and friends among other Mennonite students who attended the house church in Leonard King's parents' basement.

My second year in university was a dramatic turnaround. I excelled in math and chemistry and enjoyed a course in psychology. One of my instructors queried the 250 to three hundred students in the class about whether or not any of us organized numbers in three-dimensional space, as number lines. I immediately knew what he was referring to and put up my hand along with about 2 per cent of the class. He mentioned explicitly that if one lacks this mental elaboration it seems totally incomprehensible. "What exactly are you talking about?" my friends say when I try to describe it.

Let me try to do so here. I have always mentally visualized number sequences, say from 1 to 1,000,000 in an organized geometrical form with a quasi-exponential three-dimensional array. Similarly, I file items into time slots with specific positions of the months of the year or years of the century, or centuries of the millennium, providing a convenient way to remember ages, birthdays and the month and year of major events. I find it extremely useful in remembering the time lines of categories of things. Our professor stated at the time that the attribute he described had no correlation with intelligence, mathematical ability or any other readily identifiable psychological trait and that he simply found the phenomenon interesting. I have asked many of my friends and colleagues about it over the years. Today, experts on brain cognition call it *synesthesia*, a mixing of two usually separate brain sensory modalities (space and numbers). Others who experience synesthesia describe hearing musical notes as colors or seeing the letters of the alphabet in different colors. Synesthesia seems to be an inherited trait in some families.

In university, I was an organized and diligent student. I attended all classes and took copious notes and every evening went over them and red-lined the important points. My social life was exclusively focused on church-associated activities. I led the church choir, taught Sunday school and attended special seminars given by young seminarians who were attending school or preparing for a pastoral role. At the time, leaders in rural Mennonite churches were still appointed without formal theological training. The only seminaries recognized as practical opportunities for our members were located in Elkhart, Indiana, and Harrisonburg, Virginia, which were far away and very expensive by rural standards.

## My Last Summer as a Farmer

Like other university students from farming communities, I returned home in the spring and summer months to help with farming chores on the fifty acres adjacent to our house that my mother had inherited from her parents. One morning in July 1957, after I had completed my second year at the University of Alberta and returned to Duchess, my dad asked me to deliver some hogs to Calgary in a Fargo truck with a forty-two-foot Fruehauf enclosed trailer. This truck had come to my dad earlier that spring when he was forced to repossess it when the purchaser failed to make payments. Unable to find another buyer and being of a practical mind, he and Uncle Jim, now his business partner (after Uncle Fred had left to become a regional John Deere representative), had decided to put it to use.

I accepted the opportunity to drive the truck into Calgary with relish. I was eighteen years old and had driven many vehicles over the preceding years. I loaded the semi-trailer early that morning and set out for Calgary to deliver the hogs to their demise at the meat processing plant some 110 miles away.

The second week of July was the week of the Calgary Stampede, a rowdy rodeo that still attracts large crowds and performers who compete in bronco and bull riding, as well as chuck wagon races. I unloaded my cargo and decided to get a close-up view of the downtown in my trailer truck. By noontime, the streets were full of vehicles of all types. Thinking I was on 4th Street East, I suddenly realized, as I approached the underpass of the CPR main line, that I had entered Center Street instead. All forward motion ceased with a crashing sound as the front third of the trailer roof collapsed in accordion folds. The next few minutes are a blur, but I faintly remember that a passerby came to help and, with a roar of the engine, I extricated the truck and trailer from the bridge, backing onto 9th Avenue. I never reported the accident to the police.

I was devastated as the impact of the event settled in. I knew the reaction I'd get from my dad and even worse from Uncle Jim, who had not been enthusiastic about turning the trucking job over to a teenager. I found a quiet street near a phone booth and called my dad at the Duchess Garage. I never could tell the difference between Dad's and Uncle Jim's voices on the phone, and the plaintive appeal for mercy I thought I was delivering to my dad was actually to Uncle Jim, who greeted the news with outrage. Dad was matter-of-fact about the whole episode and never brought it up again.

The truck and trailer could no longer be used, and the unit was put in storage awaiting the insurance adjusters. That would be my last full summer working in a farming community. I retired from trucking permanently, embarrassed at what I had done. Everyone at the Duchess Garage knew I'd blown it. Somehow, over time, I recovered from the indignity of it all, and I was especially relieved when classes resumed in September and I returned to university to begin medical school.

## A Critical Year

Under the Canadian educational system at the time, only two years were spent at university as a pre-medical student, so in the fall of 1957, at age nineteen, I was ready to start medical school. My first year as a medical student at the University of Alberta was a great experience. I spent hours with the cadavers in the anatomy room, performing most of the dissections for our group of five students. I had the gift of being able to visualize anatomic features in three dimensions in almost photographic sequence, an advantage of having a synesthetic brain. I memorized whole portions of *Gray's Anatomy*, the classic textbook of the time. Biochemistry was less interesting, but I loved physiology and neuroanatomy. The beautiful descriptions and drawings by Ralph Shaner, our professor in neuroanatomy, made my first exposure to the human nervous system so vivid and real that it may have been a determining factor in my later choice of neurology as a career.

The results of my first year in medicine arrived by mail in early August, and I was delighted and astonished to discover that I led the class. There was no question that I was competitive, but I had not expected that honor, surrounded as I was by so many smart people, most of whom had come from the big cities.

What followed next came as a surprise to the dean of the medical school, to my family and even to me. I decided to leave medical school, skip the second year of studies, leave my friends in the class and go off to Eastern Mennonite College (EMC) in Harrisonburg, Virginia, to immerse myself in biblical studies, learn music and choir conducting and delve into ethics, church history and moral philosophy. The dean was gracious and assured me that I would be welcomed back on my return.

The idea was concocted with my cousin and best friend Robert Ramer, four years older than I, who was planning to go off to college in Virginia. We had both attended high school in Rosemary. Not insignificant in my decision was the growing distance I felt from my girlfriend at the time. I had trouble finding a way out of the relationship. EMC seemed like a good solution. And so it turned out to be.

EMC was an exhilarating place. I had never seen so many eligible Mennonite girls in one place. I applied my three years of university credit toward an EMC degree, registering for a BSC, with a major in Bible. My classmates were mostly seniors, some of them pre-medical students. A biology degree from EMC was excellent preparation for admission to the medical schools of Virginia and Pennsylvania. The acceptance rate for pre-med students who were recommended by Daniel Suter, professor of biology, approached 90 per cent.

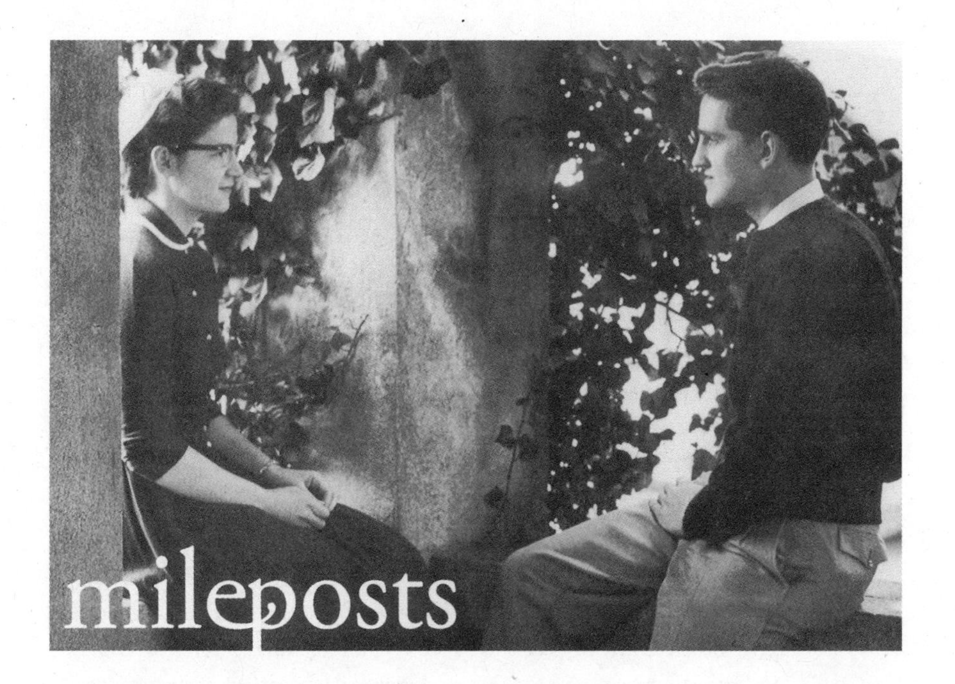


Rachel Wenger and the author on the balcony of the administration building at Eastern Mennonite College, Harrisonburg, Virginia, 1958.

My classes included Old Testament history, choral conducting, New Testament Greek, Mennonite history and Christian ethics. I mastered enough Greek to read the Gospel of John, the simplest of the New Testament gospels.

I had planned the year to be one of exploration of many things Mennonite. In addition to studies, I envisioned that my new freedom would lead to lots of dates. I met Rachel at a campus event in the basement of the chapel. It was an accidental meeting, I thought. She had heard of my arrival on campus, and when she arrived with friends, they chose the row where I was seated. We exchanged the essentials about where we came from and why we were at EMC. Her name was Rachel Ann Wenger, she came from Columbiana, Ohio, and she was in her third year on campus. That was the extent of it.

We had our first date about three weeks later, a hike up Massanutten, the highest mountain peak in the area and an easy thirty-minute bus ride from the campus. But it rained, and we sat in the bus, eventually returning to campus. After three hours of conversation, we hit on the strong likelihood that we were meant for each other. There was no turning back, and we soon became one of the established couples on campus. We were featured in the yearbook sitting on the balcony of the administration building gazing at each other.

The college's strict code of conduct made any form of intimacy on campus exceedingly difficult; all off-campus excursions were permitted only in the company of a chaperone. Fortunately, Uncle Dick and Aunt June had moved into the area. As noted previously, Uncle Dick had left Duchess to attend college in Virginia, where he met June Houser from Lancaster County, Pennsylvania. Their house was open to us for supervised dating, although they paid little attention to the rules. Not that we were prone to any substantial misbehavior. Those were days when the rules we broke were so inconsequential that no one would have noticed.

> The author's wedding portrait, June 18, 1960.

By my birthday in October, Rachel and I were seeing each other on every occasion possible. My birthday present from her was a visit to the Luray Caverns, one of the most stunning underground caves in the eastern US, in the northern Shenandoah Valley. We borrowed a car and drove with another couple to the eastern slopes of the Massanutten range.

At Christmas, I visited Rachel's family in Ohio. I did my best to convince Rachel's father, David Wenger, an electrician, that I could wire a house with minimal instructions. Despite his complaints that I always left my tools "lying around," we got on fine. He was a stern man who knew almost the whole Bible by memory; he kept questioning me about religious issues.

As I reflect on my year at EMC, I recognize that it was the most important year of my life. Without that year, my life would have followed a very different path. And I would not have met Rachel.

During the fall of 1959 I returned to Edmonton to begin my second year of medical school. After summer school at Ohio State University in Youngstown, Rachel qualified to teach elementary school in Toledo, Ohio, and we wrote each other daily. At Christmas, we met at her parent's home in Ohio, and we began plans for our wedding, scheduled for June 18, 1960.

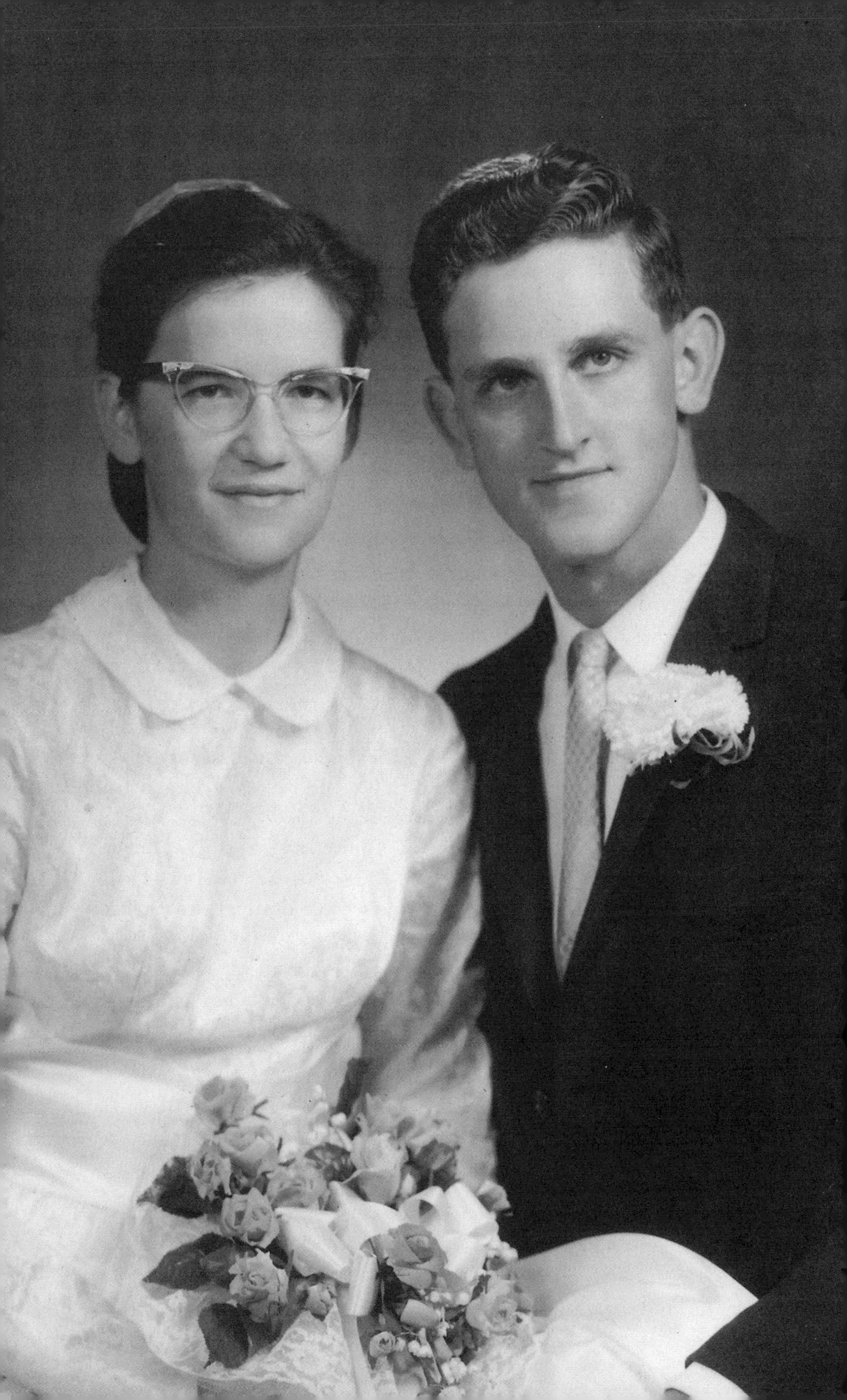

## Edmonton: Residency Training in Medicine and Neurology

After the wedding, we drove from Ohio to Alberta and set out to find a place to live in Edmonton. During the third and fourth years of medical school, we lived in rented houses where we took in boarders. Rachel completed her education at the University of Alberta, qualifying to teach elementary school. In my final year in medical school, Rachel taught third grade at the Hazeldean School in Edmonton. After graduation, we moved into an apartment at the interns' residence on the hospital campus so I could begin my internship.

I was rewarded for my studious efforts with election to the Alpha Omega Alpha Honorary Medical Society during my third year. At graduation, "with distinction," I received two gold medals (the Moshier Medal and the John W. Scott Honor Award), one for scholarship and the other for showing promise of a leadership role in medicine. I had the honor of being elected class president. Of great importance to me then and now was the appointment by the class of Dr. Lionel McLeod as our faculty honorary president. Lionel was like an older brother to me. After graduation from the University of Alberta, he had trained at the University of Minnesota in nephrology and returned to my school as a brilliant energetic role model who emerged as a major figure throughout my entire academic life.[1]

My rotating internship at the University Hospital in Edmonton began on Friday, June 15, 1962. Rachel was seven and a half months pregnant and, following school rules, had given up her teaching responsibilities in May. My first rotation was obstetrics, with a weekend call that began Friday night and continued until Monday afternoon. It was a weekend from hell, or heaven, depending on how one counted the twenty-five or so deliveries we had, which was a record for a weekend, I was told. I went to bed on Sunday night, exhausted and sleep-deprived, only to be awakened a few hours later by a call from Rachel in our apartment in the intern's residence to say that she had awakened in a pool of blood.

I admitted her to our obstetrical service under the responsibility of Dr. Brown, and we began a careful work-up to exclude the most likely diagnosis, placenta previa. No CT scans or

THE JOHN W. SCOTT HONOR AWARD
NAMED AFTER
JOHN W. SCOTT (1894 - 1982)
MD, CM (McGILL), FRCPC, FACP, LLD (ALTA)
DEAN OF MEDICINE, 1948 - 1959
UNIVERSITY OF ALBERTA
Offered to a graduating medical student who, over the 4 years of the MD Program, has evidenced to an outstanding degree those qualities of scholarship, leadership, and character that may be expected to lead to a distinguished standing in the medical profession.
RECIPIENTS
1960 LAURENCE A. HARKER
1961 NOT AWARDED
1962 JOSEPH B. MARTIN
1963 E. GARNER KING
1964 ERROL B. MARLISS
1965 DOUGLAS F. WALLER
1966 NOT AWARDED
1967 ROBERT E. MILLER
1968 RICHARD H. COMISAROW & LARRY R. PEDEGANA
1969 JAMES W. DUTTON
1970 JOHN CAMERON McINNIS
1971 LAWRENCE M. PRICE
1972 TERRY D. SOSNOWSKI
1973 JOAN RUSSEL STOGRYN
1974 ANTHONY L.A. FIELDS
1975 MURRAY G. ELLEKER
1976 GEORGE P.A. RICE
1977 RODNEY MARTIN
1978 CAROL A. SAWKA
1979 DONALD D. FENTIE
1980 NORMAN J. DAVIES
1981 HELEN F. MONTGOMERY & MAUREEN R. SHANDLING
1982 JOHN D. URSCHEL
1983 D. GORDON ALLAN
1984 SUSAN L. CAMPBELL
1985 GARY MAY
1986 DARYL S. KUCEY
1987 LOUIS HUGO FRANCESCUTTI
1988 ROBERT AGOSTINIS & FRANK BUGEJA
1989 TIMOTHY W.I. CLARK


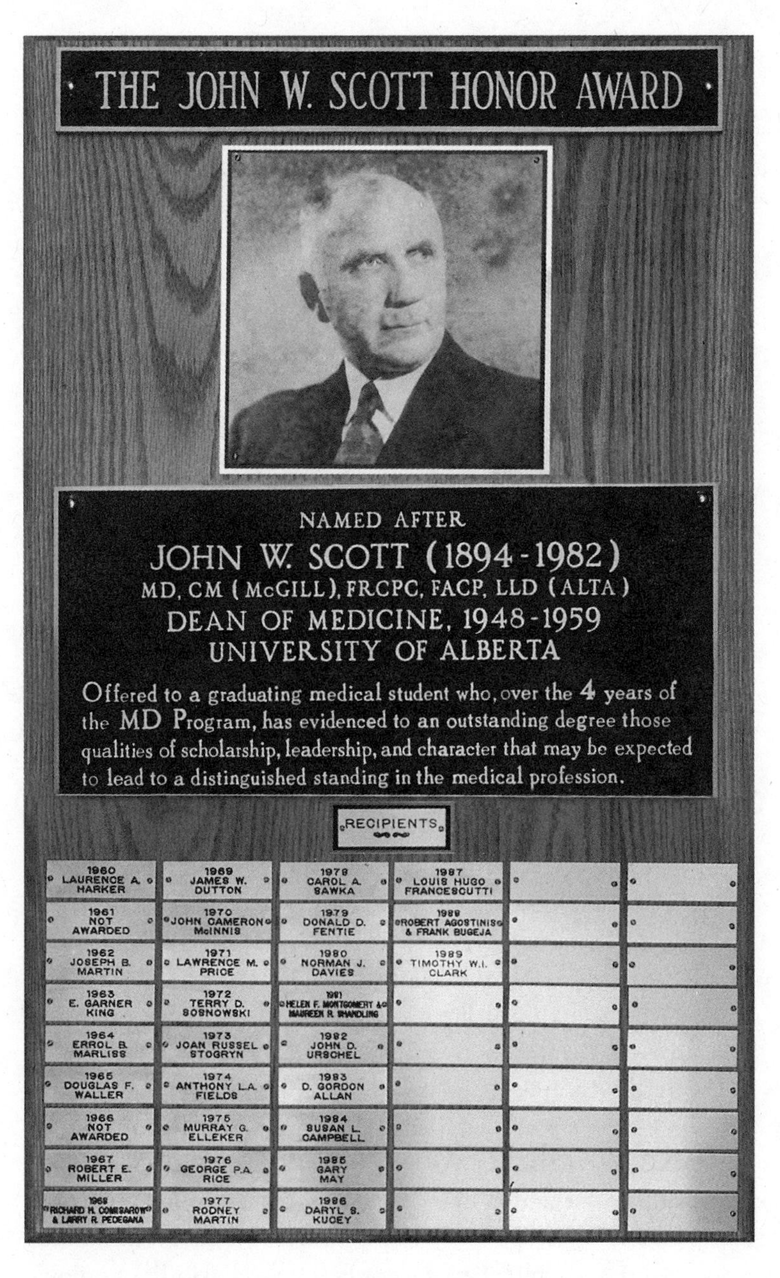

Plaque showing John W. Scott Honor Award recipients. The author was honored in 1962; first cousin Rodney Martin received the prize in 1977.

ultrasounds were available in those days, and the examination itself often made things worse. Fortunately, it turned out that the bleeding was likely from the rupture of a cervical vein, a benign event. Six weeks later, on July 27, we rejoiced in the arrival of Joseph Bradley.

We were fortunate to be allowed to continue living in the intern's residence after Bradley's birth. The remainder of the internship year was a disaster of late-night calls, frequent awakenings with the baby crying and, for my part, significant sleep deprivation. It was even worse for Rachel. Bradley contributed his share in making things more difficult. He would wake up early in the morning screaming for his bottle with the explicit demand that the milk be warm. In preparation for this daily morning call, we placed a pan filled with water on the stove the night before. At the first squeak from the crib, Rachel and I both jumped from bed: I turned on the electric burner, and she tried to subdue the outbursts of screaming to prevent disturbing neighboring interns.

As I rotated through the year, Bradley had each of the diagnoses I saw on the wards. One night, at six weeks of age, he passed blood into his diaper. I was on pediatrics then, and was sure it came from a Wilms tumor of the kidney, as sure as I had been on that frightening early admission seven weeks before delivery, that he had a small head! At that time, I had even managed to worry Dr. Brown enough to get an X-ray of Bradley's head—which appeared perfectly normal. Hopefully, the rays did no permanent damage to his young brain.

Rachel was a patient mother. With the support and friendship of my cousin Robert Ramer and his wife, Phyllis Showalter Ramer (who he also met at EMC), friends and faculty at the university and at the Holyrood Mennonite Church in Edmonton, we made it through a difficult year. In July we were required to relocate from the intern's residence and rented an apartment in the Bel Air complex a few miles from University Hospital. There, we lived close to Dr. Ben and Carol Ruether, who became and remain close friends. We were later able to re-establish our friendship with them in Rochester, New York, where Ben would arrive for a fellowship in hematology/oncology. Rachel and Carol were loyal friends and shared babysitting responsibilities, allowing one another time for shopping and some leisurely activities.[2]

The second year of residency at the University of Alberta Hospital saw me focusing on rotations in internal medicine. I loved surgery but found myself becoming more focused on clinical medicine from an internist perspective. I spent time with the chief of medicine, Donald Wilson, whose specialty was endocrinology. I also worked with Ted Bell, head of the Division of Hematology, and together we published my first paper—a case report in *The Canadian Medical Association Journal*, describing a fascinating case of splenic atrophy in a patient with non-tropical sprue, or celiac disease.[3]

That fall I was given a two-month research leave to work on a project that involved genealogical studies among the Hutterites of Saskatchewan and Alberta. The Hutterites had come to North America from their settlements in Moravia in Central Europe and were a pacifist, colony-based, Anabaptist group. The study, based on the genetic analysis of blood groups, was undertaken because colony members represented a closed genetic community. The research was supported by granting agencies in the United States, and the field work was carried out by the Department of Genetics at Case Western Reserve University. The chief aim of the research was to seek evidence of "genetic drift" to identify genetic alterations in a closed population, using as an index the variety of blood groups known at the time.

With Bradley in the safety of my parents' care, Rachel accompanied me on the project. We visited seven or eight colonies, spending about a week at each one, offering physical exams, which I did, and EKGs, which Rachel did, in return for blood and urine samples. We were joined in the study by a physical anthropologist from the US, Herman Bleibtreu, and his wife, Carol. Through their work, we came to know and appreciate the methods anthropologists applied in the field. Herman had just completed a PHD in anthropology at Harvard University, where his project surveyed the cultural aspects of family styles among the Hutterites.[4]

One colony visit provided a remarkable portent of my later interest in neuroendocrinology and would become a harbinger of things to come. Three young people—two sisters and a brother—in their late twenties and early thirties came to see me. They were about thirty to thirty-four inches in height, normal in physical appearance and intelligence but with high-pitched voices and delayed sexual development. In their colony, they were assigned the task of taking care of the poultry—chickens, ducks and geese. The furniture in the poultry barn was built to match their size.

I recognized their genetic condition, likely autosomal recessive, and thought it an opportunity for further study.

This was the fall of 1963, and little was known about their condition. I asked them to accompany me to Edmonton for further tests. But all three declined, very clearly indicating that they were quite content with the way God had made them. I was disappointed to miss a real opportunity for further study but had no choice but to respect their wishes. When we returned to Edmonton, I told the story to a friend, John Hostetler, who had grown up in an Amish family in Pennsylvania and went on to receive a PHD in sociology, becoming one of the leading authorities on Mennonite and Amish life, with an interest in the Hutterites. I took no other action beyond that and had forgotten the whole matter when, about three or four years later, I realized I had been scooped; it was my first experience with academic competition. I was glancing at a copy of *Scientific American* at a local newsstand when I saw photographs of my three subjects on the front cover and a reference to a research article in that month's issue on familial hypopituitarism. The article described the work of Victor McKusick of Johns Hopkins University. Following the scent of the trail I'd given to John Hostetler (who had assisted McKusick in meeting Amish families to study the genetics of another closed population), he had sent his team to work in the Hutterite colony. I met Victor years later, and we became close friends. When I told him the story, he chuckled, but never offered an apology![5]

Midway through the research Rachel and I were conducting with the Hutterites, I developed a severe sore throat with high temperature and enormous fatigue, and I was not able to continue my work. I sought medical consultation in Medicine Hat, a city about seventy miles east of Duchess, where the doctor examined my blood smear, found atypical monocytes and made the likely diagnosis of infectious mononucleosis. He noted, however, that the changes were sufficiently dramatic that he could not entirely exclude leukemia and suggested a follow-up in the next few weeks. Rachel and I returned to Duchess. I spent two weeks essentially inert with fatigue so severe I was scarcely able to get to the bathroom. Recovery from the symptoms, fortunately, came as rapidly as the onset, and we were able to return to the survey for the final three weeks.

It was during this stay with my parents that Joe Foley, chief of neurology at Case Western Reserve University, called from Cleveland to invite me to join him for a residency in neurology. It was the great news I'd been hoping for and probably helped my recovery. It was clear to me following advice from Lionel McLeod and other mentors at the University of Alberta (and later in Cleveland) that I should aspire to an academic career and to do so required a specialty of expertise.[6] I felt I was being encouraged to prepare for a career back in Edmonton as a teacher and scholar.

The second year of residency was great fun. The call schedule was reasonable, and I now had the prospect of going to Cleveland to train. Although I had been born a dual citizen, as we began making plans for the move to Cleveland, I discovered that since I had voted in Canada on the first opportunity I had, according to US law, I had thereby forfeited my right to US citizenship and could stay in the US only as an exchange student on a DSP66 visa. Thankfully, I could still be funded by a US Public Health Service grant because in those days, rules for training in the US made no exceptions for non-US citizens. It was a remarkably generous way to relocate, especially with a salary that was considerably higher than the $176 a month I was paid during my Edmonton internship.

The year was 1964, and little did I appreciate at the time that had I been a US citizen, I would have been required to register with the draft board and would likely have been expected to join the military or do alternative service as my uncles had done, as a conscientious objector.

## Cleveland: Neurology Residency Begins at Case Western

In a 1962 Plymouth sedan, we left Edmonton for Duchess, where we said farewell to my family, loaded our few belongings in the car and began the four-day trip to Cleveland, approximately 1,800 miles away. We arrived in time to visit Rachel's family in

Columbiana, Ohio, and to rent an apartment—the lower level of a double-decker—in Cleveland. We helped the previous tenants vacate the apartment so that we would get settled in by July 1, 1964. Our address at 2582 East 128th Street put us just inside the boundary of Shaker Heights, where we would stay for the next three years. Brad made friends with Mary Varga, who was his age and lived upstairs. I set out each day on the one and a half miles down the hill to the campus of Case Western Reserve University and University Hospitals.

The first summer was so hot I wanted to die, and some days I wished I could. The on-call room was on the fourth floor of the house staff residence, just below the roof. The minimal amount of air moving in at night through the small window under the dormer at the end of the room brought little comfort, even with a fan placed in the window. The every-third-day on-call schedule was reasonable; we always anticipated four to six admissions each night of call.

We were an interesting lot of residents. The residency program that Joe Foley developed in Cleveland accepted candidates from other countries. There were four of us from outside the United States: Vilnis Ciemins, who had arrived from Latvia a short while earlier;[7] Ingo Weiderholt, who came from Germany;[8] and Michael Swash, who arrived a year after I did, from England.[9] We joined two Americans, Mike Cohen[10] and John Conomy.[11] Michael Genco was a talented chief resident from Buffalo.[12] I also came to know and become close friends with Berch Griggs, a junior member of the medical residency program, during the second year.[13] We were an eager group and established long-standing friendships.

It was a great privilege and honor to work for Joe Foley. He had arrived at Case Western only three years earlier from the Boston City Hospital, where he worked as the neurologist/neuropathologist with the eminent and often difficult Derek Denny-Brown. Stories were legendary of Foley's good virtues as he rescued students and residents in training from the wrath of Denny-Brown. Foley was a graduate of Harvard Medical School (HMS), raised in Dorchester in the heart of Boston, and one of the few lads from this Irish neighborhood to get a Harvard education.

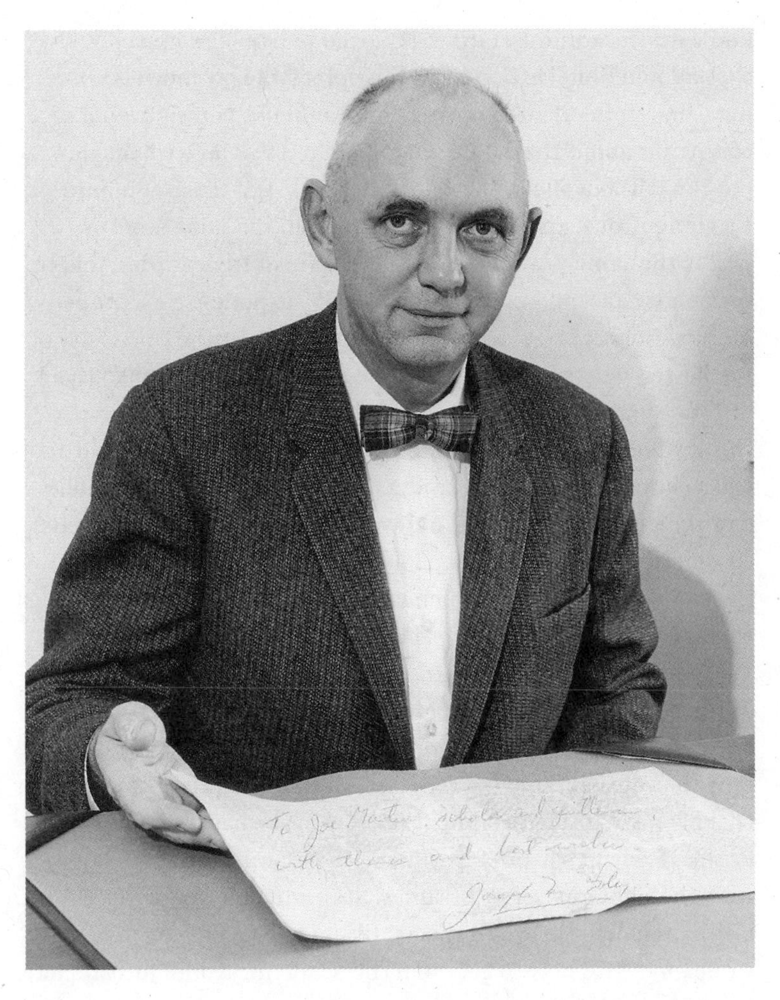

Joseph M. Foley, the author's mentor at Case Western Reserve University. The photo is inscribed: "To Joe Martin, scholar and gentleman, with thanks and best wishes, Joseph M. Foley."

Dr. Foley, as we called him out of respect, led the weekly neuropathology brain-cutting rounds. We were intimidated by his relentless insistence on anatomical detail, putting us on the spot and eagerly anticipating our failure so he could cheerfully malign us. I loved the experience and grew eager to extend my training in neuropathology.

Foley was a superb doctor who emphasized to us the importance of showing our patients the respect they deserved. He was very visible in our clinics and on the ward. He never lashed out, and I never heard him gossip in unkind or unpleasant ways about colleagues in the division or in the Department of Medicine. He was friendly with the dean, with the other chiefs and with the administration. He loved teasing the nurses, and they adored him. He taught us to appreciate how much learning came from talented nurses and would not permit a word of complaint about them. "Be nice to them. I can do without you, but not without them," he would chide us. His sense of humor was ubiquitous, and I never heard him tell the same story or repeat the same joke twice. His repertoire of Irish stories, told in vernacular accent was unmatched in my experience except perhaps by Robert Joynt, who I would meet later at the University of Rochester, where he was chair of neurology when I trained there.

Neurology training under Joe Foley turned out to be everything I'd hoped for. He recruited a formidable group of world-class neurologists to Cleveland, among them Simon Horenstein, a mischievous, demanding, old-world scholar with an enormous ego, a provocative manner and a soft heart. Everyone felt his irascibility, and his ornery behavior on occasion needed intercession by Foley to get things back on track. Then there was William Sibley, who had trained at the Neurological Institute in New York under Houston Merritt (chair of the Department of Neurology and later dean of the College of Physicians and Surgeons of Columbia University). Bill was the quickest study of the lot; his intuitive clinical skills won the day, over and over again. He spent the briefest time with patients and came out with the right answer most times. Stan van den Noort was the fair-haired one. He took a special liking to us residents and was a role model for how to get on in the academic world. Joe van der Meulen was the archetype of the successful professor, gaining in stature with his easy manner and forthright approach to clinical issues. Each of these men was a giant in his own way, and each went on to chair departments of neurology in other universities.

Despite the hectic schedule imposed on me during the residency in Cleveland, Rachel and I affiliated with and attended regularly the Friendship Community Mennonite Church a short distance outside Cleveland. I remember it best for the lunches we had with Bradley at McDonald's on the way home from church, our first introduction to the emerging American addiction to fast food.

## Cleveland Surprises

Melanie was born on July 14, 1965, at the Babies and Children's Hospital, a constituent of the University Hospitals. We welcomed a baby girl with enormous delight. But our personal delight was affected when Melanie was barely a year old and we became witness to one of the deadliest riots in the history of Cleveland. The events there were part of a national pattern of racial tension and frustration that would produce violence in many parts of the country in 1966. In Cleveland, the epicenter was in Hough, an area of the city predominantly populated by African Americans. Although there had been racial disturbances in the city earlier in the summer, the Hough events proved to be more serious and widespread. Racial violence erupted on the night of July 18, 1966, marking the start of devastating riots, with widespread destruction of property. The police lost control of the situation, which prompted the arrival of the National Guard on the morning of July 20, at the request of Mayor Ralph Locher. Four people were killed during the riots, about thirty were injured, close to three hundred arrested and about 240 fires were reported.

Although the areas impacted by the riots seemed distant from where we lived, the call-up of the National Guard brought home the seriousness of the event in full force. The tanks, armored carriers and trucks of the usually quiet National Guard were housed in an armory down the street at the end of our block, interrupting access to our street. The intensity of the riots ebbed by the end of July, but the tensions would linger in Cleveland for years to come.

As we watched the troops move in and out of our street, blockaded from resident travel for over a week, I found myself thinking of the patients from Hough I had cared for over the past year, especially a family who lived in Hough and whom I had visited the preceding summer. My relationship with the family began with an order from my neurology chief, Joe Foley, who had drilled into us the importance of always getting an autopsy when one of our patients died. The patient had been an elderly African-American gentleman with a clinical diagnosis of stroke who had died under my care. Despite all of my efforts to convince the family of the importance of a post-mortem to establish the exact cause of death, they denied us permission to perform an autopsy. Foley was ruthless in his attack of my failure to gain permission. He wanted to know if the body had been released from the hospital. If not, I was to find out where the family lived, go directly to their home and plead for permission to do the post-mortem. He recommended that I only ask permission to examine the brain, because, on occasion, that allowed the family to maintain the dignity they wished.

The family lived in the heart of Hough, the scene where riots would erupt the following summer. Rachel and I drove to the address. She waited in the car while I knocked on the door and was let in. I was embarrassed to be doing it, but I pled my case anyway. The answer from the family was unchanged: no, we don't want to trouble our dear father anymore. Let him rest in peace. Thankfully, Joe Foley accepted my predicament and the matter never resurfaced. I came away from the experience with a deep sense of respect for the concerns and wishes of patients and their families during life and after our efforts had seemingly failed.

After two years of adult clinical neurology, I made arrangements to spend the third required year in neuropathology and pediatric neurology at the Metropolitan General Hospital in Cleveland, a county hospital that was affiliated with the university, where Maurice Victor and Betty Banker, both originally from Boston, were developing an excellent neuropathology training program based on their clinical and research strengths. Maurice and Betty came to Cleveland from Boston, as had Foley, but entirely independently, establishing their own neurology training program. During my first interview with Foley when I was exploring my options, he had insisted that I cross town to meet Victor, who was a Canadian and graduate of the University of Manitoba. As I was completing a second year in the Foley program, I was encouraged to explore a third year in neuropathology, Betty's area of expertise. She was a formidable muscle pathologist and a superb investigator.

That year, I was fortunate to meet two more Canadians and an Australian, again underlining the international character of the training programs so common in the US. Garth

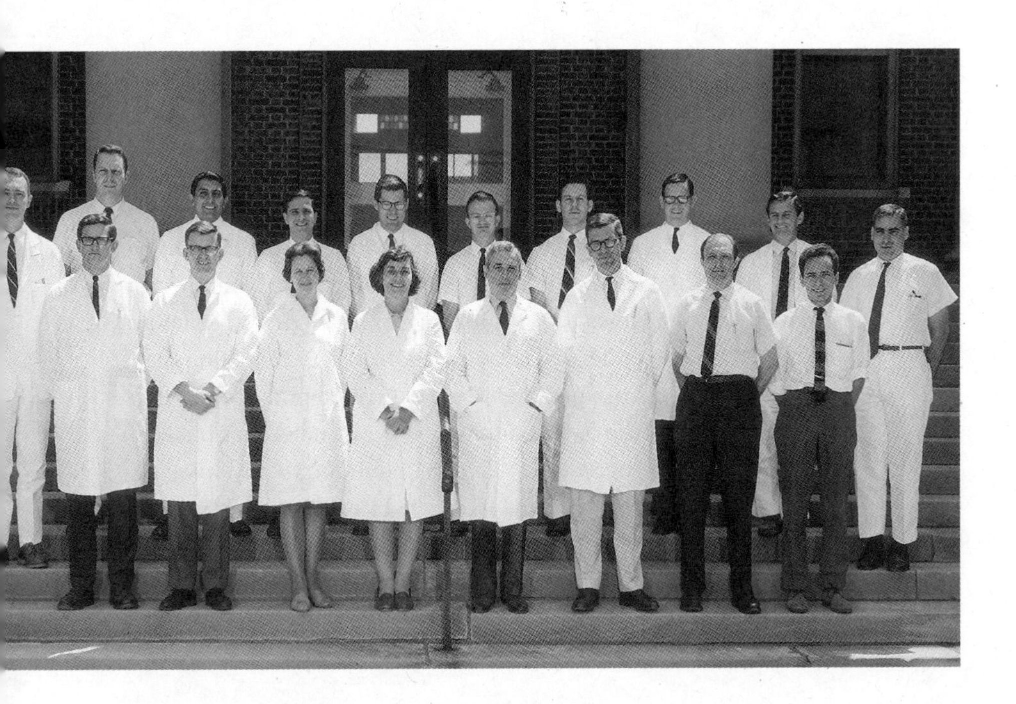

Staff and residents of the neurology division at the Cleveland Metropolitan General Hospital, 1967. Front row, left to right: the author, Garth Bray, Maie Karsoo, Betty Banker, Maurice Victor, Richard Johnson, and two other residents. Back row from left, second John Girvin, James Ferrendelli, Howard Silby, Vilnis Ciemins, Kenneth Johnson, (third from right) and Rick Burns.

Bray was a year ahead of me. He came from the University of Manitoba in Winnipeg to work with Maurice and Betty and was doing research on animal models of muscular dystrophy with Betty. His best friend from medical school, Maie Karsoo, who had immigrated to Canada from Estonia, was now working as Betty's assistant neuropathologist. We learned more from Maie's patient guidance through the microscopic assessments than from Betty. Also from Canada came John Girvin, a remarkable man who, after completing residency in neurosurgery in Canada with time abroad in England, came to Cleveland for a year of neuropathology. He was six-foot-six inches tall and an excellent athlete, having been quarterback on the University of Western Ontario football team.

But the best surprise of all was my acquaintance with Rick Burns—and Renate, his lovely wife—who arrived from Adelaide, Australia, in July 1966 for a one-year experience in American neurology. Rick had already completed training in Australia and had spent six months at Queen Square Hospital in London before completing his training in the United States. Our friendship with the Burns was the highlight of our third year in Cleveland. By sheer chance, we had rented apartments a few blocks apart and thus arranged to share the daily drive to the hospital, so Rachel and Renate could have access to a car. We still travel to Australia whenever possible to see them.

During my second year in the Foley program, I became interested in a group of patients with postural hypotension (a drop in blood pressure upon standing), some of whom had a form of neurodegeneration later known as the Shy–Drager syndrome. With Stanley van den Noort and Randall Travis, I explored the endocrine responses in these patients with disordered autonomic nervous system function. Our paper described problems in the regulation of the renin–angiotensin system and was published in *The Archives of Neurology*.[14] This introduction to physiology and the mechanisms of homeostasis led to my evolving interest in neuroendocrinology, which set the trajectory for my research experience at the University of Rochester under Seymour Reichlin.

## Rochester, New York, and a PHD

In 1967, on the occasion of the hundredth anniversary of the Dominion of Canada, the Medical Research Council of Canada announced that centennial scholarships were available for men and women of Canadian origin who wished to broaden their fields of interest. In addition to travel and other expenses, scholars were awarded support for up to three years at $10,000 per annum, and in the case of married scholars, an additional $500 for the first and $250 for each additional child. My mentors in Edmonton had alerted me to this while I was training in neurology in Cleveland and suggested that I apply. I did so with their encouragement and endorsement. I was interviewed by Claude Fortier of Laval University, one of the great Canadian fathers of neuroendocrinology, and received funding for three years. The expectation was that I would return to Edmonton at the end of the third year. Dean Walter Mackenzie and Dr. Donald R. Wilson, chairman of the Department of Medicine in Edmonton, congratulated me in April 1967 and stated that on the successful completion of my work in Rochester, I was guaranteed an appointment in neurology in the Department of Medicine at the University of Alberta.

We arrived in Rochester in July 1967 to occupy a house we had rented a mile from the University and Strong Memorial Hospital. I registered as a graduate student, took the requirements for a PHD and graduated in 1971. Douglas Richard was born on October 26, 1968, on a Saturday morning at Strong Memorial Hospital—in total darkness. Power had failed while Rachel was straining in the labor room, and Douglas arrived into this world under flashlight guidance, howling the first of many frustrations at his moment of birth. We still tease him that the event must have been so momentous that simultaneously a catastrophe befell the Wenger chicken house in Columbiana, burning it to the ground.

Life in Rochester was hectic, to put it mildly. I worked in the lab day and night learning a whole world of brain/body interaction and all the different ways of studying it. Then, in the third year of my centennial scholarship, my mentor, Seymour Reichlin, took a position as head of the new Department of Medical Specialties in Farmington, Connecticut, outside Hartford. I, with my family, followed him there to complete my research. That third year proved to be most productive. Pending the completion of a new medical school, my lab was in a temporary space by the Newington Veterans Administration Hospital.

The appeal for me at the University of Rochester was embodied simply in the remarkable man I met there on my first visit, Seymour Reichlin. Si, as he insisted on being called, was the American godfather of the field of neuroendocrinology. He had spent time at Oxford with the venerable Geoffrey Harris, whose observations *in vivo* had demonstrated unequivocally that blood flowed from the hypothalamus to bathe the anterior pituitary in releasing factors that controlled the endocrine symphony. Harris once visited the lab, and I had the experience of an hour with an Oxford "don" as he grilled me about my knowledge of the brain, endocrine glands and reproduction.

Reichlin was the quintessential physician-scientist, equally at home in the clinical trenches, where he conducted ongoing clinical trials and translational research, as he was in the laboratory. He was a polymath, and time was often wasted, it seemed to me, musing about things having little to do with my research. And to make it more challenging, he arrived almost every day with

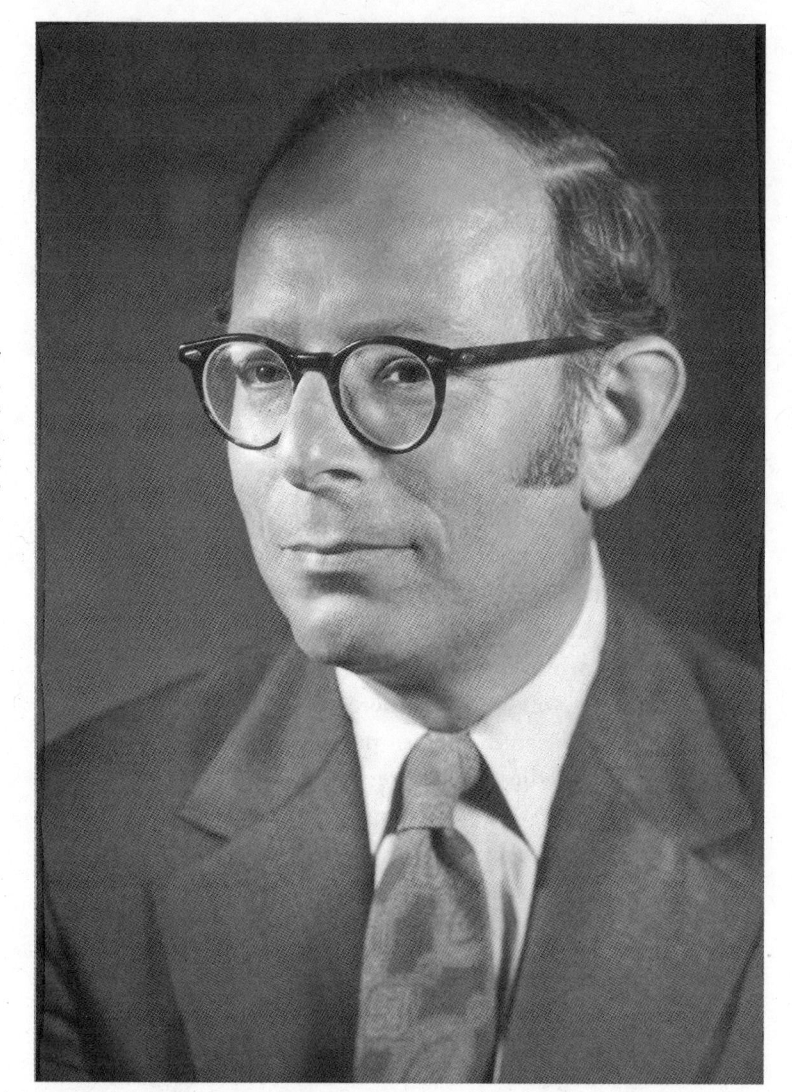

Seymour Reichlin, the author's research supervisor at the University of Rochester.

a new idea about the next experiment before I had finished the last. His own research work, accomplished largely by his senior technician, Rita Boshans, and more junior technician, Judy Bollinger, was often left partly done. There seemed to be many laboratory manuals of unpublished research as older ideas were supplanted by better ones. All of this I simply accepted, believing firmly that these were the traits of genius.

As remarkable as his broad insights into biology and medicine (and psychiatry, where he had spent a couple of years in training) were, his political skills in the academic marketplace were even more spectacular. He was friends with everyone. I watched with amazement as the enmity between the scientists Roger Guillemin and Andrew Schally, both at different institutions, escalated as they tried to outdo each other in identifying hypothalamic regulatory (releasing) factors—for which they would eventually share the Nobel Prize. Si got on with both, and they greeted him (separately) with great affection at annual endocrine gatherings.

Si's intimate knowledge of the entire landscape of internal medicine, neurology, and indeed also psychiatry, made him a formidable presence in any conversation we had. The opportunity to work with him was one of the great experiences of my life.

Rachel, however, remembers that year in Connecticut as a total washout. We had settled in New Britain. She was pregnant with our fourth child, Neil, while I was moving a lab, trying to get my final research completed, writing a thesis and trying to finish everything—before our next move, which was to be to Montreal. Neil was conceived sometime in July of 1969. We celebrated his conception by naming him for Neil Armstrong, who was exploring the moon while we were making a new baby. The spring months of 1970 were occupied, on my part, by a dawn to midnight attack on writing my thesis and preparing papers for publication.

My work with Si Reichlin focused entirely on measurements of thyroid stimulating hormone (TSH) by a new radioimmunoassay I'd developed. I examined fluctuations in circulating TSH levels during manipulation of the hypothalamus-pituitary-thyroid axis, which is important in regulating the body's metabolism.[15] I was able to show that hypothalamic electrical stimulation with implanted electrodes placed at selected sites produced TSH release, mapping the distribution of positive response sites to an area that later was shown—following the discovery of thyrotropin-releasing hormone (TRH) by Roger Guillemin and Andrew Schally, in separate laboratories—to correspond closely to the anatomic localization of TRH neurons.[16]

I was fortunate during these years to work with Gregory Brown, a fellow Canadian and a psychiatrist, who had also registered for a PHD. We took coursework together, engaged in remarkably productive discussions of our research, and I found that many of the sustaining concepts and ideas that influenced my later work came from those conversations. Greg returned to the Clark Institute of Psychiatry at the University of Toronto, where he had a distinguished career. Reichlin, Brown and I published together the first comprehensive book on our field, which we entitled *Clinical Neuroendocrinology*, an effort to blend the compelling ideas of clinical endocrinology and the research field of neuroendocrinology.[17]

# FOUR

## *Montreal*

THE PURPOSE OF OUR FIRST VISIT to Montreal, soon after our arrival in Rochester, New York, was to attend Expo 67, judged by many to have been one of the most successful world's fairs of the twentieth century. Rachel and I fell in love immediately with the city but had no inkling whatsoever that we might one day be blessed by living there. My earliest sentiments for Montreal came early in childhood when I found myself cheering for the Montreal Canadiens—one of only six original teams in the National Hockey League—instead of the Toronto Maple Leafs. I was so enamored of Maurice "The Rocket" Richard that I even thought he had the same square face, high forehead and prominent jaw as my father.

In June 1970 we packed up to move to Montreal. I had finally taken a "real" job, at McGill University. We arrived with four children. Brad was seven years old and about to start third grade, Melanie was four, ready to enter kindergarten, Doug was eighteen months, and Neil, our baby, was a scant six weeks old. Just as we were busy unloading the truck at 131 Brock Avenue South in Montreal West, we realized that Doug had walked away from the chaos. Fortunately, he was found by a postman a few blocks away and was returned to our care.

## Appointment at McGill

The invitation to join the faculty at McGill had come during my second year at Rochester from Don Baxter, head of neurology at the Montreal General Hospital, who had convinced me that the opportunities at McGill would be more favorable to my academic pursuits than my original plan to return to the University of Alberta in Edmonton. Rachel and I were both delighted to have been offered the opportunity to settle down in a big city like Montreal after a somewhat isolated life in 1960s Edmonton. The offer was especially exciting to me because I could now pursue the academic interests and research I had developed in Cleveland and Rochester in an academic setting where research and clinical work in neurology offered great promise. The decision to return to Canada had not been an issue—I felt obligated to the Medical Research Council of Canada to do everything possible to repay the generous fellowship support I'd enjoyed at the University of Rochester. And Montreal and McGill seemed the right decision. At the time, I reasoned that I had not received a formal offer from Edmonton, which made it easier to take the offer from McGill.

But my decision to go to McGill rather than return to Edmonton was not received well by Dean Mackenzie of the University of Alberta Medical School. Indeed, one of the memories deeply sequestered in my hippocampus is of a midday phone call from Dean Mackenzie while I was at work in the laboratory at Rochester. He was calling to find out if the rumors he had heard that I would not be returning to Edmonton were true. I remember pausing a moment and then admitting that I planned to go to Montreal. Dean Mackenzie became acerbic, impatient and petulant, and his tone turned sharp as he reminded me that I ought to keep my commitment to return to Edmonton. The dilemma was real. I had appreciated the support of Don Wilson and George Monckton, the head of the Division of Neurology at the University of Alberta. George had taught me in medical school. But while I was fond of Professor Monckton, a tall, spindly, Ichabod Crane-like, British, Queen Square–trained neurologist, I was very concerned that my assignment there as the second full-time staff member in clinical neurology in a 1,200-bed hospital, would virtually extinguish my ability to establish a viable experimental laboratory operation. I never spoke to Dean Mackenzie again. Only some time later, after I had gone to Montreal, did I come to hear that the University of Alberta's new clinical research building had been completed and that my name and laboratory assignment were displayed prominently on the directory inside the main entrance along with that of Monckton.

In reality, what had most affected my decision to take the position at McGill was the commitment I received from Don Baxter that the clinical activities required of me would be limited in order to give me the time I needed to initiate an independent research program. Today I regret that my deliberations were not more transparent, but I know that the choice was right.

Our house in Montreal cost $30,000. To buy it, we borrowed $4,000 from Rachel's cousin and her brother, Glen, and took out a mortgage for the rest at 7.75 per cent. My starting salary was $28,000. Our home was a beautiful place to begin part three of the Martin Family Saga. I felt very grateful for our good fortune. Rachel and I had been married ten years, we had four wonderful children, each of whom had been born in a different city, and we had moved ten times. Small wonder that neither Rachel nor I remember the addresses and telephone numbers of each of the places we have lived.

## Our First House and the Montreal General Hospital

Our first owned home was a remarkable 1920s-vintage dark-brick colonial. It had been the home of a distinguished family, the Frank Shaughnessies. He had moved his family to Montreal from the US at the beginning of World War I and became a legendary McGill Redman football coach. We purchased their furniture, most notably a 1906 Arts and Crafts dining room set manufactured in Cincinnati. It was dark and ugly and the veneer had nearly blackened with age. Rachel set about a year-long effort of stripping the outer layer, applying a new lacquer and in the process devaluing what we came to learn was a museum-quality piece. Some years later when we had moved the set to Boston with us, friends visiting our home in Belmont one evening noted its similarity to articles at an Arts and Crafts exhibit at the Boston Museum of Fine Arts. From the exhibit we purchased a copy of the 1906 catalog of Shop of the Crafters, illustrating the works of a German furniture maker based in Cincinnati, whose shop and manufacturing operation had lasted a mere ten years or so at the beginning of the twentieth century. Suddenly aware of its value, we made certain that it accompanied us in our subsequent travels to San Francisco and then back to Boston where it is now placed in a perfect setting in our Brookline home, nestled in an oval-shaped dining room with bay windows and an alcove perfectly shaped for the largest of the set, a buffet measuring sixty-four inches wide and sixty-seven inches high.

I spent long hours at my new laboratory getting established in the University Medical Clinic at the Montreal General Hospital, the MGH North as I came to call it in retrospect, especially after my subsequent association with the Massachusetts General Hospital in Boston, which I called the MGH South. The Montreal General was the second hospital established in Montreal. The first, the Hôtel-Dieu de Montréal, had been founded in 1645 by Jeanne Mance, the first nurse in New France, soon after the French had arrived on the Island of Montreal. This hospital remained the only francophone hospital in Montreal during the two centuries after the conquest of New France by the British.

The Montreal General, established in 1821, was the first hospital for the English-speaking population in Montreal. One year later, in 1822, the doors were opened with a capacity of seventy-two beds, four Edinburgh-trained physicians and a navy-trained surgeon, just one year after the famous Bulfinch Building opened at the MGH South. A medical school, the Montreal Medical Institute, opened next through the initiative of the hospital's medical staff. Classes were first held during 1823–24, and the hospital became the first in the North American continent to allow students on the wards.[1]

About ten years earlier, in 1813, businessman and philanthropist James McGill of Montreal had died leaving a will in which he bequeathed his forty-six-acre farm, known as Burnside, to

The Royal Institution for the Advancement of Learning to establish, within ten years of his death, a university or college in his name. McGill also bequeathed £10,000 for the expenses associated with the establishment and maintenance of the college. The will stipulated, however, that if the college was not established within ten years of his death, the property and funds would revert to James McGill's heirs. In 1828, in order to meet the deadline and save the bequest, the Montreal Medical Institute was asked to become the first faculty of McGill University with Andrew F. Holmes as dean, and thereby become the instrument by which the university justified its existence. Additions to the hospital were built in 1884, and a hospital for infectious diseases opened in 1888. Quality of care improved at the Montreal General by the arrival of new physicians from Europe, especially under such legendary figures as Thomas Roddick, who had studied antiseptic methods under Joseph Lister and introduced antiseptic surgery at the Montreal General Hospital and throughout Canada; William Osler, a McGill graduate who returned to the Montreal General in 1874 after two years of study in Europe, where he served as a pathologist and physician, and later throughout his illustrious career would revolutionize American medicine; and James Stewart, with a major interest in neurology and psychiatry.

In 1903 the Montreal General was the first hospital in the Province of Quebec to recognize neurology as a specialty. This movement was initially led by David Alexander Shirres, a neurologist from Aberdeen with an interest in neuropathology. Between 1904 and 1920, Shirres served as lecturer in neuropathology at McGill, neurologist to the Montreal General Hospital and professor of neurology at the University of Vermont, which he visited regularly. His successors at the increasingly busy service at the Montreal General included neurologist Fred Holland MacKay (1920–47), Francis McNaughton (1947–51) and Preston Robb (1951–54). One of the members of the neurology service was C. Miller Fisher who, after being a prisoner of war in Germany from 1943 to 1945, had come for training in neurology at the Montreal Neurological Institute (1945–48), after which he engaged in a period of study in England. He returned to McGill and the

Montreal General, as well as the Queen Mary Veterans' Hospital affiliated with McGill University Faculty of Medicine, where he furthered his interest in stroke patients. Miller was subsequently invited to join the staff of the MGH South, becoming the foremost authority on cerebrovascular disease in the world.[2]

Over the years, the McGill University Faculty of Medicine established other affiliations with hospitals in the Montreal area, notably the Royal Victoria Hospital (RVH), the Montreal Children's Hospital (MCH) and the Jewish General Hospital. Each of these hospitals had independent governing boards, creating a model of medical complexity that I learned to navigate in 1970, knowledge of which would serve me in good stead later when I joined the Harvard medical community.

## The FLQ Crisis

Rachel settled our family into the new home in Montreal. Patient and unselfish, she navigated the preparations for school for Brad and Melanie, met neighbors, planned car pools and arranged our few belongings. All seemed to be progressing smoothly, but by October, the political situation in Montreal had become critical.

In a city with so many immigrants from all over the world and a minority of English Canadians, the French Canadians constituted the majority, but only in numbers—not influence. The French separatist movement in Quebec, which had started several years earlier, demanded sovereignty for Quebec and independence from Ottawa and the economic, linguistic and political dominance of the English minority. Violence had not been uncommon during the preceding years, but in October 1970, the Front de libération du Québec (FLQ) kidnapped James Cross, the British Trade Commissioner, and Pierre Laporte, a Quebec cabinet minister, thereby triggering a series of events that ultimately culminated in the only peacetime use of the *War Measures Act* in Canada's history. Canadian forces were deployed throughout the province of Quebec. The police, who arrested and detained, without bail, 497 individuals, were given far-reaching powers by Prime Minister Pierre Trudeau's Liberal government. Of the two kidnapped government officials, Laporte was found murdered by his captors, but James Cross, who lived not too far from the Montreal General where I worked, was freed through negotiations sixty days later.

During most of our stay in Montreal, the city remained in turmoil, with invisible lines separating the French and English Canadians, including in the area of higher education. McGill was the privileged academic bastion of the English Canadian minority in a predominantly French-speaking city, an island removed from its immediate environment. In a university that received the lion's share of government funding paid by a taxpayer base that was largely francophone, only 3 per cent of the student population was francophone. A little less than one year before I joined the faculty at McGill, over 10,000 peaceful demonstrators led by Stanley Gray, a professor of political science from Ontario, had marched to the gates of the university demanding, among other things, that the institution conduct instruction in the French language. The marchers were met at the school gates by hundreds of police and security guards. The majority of McGill's students and faculty opposed such a position, and many of the protesters were arrested.

Tensions continued as the Parti Québécois, led by René Lévesque, was elected to form the government of Quebec in the 1976 provincial elections, with the political, social and economic independence of the province as its primary goals. An especially significant, and perhaps the most prominent, legacy of the Parti Québécois was the *Charter of the French Language* (Bill 101), which defined, among other things, the linguistic primacy of the French language and sought to make French the common public language of Quebec. These changes would ultimately cause an accelerated exodus of the English-speaking population of Quebec and related economic activity to Toronto and farther west, and a significant degree of uncertainty about the future of those English speakers who stayed in Montreal, among them our family.

## Research Collaborations

During my first five years at the Montreal General Hospital, I spent one full month out of the year on the wards with residents and students and held a clinic for half a day each week, seeing follow-up and new patients and teaching students and residents. I soon began to learn conversational French to be able to communicate with my French-speaking patients who wanted to see "le docteur anglais." My laboratory was near those of Carl Goresky and Harry Goldsmith, both of whom were professors of medicine and skilled in the business of laboratory management, academic politics and the anomalies of McGill administration. The Department of Medicine, led by Doug Cameron, was making strides in moving the Montreal General toward a stronger competitive position vis-à-vis the Royal Victoria Hospital, where John Beck, a large man with enormous ambition, chaired a more nationally and internationally recognized Department of Medicine in an expanding academic venture. Doug Cameron was a ruthless, but fair and loyal, leader, well versed in the art of politics. I found out years later that when I was being recruited to the Montreal General, Doug had suggested that Don Baxter attend to the task of persuading me to come to McGill, while he would look after the "politics" concerning the University of Alberta.

> The author in his laboratory at the McGill University Medical Clinic, Montreal General Hospital, 1971. The stereotactic instrument was used to place electrodes into rat brains to determine the effects of stimulation on growth hormone secretion.

The Division of Neurology at the Montreal General was given favorable status in the Department of Medicine. My laboratory in the McGill University Clinic at the Montreal General consisted of one room, measuring about four hundred square feet, where I established my laboratory team with two technicians and proceeded to develop methods to deliver brain stimulation in rats with implanted electrodes in hypothalamic and extra hypothalamic sites while measuring, via a newly developed radioimmunoassay for rat growth hormone, the minute-to-minute changes evoked by stimulation. This work was published in *Endocrinology* and helped establish me as an independent investigator.[3]

Soon after my arrival, the administrators at the MGH North set about constructing a new research building. The Division of Neurology fared well in the allocation of new, modern and bright laboratory space. With the recruitment of two electrophysiologists, Leo Renaud and Mike Rasminsky, and the establishment of laboratories in experimental neuropathy by Albert Aguayo and Garth Bray, we formed a growing, interactive and collaborative group. As noted previously, I had met Garth four years

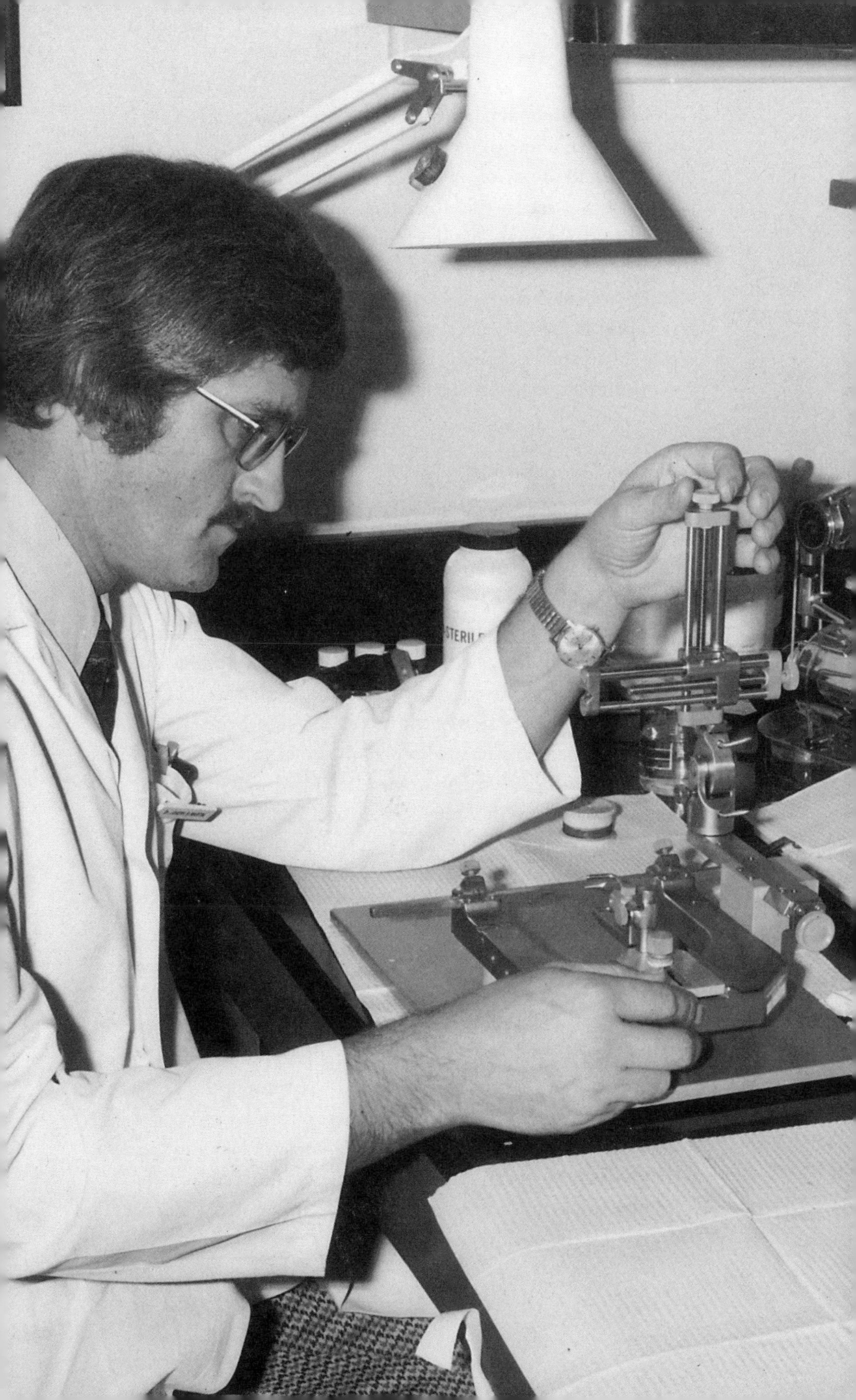

earlier in Cleveland during my residency training, while he trained with Maurice Victor.

As he had promised on my recruitment, Don Baxter worked long hours to secure the clinical base of our emerging enterprise in the Department of Medicine. Don had arrived at the Montreal General from Saskatchewan with Joe Stratford, a neurosurgeon and close friend, and together they had established an outstanding clinical neurosciences group. Our clinical space was developed in a portion of the recently vacated School of Nursing, and we shared offices there for consultative and diagnostic services.

## The Hard Work Begins

When I arrived at the Montreal General Hospital in June of 1970, I had been awarded a Medical Research Council of Canada scholarship for salary and an additional grant for research support. With this funding, I set out to pursue neuroendocrine research on brain hormones, specifically the hypothalamic regulation of growth hormone (GH) secretion, which we now know affects body growth and maturation and a number of other metabolic processes. The secretion of GH was clearly under the precise control of the brain; it was known to be secreted in large surges during deep sleep. Its absence resulted in growth impairment, as I had witnessed in the three Hutterites I met during my research at the colonies in Alberta. I was interested in learning about the influence the brain had on this hormone.

Thyrotropin-releasing hormone (TRH), the first of the hypothalamic releasing factors to be isolated and purified, was discovered in 1971. It was followed in 1973 by the discovery of somatostatin, a powerful inhibitor of GH secretion. Somatostatin was found in abundance in sheep hypothalamic extracts that Roger Guillemin at the Salk Institute for Biological Studies in San Diego was extracting for active hormones. Paul Brazeau, a French-Canadian post-doctoral student in Roger's lab, had been the key person in development of bioassays for the inhibitory peptide, which permitted its purification and sequence determination. Paul was first author on a science paper describing the discovery, and I set out to recruit him to join our new laboratories, knowing that he might consider an offer to return to Quebec.

Don Baxter was optimistic and supportive and found the necessary resources to complete a recruitment package, even though Paul was not clinically trained and would need to rely on salary support from grants. Paul joined Leo Renaud and me in 1973, and the three of us formed a productive interactive trio over the next three to four years. Paul would later show his Québécois loyalties when he appeared at meetings in the Department of Medicine wearing a Parti Québécois button! I was proud of him for "showing the flag" in this way.

Leo's electrophysiology experience with microiontophoresis, a technique used in neuroscience research, provided a way to show that the neuropeptides TRH, somatostatin and the subsequently indentified luteinizing-hormone-releasing hormone (LHRH) were each active in modulating neuronal excitability. Administration of other small hormones as controls was without effect. We published our findings, in the journals *Nature*[4] and *The Lancet*,[5] showing potent effects on neuronal firing rates. These observations were greeted with considerable enthusiasm at a time when anatomists were tracing neuronal peptide–containing pathways in the brain outside those involved in pituitary regulation. These electrophysiological effects opened up the possibility that these small peptides might function at synaptic connections as neurotransmitters or neuronal modulators.

I have often thought back to those days in Montreal and realize how fortunate I was to forge these research collaborations. As a result of them, my own work evolved into an analysis of the dynamics of GH changes in peripheral blood. Some of the methods we used seem rather crude in retrospect, but they allowed us to make minute-to-minute measurements of brain control over the endocrine system. A frustrating aspect of studies in anesthetized rats was the low levels of plasma GH compared to a striking variation in the levels found in blood from cranial arteries after decapitation. The commonly accepted approach to obtaining baseline "non-stressed" hormone levels was the collection of blood from the rats' cranial arteries. GH levels obtained by this method varied enormously from undetectable values of < 1 ng/ml to values that exceeded 400 ng/ml. It seemed likely that these striking variations represented dynamic surges of GH secretory activity. To test this hypothesis, we developed an isolation box strategy, employing a chronically implanted jugular venous catheter attached firmly to a cranial cement cast that permitted intermittent sampling in freely moving rats over many hours. Small samples sufficient for duplicate determination of GH by radioimmunoassay were obtained at fifteen-minute intervals, and the blood volume was replaced by saline.

The results were astonishing. With the careful work of graduate students Gloria Tannenbaum[6] and John Willoughby,[7] we determined an episodic pulsatile pattern of secretion, closely entrained by the light–dark circadian cycle. Subsequent experiments using stereotactically placed lesions of key areas of the hypothalamus showed the hypothalamic origin of these secretory bursts; they were completely abolished by prior administration of somatostatin. These physiologic findings were later reinforced when the growth-hormone-releasing hormone (GHRH) was identified, first from pancreatic endocrine tumors and then in hypothalamic extracts.

In July of 1976, at age thirty-seven, I was promoted to professor of neurology at McGill University. I had received national recognition as secretary of the Canadian Society of Clinical Investigation and had begun to enjoy the privilege of academic travel abroad. My work on GH prompted my first visit to Europe: to Milan, Italy, in 1973, for an international conference on GH regulation. Although our children were young, I convinced Rachel to join me at the end of the conference for a tour of northern Italy, just the two of us. As on previous occasions, my mother was willing to watch the children while Rachel and I were away. She boarded the train in Brooks, Alberta, and forty-eight hours later arrived in Montreal West.

When Rachel arrived in Milan, we rented a small yellow Fiat and began our ten-day adventure. We took time to view Leonardo da Vinci's *Last Supper* in Milan, traveled to Verona, where the love story of Romeo and Juliet had unfolded, then moved on to Bologna and Venice, Florence and Genoa before returning to Milan. It was a spectacular time for Rachel and me: our second honeymoon. Since then we have uprooted ourselves many times on the slightest excuse for international gatherings—to Europe, Asia, Australia and South Africa. My work has certainly allowed us to enjoy some remarkable tourist experiences.

When we returned from Italy, a review of my work in GH regulation published in the *New England Journal of Medicine* put a certain capstone on my early academic efforts.[8] Rachel remembers the return trip from Boston when the imminent publication of the article led us to divert to a medical library in Burlington, Vermont, to see if the publication had arrived. We—actually, I—was disappointed and had to await its arrival in Montreal some days later.

## Expanding My Research Portfolio

When I arrived at Montreal General Hospital in 1970, Charles Hollenberg was head of the Division of Endocrinology. Together with Carl Goresky, he had recruited me to become a member of the McGill University Clinic at the Montreal General. Not long after I arrived, to my chagrin, he announced his imminent departure to Toronto to become chair of the Department of Medicine at the University of Toronto Medical School.

The endocrine group at the Montreal General was not strong in laboratory work, so I sought out Henry Friesen at the Royal Victoria Hospital to establish research connections with him and his laboratory group. Henry graciously welcomed me, and within a short time we were collaborating on the role of neurophysin in vasopressin secretion, a hormone that plays an important role in ensuring that your body does not lose too much water. I provided rat physiological models, Henry's group provided the measurement, and we published several papers together.[9] I was grateful to him for providing intellectual guidance at a stage of my career when the development of the physician-scientist required time to think about research, and friends to talk to about it. Not surprisingly, Henry was focused on his great contributions to prolactin research: identifying and sequencing the hormone, developing radioimmunoassay in the human and establishing some of the earliest clinical trials on prolactin suppression in the human with bromocriptine. These enormous contributions led to his receiving many awards, among the most important being the Gairdner International Medical Research Award.

### The House of Friendship (La maison de l'amitié)

While my work engaged me intellectually and I made good friends in my colleagues, Rachel and I continued to maintain close contact with the Mennonite community. A good portion of our social life in Montreal centered on helping establish a community service center for the large Portuguese immigrant community. Discussions for a center first came up at meetings with a few other Mennonite couples who met at our home one Sunday evening each month. Later, the group included people who had lived in the area longer than we had, some of whom were not Mennonites. Our plans received financial support from Mennonites in Ontario and from the Mennonite Central Committee of Canada, allowing us to purchase in 1973 an old Jewish schoolhouse at 120 Duluth, which we called The House of Friendship. A board of councilors, which I chaired for a few years, oversaw the various projects and operations of The House, which was open to the entire community. It also became home to our church, where we held Sunday morning services for the small community of Mennonites in greater Montreal.

The House of Friendship continues to provide vital community services to this day, having gone through transitions over the decades and adjusting its programs to new needs. Over the years, it has offered intervention programs for refugees with legal problems, classes in English and French, a daycare and community activities to provide newly arrived refugees a chance to meet local people to minimize their isolation. The House continues as a community center that houses visiting university students who commit to community service during their stay there.[10]

### The Montreal Neurological Institute



By the fall of 1975 an unexpected opportunity arose within the McGill academic community. The position of neurologist-in-chief at the Montreal Neurological Institute (MNI) and Hospital (MNH), which included responsibility for neurological consultations at the Royal Victoria Hospital, opened up when Preston Robb announced his plan to retire.

The origins of the MNI were legendary in the McGill orbit. To address the urgent need for a neurosurgeon in the expanding world of neurology at McGill, Wilder Penfield, a neurosurgeon from the New York Neurological Institute and Columbia University, was recruited to Montreal in the fall of 1928, with his colleague, William Cone. It wasn't long before young scientists, including Dorothy Russell, a British neuropathologist, had joined them, and by 1931 the group had outgrown the allocated space. Edward Archibald, surgeon-in-chief at the Royal Victoria Hospital, and Charles Martin, dean of the McGill Faculty of Medicine were able to convince Alan Gregg of the Rockefeller Foundation to visit Montreal and consider supporting a neurological institute under the direction of Wilder Penfield. The foundation obliged, and the Montreal Neurological Institute was formally opened on September 27, 1934. One of the opening addresses was given by Penfield himself, who concluded:

> *...The building is only a shell. Within the shell should lie a living mollusk, a collective creature that is expected from time to time to form a pearl of great price. If this pearl can only be secreted within the protective covering of the shell and not without it, then the Institute achieves its purpose....The doors of the Montreal Neurological Institute are open to stimulation and guidance...*

This encapsulation of the functions of the "Institute" accurately captured what the MNI became over the decades that followed.[11]

The institute and hospital were both located within a single building directly across from the Royal Victoria Hospital. They were connected by an overpass that crossed over busy University Street, making consultative work in neurology at the RVH very convenient. The RVH did not have its own department of neurology and neurosurgery but instead used the facilities and consultations of the MNH and its staff. In turn, the staff of the RVH provided consultative support in medicine, surgery and the other specialties of a general hospital.

When the career opportunity arose at the MNI, I was intrigued. I felt I was qualified to be considered for the position as neurologist-in-chief at the institute.

I had previously interacted with several of the scientists at the MNI: Peter Gloor, a distinguished electrophysiologist who had defined the functional relationships of several structures of the limbic system and had served as a thesis research sponsor for my colleague Leo Renaud; Leon Wolfe, an accomplished neurochemist; Brenda Milner, whose work on the neuropsychological aspects of memory became legendary; and George Karpati, who worked on muscular dystrophy. Through my collaborations with the Friesen Laboratory at the RVH, I had also been introduced to several junior workers in Henry Friesen's unit.

> Map 4: McGill University, Montreal, and vicinity hospitals.

I also saw new opportunities for collaboration in clinical research with George Tolis in endocrinology and Sam Lal in psychiatry. The study of the regulation of prolactin secretion in human subjects nourished my own curiosity regarding the clinical investigation of the functions of the pituitary gland. These new affinities were attractive to me. New developments in pituitary surgery, focusing on the trans-sphenoidal route, led by Jules Hardy at the nearby Notre Dame Hospital showed great promise.

After extensive discussions with these and other members of the MNI and RVH, I was offered and accepted the position of neurologist-in-chief, effective July 1, 1976. By that time, my skills in clinical neurology had been rekindled, and I was excited about bringing more science to the neurology group.

There was one problem, however; research space was not available at the MNI or RVH. I was given permission to maintain my close links with the neuroendocrinology group at the Montreal General, where I was fortunate to be able to stay in contact with Leo Renaud, Paul Brazeau and Gloria Tannenbaum. Soon thereafter, Gloria took a position in endocrinology at the Montreal Children's Hospital. Gloria's career surged, and she established the endocrine and neural feedback dynamic of GH regulation in detail, contributing more than anyone else in that field. She was promoted to professor of neurology and pediatrics a few years later.

During this time I began to see patients with neuroendocrine problems. Many had pituitary tumors, some secreting abnormal levels of growth hormone (acromegaly), prolactin (causing galactorrhea, a milky discharge unrelated to breast feeding and amenorrhea, the absence of a menstrual period)

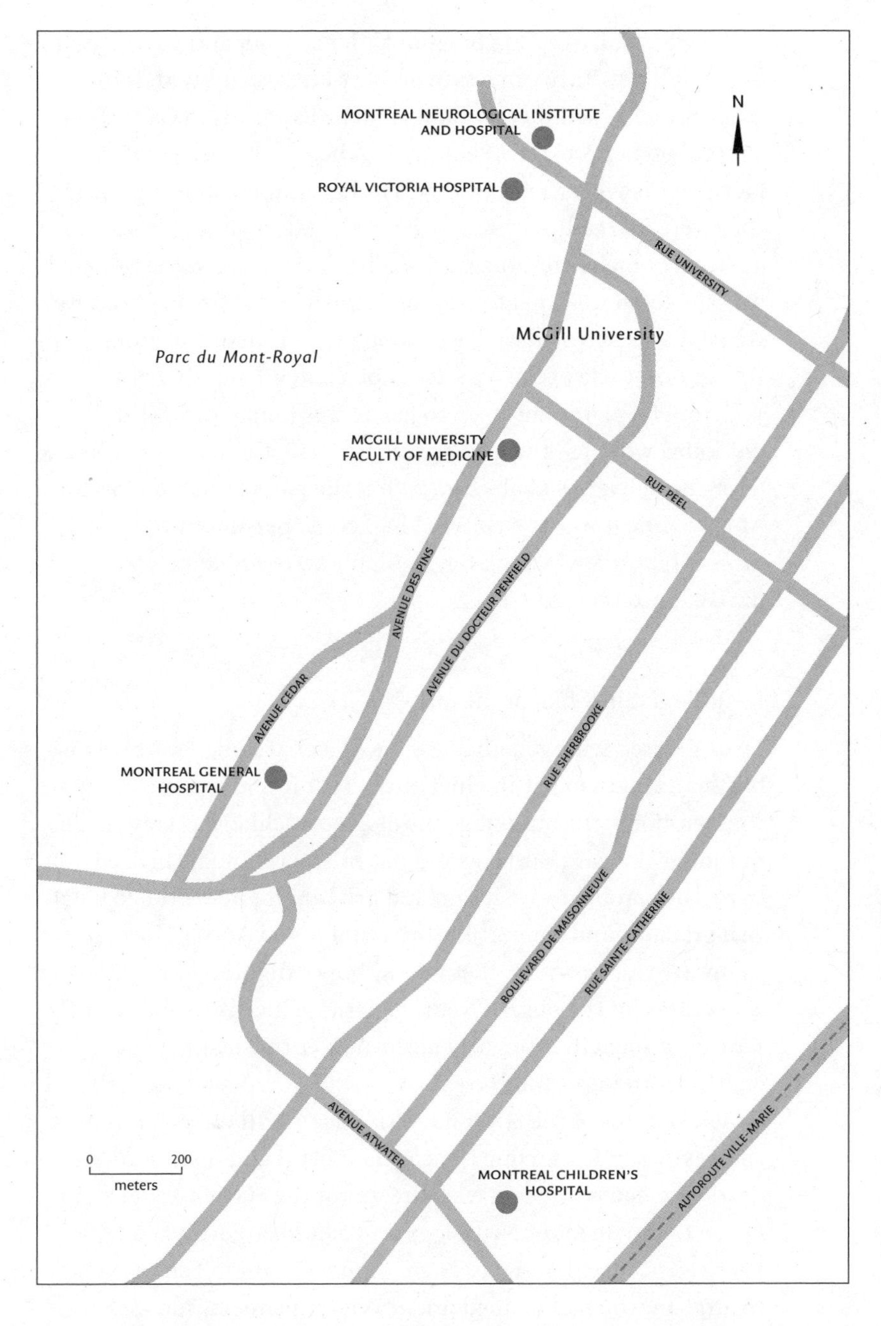


and adrenocorticotropic hormone (resulting in Cushing's disease, with increased secretion of cortisol caused by a tumor in the pituitary gland). One of my patients was the wife of a legendary hockey player for the Montreal Canadiens, who was having difficulty getting pregnant. Her amenorrhea was caused by a small pituitary tumor amenable to treatment with bromocriptine, which was available for clinical trials in Canada for suppression of prolactin secretion. When I measured her prolactin levels with Henry Friesen's radioimmunoassay, I noticed they were markedly elevated, and we began treatment awaiting a return of menstruation. Cycles reinitiated early in the fall, and we scheduled treatment to coincide with her husband's hockey schedule. As she ovulated, we stopped administering bromocriptine at mid-cycle of the first attempt at pregnancy. It worked. We stopped giving the drug to her at this point since we did not know whether it would be safe for the fetus. Nine months later she delivered a baby boy, whom the parents named Joseph. At that time it was the closest I had come personally to hockey fame. Then, a few years later, my nephew, Jeff Shantz, was drafted into the NHL.

## Neurologist-in-Chief at the MNI–MNH

I was greeted with generous good will as I assumed my responsibilities as neurologist-in-chief at the MNI in the summer of 1976. Preston Robb, the outgoing neurologist-in-chief was staying on but made it clear that he would not interfere, and he invited me to discuss problems with him and ask him for help if I needed it. In a gracious and congratulatory letter dated April 9, 1976, prior to my arrival, he wrote, "Let me say how delighted I am with your acceptance of the post of Neurologist-in-Chief at the Institute. I am sure you will bring new ideas, new enthusiasm, and new energy to an important post."

The politics of the MNI and MNH became all too obvious over the next year. Ted Rasmussen, a thoughtful and distinguished academic neurosurgeon, was director of the MNI and chairman of the Department of Neurology and Neurosurgery when I arrived at McGill in 1970. Then, in 1971, William Feindel, a neurosurgeon who had trained under Wilder Penfield, succeeded Rasmussen in both these positions. More than any other single individual, Feindel sought to move the institute toward a veritable shrine in honor of his mentor Penfield, who died in 1976.

Feindel was a formidable intellect, endowed with an ambition to maintain the prominence of the MNI internationally. He was successful in securing one of the first CT scanning machines manufactured by the EMI Corporation in England in the 1970s, and he placed enormous emphasis on the power of imaging, including the early introduction, some years later, of positron emission tomography (PET scanning) and magnetic resonance imaging (MRI).

Bill Feindel's appointment as MNI director was renewed in 1976. After I became neurologist-in-chief in July of that year, the Faculty of Medicine also reviewed his position as chair of the Department of Neurology and Neurosurgery. The dean at the time was Patrick Cronin, a cardiologist and the son of the author and physician A.J. Cronin.

Dean Cronin carried out a formal search for the position of chair of the Department of Neurology and Neurosurgery. Propelled by a deep concern about the critical issues that neurology faced within the McGill orbit at that time, I presented the search committee with a personal perspective, including comments and suggestions to remedy the situation. I pointed out that the emerging strengths in neurology at McGill's teaching hospitals in the course of the last ten years had made it imperative that neurology consolidate its expertise and talents if it were to achieve major objectives in academic neurology. To this end, I suggested, it was essential to explore and institute avenues of collaboration and coordination and to create a unified administrative structure that functioned on clearly defined and transparent procedures for faculty appointments and promotions, departmental reviews, teaching responsibilities, recruitments and the disbursement of departmental and special endowment funds to the faculty.

My report also focused on the MNI and its arbitrary and hierarchic administrative style, whereby decisions concerning appointments, use of endowment funds, use of space and budgetary allotments were made solely by the director with no recognized form of consultation. I concluded that unless substantial changes were made, we stood to lose some of our best faculty. My own concerns reflected those voiced by other colleagues in the McGill neurology community. One letter from Garth Bray, addressed to me in November 1976, is especially revealing. It read, in part:

*You are well aware of the generally low regard for which most Canadian and American neurologists have held the MNI as a neurology training center. However, general respect for the McGill Department of Neurology and Neurosurgery has been steadily increasing in the past few years, largely through the efforts of D.W. Baxter at the MGH and Gordon Watters at the MCH. It is my sincere hope that, through your own position within the MNH, it will be possible for you to exert influence towards the development of a true partnership within the department and not just the Head-Office-Branch-Plant attitude that obviously continues to exist...*

Patrick Cronin proved to be a great ally in the ongoing proceedings. He recognized, I believe, that neurology was on the threshold of a major surge in scientific discovery. Etiologic diagnoses were emerging for the lipid storage disorders, brain transmitters relevant to the treatment of Parkinson's disease (dopamine) and depression (serotonin) were leading to new drugs, and neurochemical identification of brain pathways promised new methods for unraveling a host of disorders.

When I wrote the report to Dean Cronin's committee, I had been neurologist-in-chief at the MNH for six or eight months. On the one hand, it seemed too early to take on another academic appointment. But support for my candidacy to the position of chair was strong throughout the university, and I was invited by the dean that spring to assume the position of chair of the Department of Neurology and Neurosurgery at McGill effective July 1977, in addition to my continuing role as neurologist-in-chief at the MNH. The news drew letters of congratulations from colleagues. I was particularly grateful for a letter of congratulations I received at the end of July from Dr. Maurice McGregor, chairman of the Department of Medicine and a former dean of the Faculty of Medicine.



The dean's move to have me appointed chair of the McGill Department of Neurology and Neurosurgery in addition to my position as chief of neurology at the MNH generated enthusiasm in many quarters of the McGill orbit—but not all. What followed in the summer and fall of 1977 was one of the most stressful experiences of my entire academic life. But to appreciate the drama of the episode, it is essential to consider related events in the academic world of neurology, particularly south of the border in Massachusetts.

In 1977 Dr. Raymond Adams, who was and remains, arguably, the single most influential figure in the entire field of neurology in the second half of the twentieth century, announced his intention to retire as chief of the neurology service at the Massachusetts General Hospital in Boston—the MGH South. Dr. Adams had arrived at the Massachusetts General Hospital in 1951 from the Boston City Hospital, where he had worked with Derek Denny-Brown. Later, Maurice Victor, who had attended medical school at the University of Manitoba, and Miller Fisher, coming from McGill and the Montreal General, joined him. Adams forged the leading efforts in modern neuropathology in close collaboration with vigorous scientific and clinical activities in neurosurgery. Over the next twenty-five years, the department surged into areas of experimental neuropathology, contributing more leaders to the academic neurological community than any other: Arthur Asbury, who became chair of the Department of Neurology at the University of Pennsylvania; Richard Johnson, who went on to a distinguished career at John Hopkins, eventually becoming chair of the department; Richard Barringer, who, following a stint in San Francisco, went on to become chair at the University of Utah; and many others.

Adams was sixty-six years old at the time. While he remained very active in both clinical and neuropathological efforts, he had to step aside as chief because of mandatory MGH regulations. The search committee to find a successor to Adams was formed and chaired by Dr. Seymour Kety, a renowned neuroscientist whose work had resulted in the clinical applications of PET scanning. The search for Adams's successor became a turning point for me during that stressful fall of 1977.

Dean Pat Cronin called me in to his office early in June of 1977 to say that my appointment as chair would need to be delayed until September because of some administrative details that he needed to work out. I was unsuccessful in querying him for more facts. So far as I was concerned, there were no remaining issues to negotiate, and I began to sense that something unpleasant was brewing at McGill.

Virtually simultaneous to receiving this notice from Dean Cronin, I received a call and an invitation to visit the Massachusetts General Hospital to provide advice and consultation to a committee there examining the future of neurology at the hospital. The call was from Dr. Kety, the committee chair. I was both flattered and perplexed by the significance of this development. I learned later, of course, that consideration for an appointment to leadership positions at Harvard Medical School commonly led to an invitation in consultative mode to give the committee an opportunity to meet and scrutinize a candidate.

At this point, I checked in with my mentor, Seymour Reichlin, who had by then relocated to Tufts University School of Medicine in Boston. Si gave me a background briefing on the Boston medical scene and alerted me to the fact that Nicholas Zervas, who had recently been appointed chief of neurosurgery at the MGH South, had a great interest in pituitary adenomas and their surgical treatment. Si also remarked on a truly remarkable individual in the Boston neurological scene, Dr. Norman Geschwind, who had moved from Boston City Hospital to the Beth Israel Hospital (BIH) in Boston and had an interest in the relationship of brain function to autoimmune disorders of the body.

An appointment with the twenty-member search committee in Boston was scheduled for July 1977. Zervas served as a member of the committee, as did Alex Leaf, chair of medicine, and Jerry Austen, chief of surgery. Although I no longer have the notes I had prepared for that meeting, I remember speaking about the importance of neurology in the setting of a general hospital and about the importance of collaboration with the Department of Medicine. I specifically addressed the challenges of neurological complications of diabetes mellitus, the importance of the nervous system in regulation of homeostasis and the future promise of neurotransmitter research and brain imaging.

I was left with the impression that the group was engaged, interactive and seriously curious about my thoughts and predictions. With the meeting over, I joined Rachel, Doug and Neil, all of whom had accompanied me on the trip, for some tourist experiences in Boston, and then we proceeded to drive home to Montreal. I received no feedback whatsoever following the Boston visit but did learn, during a conversation with Dick Johnson (who had been in Maurice Victor's department at the Metropolitan General Hospital in Cleveland at the same time as I and was now a rapidly rising star in neurovirology at Johns Hopkins) that the MGH committee was likely to offer the position to Barry Arnason from the University of Chicago. Barry, who had accepted the position of chair of neurology at the University of Chicago not long before, was a Canadian from Winnipeg and had stayed on at the MGH with Ray Adams after completing his residency. He was emerging as an international figure in the relatively new discipline of neuroimmunology, with a particular focus on the mechanisms of disease that caused multiple sclerosis.

## The Summer of 1977, and a Trip to Europe

Rachel, the kids and I spent much of August in extended weekends at our farm in Chateauguay, New York, which we had purchased in 1973, and where we spent many weekends year round. I gave little further thought to the Boston visit. I was anticipating taking on my duties as chair of the department at McGill and looking forward to upcoming meetings in Bordeaux, Paris, Amsterdam and Copenhagen. Fifteen at the time, our son, Brad, was to accompany me on the trip. He had saved his earnings as a paperboy for the Montreal *Gazette* for four years and would pay his own way. Unfortunately, while my perks granted me first-class status on many of the train routes through France, Holland and Germany, Brad was traveling on a Eurail student pass. He did join me in my compartment for a portion of one day's voyage, only to be ignominiously removed to second class by an unfriendly conductor.

The trip with Brad, like the trip Rachel and I had taken to Italy four years earlier, was a remarkable experience. It began in Bordeaux at a meeting on neuroendocrinology. The meeting had been organized by a Frenchman, Jean-Didier Vincent, a friend of Leo Renaud, who, like Leo himself, worked on electrophysiological studies of the hypothalamus. Brad was invited to stay at the Vincent home while I stayed at the dormitory at the meeting site.

I had been to Paris on several occasions before to visit with and establish Quebec–France collaborations in neuroendocrinology with Professor Claude Kordon of the Institut national de la santé et de la recherche médicale (INSERM), who had arranged for several postdoctoral fellows to come to my laboratory from his group, most notably Jacques Epelbaum and Dominique Durand.

The meeting in Bordeaux was a blast, with serious scientific discussions during the day followed by late-night parties at the beach or in the chateaus of the region. On the last night of the meeting, we convened at the Château Beychevelle for a banquet. The chateau, dubbed the Versailles of the Médoc as a tribute to its elegant classical architecture and French gardens, had a winegrowing tradition that dated back to the Middle Ages. According to legend, ships sailing in front of the chateau had to lower their sails as a sign of respect to its owner, hence the name Beychevelle, which derives from *baisse voile*, the French term for the lowering of sails.

Our evening at Beychevelle began in the expansive wine cellars, with induction of the guest lecturers into French wine society. The feast consisted of seven courses of fine wine and food and ended with me snake-dancing through the chateau, followed by an inebriated trip back to the hotel, during which I succeeded in misplacing the medal I'd received during the ceremony. To my deep regret, I never recovered it. I collapsed in bed at 3:30 a.m. with a 5 a.m. wake-up call to catch the train to Paris where I was to join Brad and Jacques and his wife, who had returned to Paris the day before. The train trip to Paris seemed endless, and I feared I might go into ventricular fibrillation or have a cardiac arrest. I learned later of what cardiologists refer to as "holiday heart," and I'm certain I was in and out of atrial fibrillation. I was too sick the next day to tour Paris with Brad. I convinced him that I had the "flu."

After Paris, Brad and I took the train to the World Congress of Neurology in Amsterdam and then on to the International Neurochemistry meetings in Copenhagen. From there, we traveled to Stockholm, where we were hosted by a dear friend, Tomas Hökfelt of the Karolinska Institute, and then on to Gothenburg, where I spent time with Stéphan Eden, who became a collaborator on our work of regulatory patterns of GH secretion, in particular the influence of sexual dimorphism. We ended our journey in Oslo, visiting Mrs. Reiko Tveitan, whose husband had died of ALS (Lou Gehrig's disease) while under my care in Montreal. Mrs. Tveitan took us to the site of the Winter Olympics in Oslo and to the Edvard Munch Museum, which exhibited the works of Norway's most famous painter and printmaker. We flew home via London, reaching Montreal in mid-September.

## Return to Montreal

My return to Montreal proved traumatic in the extreme. Waiting for me was a message to contact Dean Cronin immediately. Then, in my mailbox I found a copy of a petition prepared by William Feindel, director of the MNI, and sent to many of the members of the Department of Neurology and Neurosurgery, including the MNI, the Montreal General Hospital and the Montreal Children's Hospital. In the petition, dated July 27, 1977, Feindel objected to a memorandum from the dean's office regarding the ad hoc committee's "unofficial proposal for separation of the Direction of the MNI from the chairmanship of the Department of Neurology and Neurosurgery," and thereby to my appointment to the position of chair of the department which had, since 1930, always been occupied by a neurosurgeon. "Such a proposition," Feindel wrote, "would obviously involve a major departure from our long established administrative structure." In the last paragraph of the petition, he announced to his readers that he had been instructed by the principal (McGill University's president) "to carry out the duties and responsibilities of the Chairman and Director." Feindel had never made an effort to discuss the matter with me, nor had I been aware of his campaign to reverse the dean's decision, although I had always suspected that he wanted to continue to occupy both positions. Now I understood the dean's delay in my appointment, although he reassured me firmly that he remained in support of me taking the position.

Rachel and I felt vulnerable. My friends at the Montreal General, although still cordial, had never fully accepted my move to the MNI. There certainly was no question about returning to the Montreal General, and I found few colleagues in neurology at the MNI willing to share their views or give advice. A distinguished neurological clinician at the MNI, Francis McNaughton ("St. Francis," as he was affectionately called) was visibly shaken by the power play from neurosurgery, but he was too kind and gentle to offer any substantial advice.

After about ten days, and despite the dean's reassurances, I decided to call Seymour Kety to inquire about the status of the search in Boston. He responded at once. In his view, my visit in July had gone well and, he said, the committee would be convening again shortly. He promised to relay my inquiry of continued interest to the committee. I later learned that members of the committee, particularly Nick Zervas, the head of neurosurgery, had doubted that I could be recruited away from the MNI. Within a week, I was invited for a second meeting with the committee in early November. I traveled to Boston alone, spent another hour with the group and was invited to remain outside the chamber and await the outcome of their discussion. After thirty minutes or so, Seymour Kety invited me back into the room to say that the committee was prepared to recommend unanimously my appointment to the Bullard Professorship of Neurology at HMS. (The position of chief of the neurology service at the MGH was supported by an HMS chair allocated by Dean Daniel C. Tosteson of HMS.) Nick Zervas was enthusiastically supportive as was Alex Leaf.

Seymour Kety called a cab, and we went across town to the Longwood Medical Area to the office of the dean in Building A on the HMS campus. I was ushered into a rather spartan, dark office on the first floor of the building. Dan Tosteson was somewhat reserved and struck me as a bit shy and perfunctory. I learned later that he had assumed the deanship only in July of that year and that I was the first new chair recruit that he interviewed. Seymour Kety gave an account of my background and research interests to Tosteson, and he told him of the search committee's unanimous recommendation of my appointment.

I remember little of the next two months back at McGill. About a month before my November 1977 trip to Boston, I wrote Dr. Samuel O. Freedman, who had succeeded Dr. Cronin as dean of the Faculty of Medicine at McGill, about my intention to withdraw my candidacy for the position of chairman of the Department of Neurology and Neurosurgery at McGill. I ended my letter with a list of conditions which, if met, might make me reconsider my position. As I waited for more specifics about the potential position in Boston, it soon became known in my circle in Montreal that I was under consideration for the job at Harvard. Bill Feindel remained cordial and warm, as he had always been since my arrival at the MNI eighteen months earlier. He made no gesture to assure me of my position at the MNI, and I sensed that my departure, if it were to take place, would not cause him any remorse.

My second interview in Boston occurred just a few days after McGill's board of governors approved the principal's recommendation for my appointment as chair of the Department of Neurology and Neurosurgery effective November 1977. I sought the counsel of Joe Stratford, who was chief of neurosurgery at the Montreal General Hospital and someone who knew Bill Feindel very well. I asked Joe whether any potential outcomes of the situation would make my stay at the MNI feasible and palatable. I explained that I had personally reached the conclusion that the Boston offer was too attractive and compelling in view of the circumstances I was now facing at McGill. He recorded our conversation in a long handwritten note that was recently given to me. In the note, he sensed that I had firmly decided to move to Boston, that he quite clearly appreciated the dilemma I faced and that he was not able to reassure me otherwise. I valued his opinion a great deal and felt better about my decision after the conversation with him. By January Rachel and I had resolved to explore all the implications of the Boston offer. I visited Boston in February once more, a week after the great blizzard of 1978 that had paralyzed the entire city for most of a week with a snowfall of thirty-six inches and strong winds that piled snow high across the entire landscape.

I soon came to appreciate that my future plans, should I choose to take the job in Boston, depended on the hospital chief, Charles Sanders, and whether he could locate space for my lab and provide sufficient resources for me to recruit other scientists. I learned that the HMS budget for the department was about

$50,000 annually, plus the Bullard Professorship, an endowed chair, which was the only one in the department. I negotiated with the dean to double the annual department budget, although I had no idea what that meant. As for the hospital, my laboratory space would be the one recently vacated by none other than Seymour Kety himself, who had recently moved his research to McLean Hospital in Belmont. My "package" for the scientific expansion of the department was $1 million over five years. The lab space would be renovated for my purposes with completion planned for the fall of 1978.

Many colleagues in Montreal were sorry to see me leave for Harvard and the MGH and wished me success, among them Bill Feindel. "Dear Joe," he wrote in his letter of April 4, 1978,

*As you can appreciate, it was a shock to all of us that you have decided to move to Harvard, as you announced last week at our Professional meeting. We all regret you are leaving particularly after such a short few months as our Chairman....Let me say how much I have appreciated working with you over the past year and a half since we appointed you Neurologist-in-Chief.... You know that your colleagues here wish all success and good fortune for you and Rachel and your family in this new venture. If there is anything I can do personally to smooth over the transition for your move, please do not hesitate to ask me. We shall follow your career with great interest and satisfaction.*

Although we met from time to time at various meetings in Canada and abroad over the next thirty years, Bill Feindel never brought up the controversy on any occasion. After my departure, Preston Robb stepped back into his old position as neurologist-in-chief and chaired the Department of Neurology and Neurosurgery for a year.

Unlike Feindel, Robb was quite upset at these developments. Years later in his history of neurology at McGill University he wrote:





*I should go back a bit. Since the days of Dr. Penfield, traditionally the director of the Institute acted as chairman of the McGill Department. When Dr. Martin was appointed as neurologist-in-chief, the dean, Patrick Cronin, decided to separate the posts of director and chairman. Most of the undergraduate and graduate teaching was done by neurologists. It made sense*

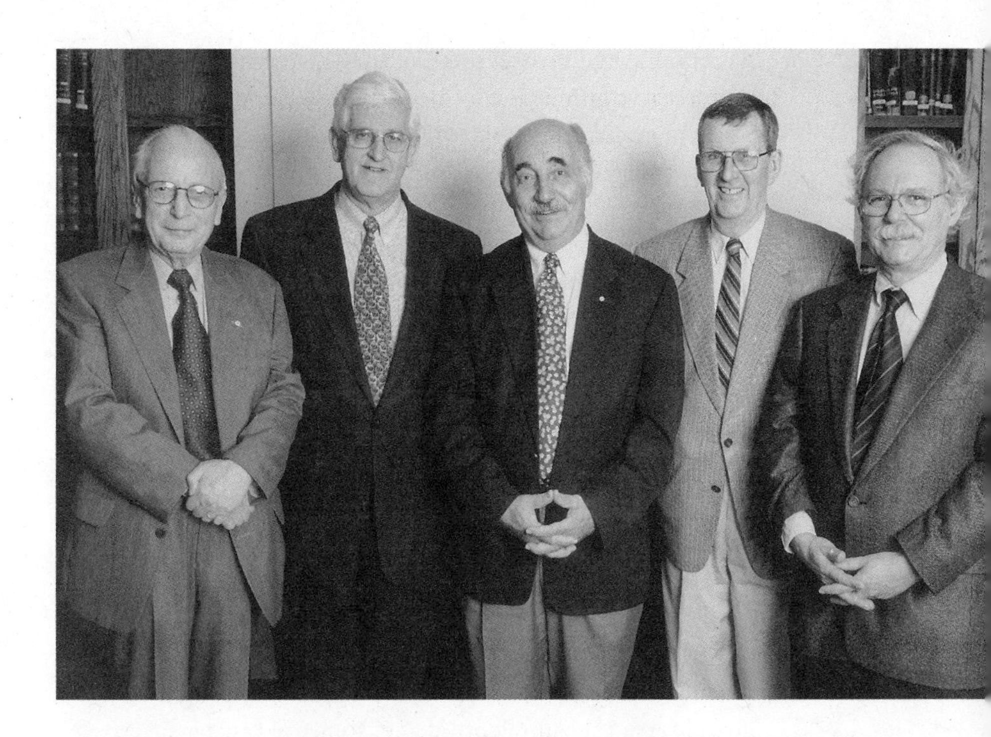

Montreal General Hospital neurology group at the Donald Baxter Lecture given by the author, Montreal Neurological Institute, 2000. From left: Donald Baxter, the author, Albert Aguayo, Garth Bray and Michael Rasminsky.

*that the two jobs be separated but that a neurologist act as chairman of the McGill department of neurology and neurosurgery. Dr. Feindel strenuously objected to this change, which delayed its implementation. By the time it took effect, Dr. Martin had decided to accept the position in Boston, and I returned to the Institute with all the related problems.*[12]

Robb was succeeded by Don Baxter who held both the chief of neurology and department chair positions from 1979 to 1984. In 1984 Don was appointed director of the MNI, the first non-surgeon to head the institute, to replace Bill Feindel. Don was a strong and uncompromising leader, supportive of coupling basic science and clinical care. He was followed by Richard Murphy, who led the MNI from 1992 to 2000, when he left to be the president of the Salk Institute for Biological Studies in La Jolla, California.

Years later, in May 2000, when Rachel and I were on our way to Montreal after an invitation to give the Donald Baxter Lecture at the MNI, we reminisced about our time in Montreal, how it had touched our lives in so many ways and the wonderful friends we had made and kept in touch with.

Our family had thrived there, with the older children taking advantage of a bilingual education. Rachel had taught in a pre-school program in Montreal West; it was time away from home that she enjoyed, and it served as a venue to connect with the community. We continued our close associations with our dear friends at The House of Friendship and watched it grow in influence and support of the local Portuguese community. And although the political circumstances that had unfolded during our stay in Montreal brought us concern and uncertainty, it never played a significant role in our decision to leave the city. I would have been very pleased to continue my academic role there.

My decision to leave McGill was very difficult. I sensed no personal animosity from the opposition I'd encountered at the MNI. For those deeply ensconced in the traditions of the MNI, reaching out to a more generous collaborative effort to develop neurology and neuroscience at McGill was not a priority. On my frequent visits back to McGill over the subsequent three decades, I have observed the unrelenting persistence of this perspective with sadness. While strong in basic neuroscience, guided by Richard Murphy and the current director, David Colman, the MNI and MNH have not excelled in most areas of neurology and neurosurgery.[13]

As I began my lecture that eighth day in May 2000, I thanked Don Baxter, who was in the audience, for his support in providing the framework for me to establish an independent research career. The influence he and my colleagues at McGill had on my maturation and academic evolution cannot be overemphasized.

Friends have asked whether I left because I felt encumbered by the traditions of the MNI and McGill or whether I was simply opportunistic in taking another job. I'll never know for sure which it was, but I'm thankful that we chose to move on.

# FIVE

# *Boston: The MGH Years*

THE MASSACHUSETTS GENERAL HOSPITAL was founded in 1811. John Warren, professor of anatomy and surgery at Harvard Medical School (one of the original three founders of Harvard Medical School in 1782 together with Benjamin Waterhouse and Aaron Dexter), spearheaded the move of the school from Cambridge to Boston in order to place opportunities for clinical work closer to the main population of the region. Warren's son, John Collins Warren, along with James Jackson, led the efforts in planning for the MGH, which would become the principal teaching hospital. The guiding principle behind formation of the MGH was to provide care for the poor of Boston, who could not afford to receive medical care at home, as was the standard of the day for the wealthy. The hospital, designed by famous American architect Charles Bulfinch, and placed strategically on the bank of the Charles River, provided access at high tide to boats that brought patients by water. During the mid-to-late nineteenth century, Harvard Medical School was located adjacent to the MGH.[1]

Rachel and I were excited about moving to Boston and becoming a part of the legacy of the MGH. Planning for the relocation to Boston posed several challenges, however, one of the most significant of which was finding a public high school for the children. Brad, a bright lad who underperformed in Montreal West High School and, we feared, was developing some unsalutary friendships, had just finished grade ten and would be turning sixteen over the summer. Melanie had attended French immersion in the Protestant school system in Montreal, beginning in kindergarten, and had just finished a year at Sacred Heart Academy. She was remarkably fluent in both spoken and written French but wanted to finish high school in English. Doug was starting the fourth grade and had taken a few years of French but not enough to want to continue, and Neil, at age eight, was ready to start third grade.

While we searched for a town with excellent public schools, we also had to consider real estate values and what we could afford for a home. Other than a modest McGill pension (that necessarily had to remain in Canada, until I reached retirement age) we had no savings. The farm we owned in Chateauguay provided us with a wonderful setting for weekends with the family—gardening, hiking and cross-country skiing—but no financial advantage. We loved the farm and the time we spent there but eventually gave it up because of its distance from Boston.

## Harvard Red Tape

As we were planning the relocation in the spring of 1978, a truly remarkable Harvard academic procedural matter caused great uncertainty and considerable angst for Rachel and me. I had concluded negotiations with Harvard Medical School and the MGH in early March and announced our intention to move to Boston to colleagues in Montreal when Dan Tosteson, somewhat new to the dean game and perhaps not particularly sensitive to our predicament of relocating a large family, called to tell me of the process involved in my appointment. In retrospect, after a decade as dean at HMS, I appreciate his dilemma to a degree. Dan explained that the paperwork for my appointment as professor was slowly finding its way from Seymour Kety's ad

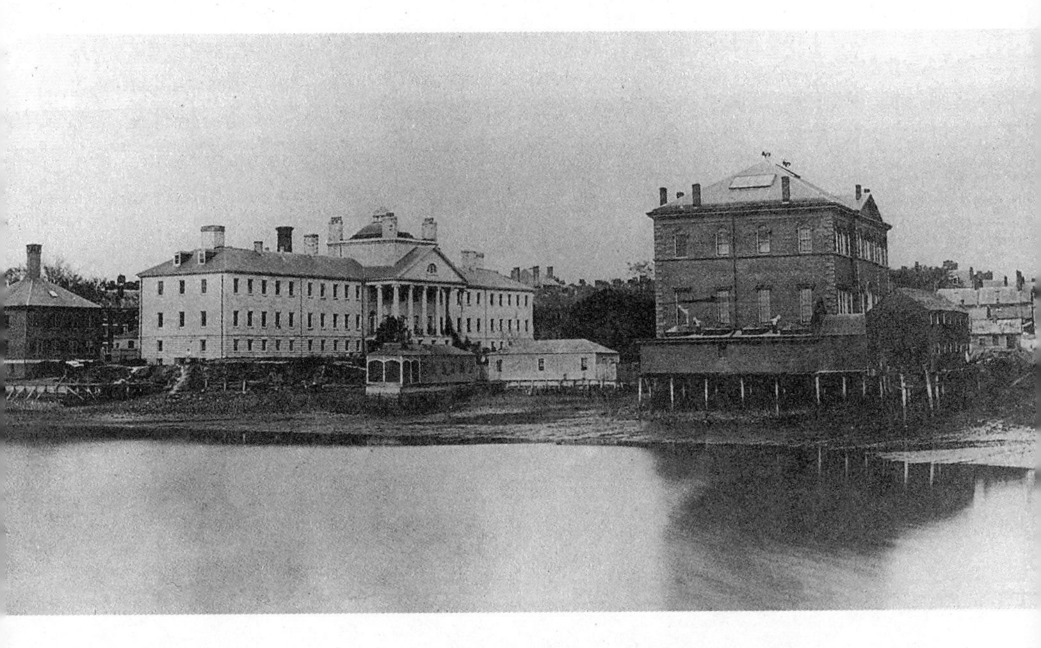

hoc committee to the Subcommittee of Professors, a group of thirty senior faculty members appointed to oversee the tenure process by serving rotating terms of three years each. That process, said the dean, would not be completed until late April. But that was not all. The final stage required the approval of the Harvard Corporation, represented by the president and fellows of Harvard College. President Derek Bok would not be considering the matter until mid-May. I learned later that Bok personally reviewed each tenure case from the medical school and that there was indeed no rushing him in these deliberations.

Rachel was very upset. We had seen several houses in the Boston area that offered the amenities we wanted. But the market was tight, and with the busy springtime and early summer season coming on, arrangements needed to be made for a moving company. My appeals to the dean at Harvard Medical School did not relieve our anxieties. Eventually, a favorable adjudication from Harvard came in May. We traveled to Boston over the Memorial Day weekend and purchased a house in Belmont for $105,000, available for a move-in day in late June but without any chance of renovation or interior painting. Belmont, we were told, had a good school system, and the house was located such that each of our children could walk to their respective schools.

Massachusetts General Hospital, 1853, when Harvard Medical School was located adjacent along the banks of the Charles River. Patients were ferried to the hospital at high tide and local legend has it that cadaver remains from dissections in the school were tossed from windows into the river.

Subsequently, all four children graduated from Belmont High School, which provided them with quite a satisfactory education and the prerequisites for admission into excellent universities.

A third factor relevant to our move beyond schools and the purchase of a home was my efforts to plan ahead for the transition of my laboratory and to initiate efforts at recruiting other scientists—either from my contacts at McGill or elsewhere. I was unsuccessful with the former. Neither Leo Renaud nor Paul Brazeau was interested in moving to the US. They had received significant research support from the Medical Research Council of Canada, as well as the Quebec government, and were not interested in the process of applying for new support from the US National Institutes of Health (NIH), where initial support was considered difficult to obtain. My next step was to explore possibilities for recruitment of talented individuals in Boston and beyond.

## Lessons from an Obstacle Course

On one of my visits to the MGH earlier in the spring, I had asked to meet with Susan Leeman, who was then an associate professor in the Department of Physiology at HMS. Susan was an outstanding scientist who, in 1971, achieved the first isolation of the neuropeptide substance P, a molecule later shown to be important in the pathway of pain modulation. We had met at neuroendocrine meetings in the past and had heard each other's presentations. I wondered whether she might be a potential colleague for collaborative work at the MGH. The discussions with her seemed promising, and, during the summer months, I explored with Charlie Sanders, the general director of the MGH, the possibility and feasibility of relocating her research group from the HMS Quad to my department at the MGH. Susan was pleased with the possibility, and meetings were arranged with Dr. John Potts, then head of endocrinology in the Department of Medicine, who was supportive. Shortly after my arrival that summer, we began to make specific plans for her move.

Susan Leeman's proposed appointment appeared to generate opposition at the MGH, however, and became an obstacle course of the first degree. Basically optimistic by nature and perhaps overly self-assured about my ability to convince others of a course of action, my first instinct was to fight the issue to the end. Susan trusted my judgment and continued her plan to move her lab. I pressed forward with a series of meetings with Charles Sanders, Dean Tosteson and Tom Wilson, who chaired Susan's department at HMS.

A long conversation with Tom to resolve the matter was not helpful. From his perspective, he was fully supportive of Susan's citizenship in his department. She was an excellent teacher, had superb graduate students and was well funded. The dean, for his part, finessed the situation, saying that it was really a matter for the MGH community. Charlie Sanders listened but offered no advice on how to proceed. I then asked my friend Si Reichlin, who knew Susan well, for his advice. He thought the idea of Susan joining my group made a lot of sense and urged me to continue my efforts to get her appointed at the MGH.

The matter dragged on for another two months and impacted every aspect of my life. I became insomniac, lost ten to fifteen pounds and, for the first time in my life, I felt powerless and impotent. I found myself lamenting having left McGill. Susan, on her part, grew impatient. Finally, she confronted me in my office and I described the reality of the situation: I could not get sufficient support from the parties involved to make her life bearable at the MGH. Perhaps the reluctance at the MGH was simply over allotting a tenured slot to her. I will never know.

After we moved to Boston, I started keeping a journal of important events. Over the years, the journal served as a mechanism to vet my inner feelings and frustrations, and in which I have continued to add entries over the years. My journal reflections were infrequent, approximately once every four to six months, usually triggered by pensive moments rather than momentous events. The earliest entries in my diary relate to the events surrounding Susan's recruitment. As I review them now, more than thirty years later, I can appreciate how toxic the experience of those first few months in Boston was.



September 24, 1978: *Many of the real agonies of middle life have unfolded during the past few months...There is guilt about the dislocation of a family... The issue with Leeman has been the most distressing...the guilt that she has been personally hurt through it all...Never before have I experienced the devastating swings in hope and panic.*

September 30, 1978: *The issues remain unresolved. Leeman is very upset... She has spoken to the dean and to Adelstein [dean of academic affairs at* HMS*]. The latter has talked to Sanders. In general, feelings about work are positive but there are doubts about recruiting. Why is it so difficult to get anyone to come? There has to be a breakthrough soon.*

October 18, 1978: *Two days to my 40th [birthday]. Events have not resolved but there is less tension. Nights still tend to be long and it's very easy to feel anxious and discouraged. The family is settling well...*

November 26, 1978: *There has been little real progress in the last month. At least I'm sleeping better. But there are still moments (and hours) of overwhelming anxiety and depression. At times it drains everything away—usually while at work...Leeman talked to John Potts last Wednesday—that seemed positive. She won't come without more reassurance...*

December 24, 1978: *Today is Sunday—before Christmas. The sky is clear and the air still. The children are excited and happy. Rachel has inspired us all with Christmas—even I have begun to feel the mood. Things are the best since our arrival. Leeman will not come—but we have preserved our friendship and I, my integrity—I think.*

But Susan never entirely forgave me, nor did she forgive the leaders at Harvard Medical School or the MGH. After a few years, she left HMS for a senior position at the University of Massachusetts Medical School and later moved to Boston University School of Medicine, where she remains active in research in 2011. I have never been able to completely resolve the tremendous disappointment I felt at the failure of the leadership in the HMS community to step up to the plate and participate in an equitable outcome. Susan was the one most hurt by the debacle. I recovered from the incident over the next few months but came away from the episode much more aware of the internecine and often unforgiving warfare that too often characterizes our academic institutions.[2]

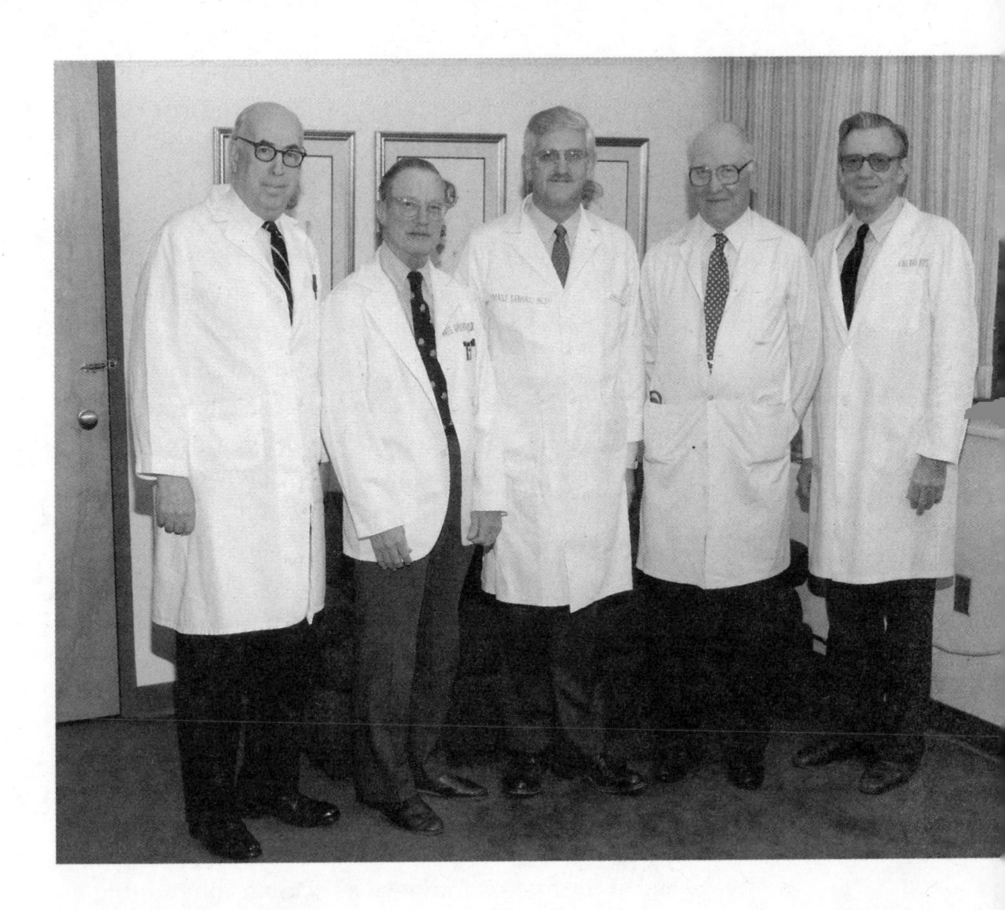

## Settling in at the MGH

Massachusetts General Hospital neurology senior leaders, 1980. From left: C. Miller Fisher, E. Peirson Richardson, the author, Raymond Adams and Verne Caviness.

Despite the problems I encountered in trying to recruit Susan Leeman, by July 1, 1979, I perceived that my first year had been a good experience overall. I sensed some remorse among the MGH leaders about the Leeman affair and an attendant willingness to help me succeed. My greatest challenge was to reorganize the neurology department and put in place a business plan with a balance sheet and profit and loss assessment, as well as to determine whom among the quite capable clinicians I could call upon to perform full-time roles in educational and clinical leadership.

Allan Ropper, who after completing the requirements for his residency stayed on an extra year to serve as my chief resident, helped me enormously during that first year. He was an outstanding clinician, skeptical about science adding much value to clinical neurology, but highly respected by the staff of the neurology, neurosurgery and medical departments, as well. Over the next decade Allan went on to establish the first neurological–neurosurgical intensive care unit in the US within the clinical neuroscience departments at the MGH.

Allan's critical role from my perspective as chief of neurology was to guide me through the clinical warrens of the MGH and to help me earn respect as a clinician. The majority of the clinical faculty was suspicious of this new "MD/PHD" and they still sought out the opinion of Ray Adams and Miller Fisher before approaching me. That didn't bother me because I, too, admired and respected both men, but I knew it was necessary to show my own ability and develop a new game plan. To do so, we put on superb grand rounds in the historic Ether Dome, where we presented patients with difficult clinical syndromes. I queried the patients and examined them in the presence of the faculty, residents and students in well-attended sessions and often called on other faculty members for their opinions. My particular area of specialty was also a benefit since I was the only neuroendocrinologist in the department. I worked with Nick Zervas and Peter Black, members of the neurosurgery department, and with endocrinologists like Ann Klibansky and Gil Daniels in John Potts's endocrine unit to establish a neuroendocrine clinic.

> Annual photo of the MGH Department of Neurology staff and residents, 1982. Front row, left to right: Raymond Adams, Vincent Perlo, the author, James Lehrich and Shirley Wray.

By the end of the first year my own lab was up and running. Residents in the neurology program, who would stop by to see what we were up to, soon joined our efforts. Steve Sagar, Flint Beal and Peter Riskind, each now distinguished professors of neurology in institutions throughout the United States, came to work in the lab. My first NIH grant had been funded with a high-priority score, and I was optimistic about putting together a productive research group.

## Editorship of Harrison's Textbook of Medicine

Not long after my arrival at the MGH, I was invited to the office of Kurt Isselbacher, chief of the gastrointestinal service, to discuss the succession of editors of *Harrison's Principles of Internal Medicine* (HPIM). The current editors were seeking a new editor for the neurological section of the text and wanted to have my ideas about the future of neurology, especially as it related to

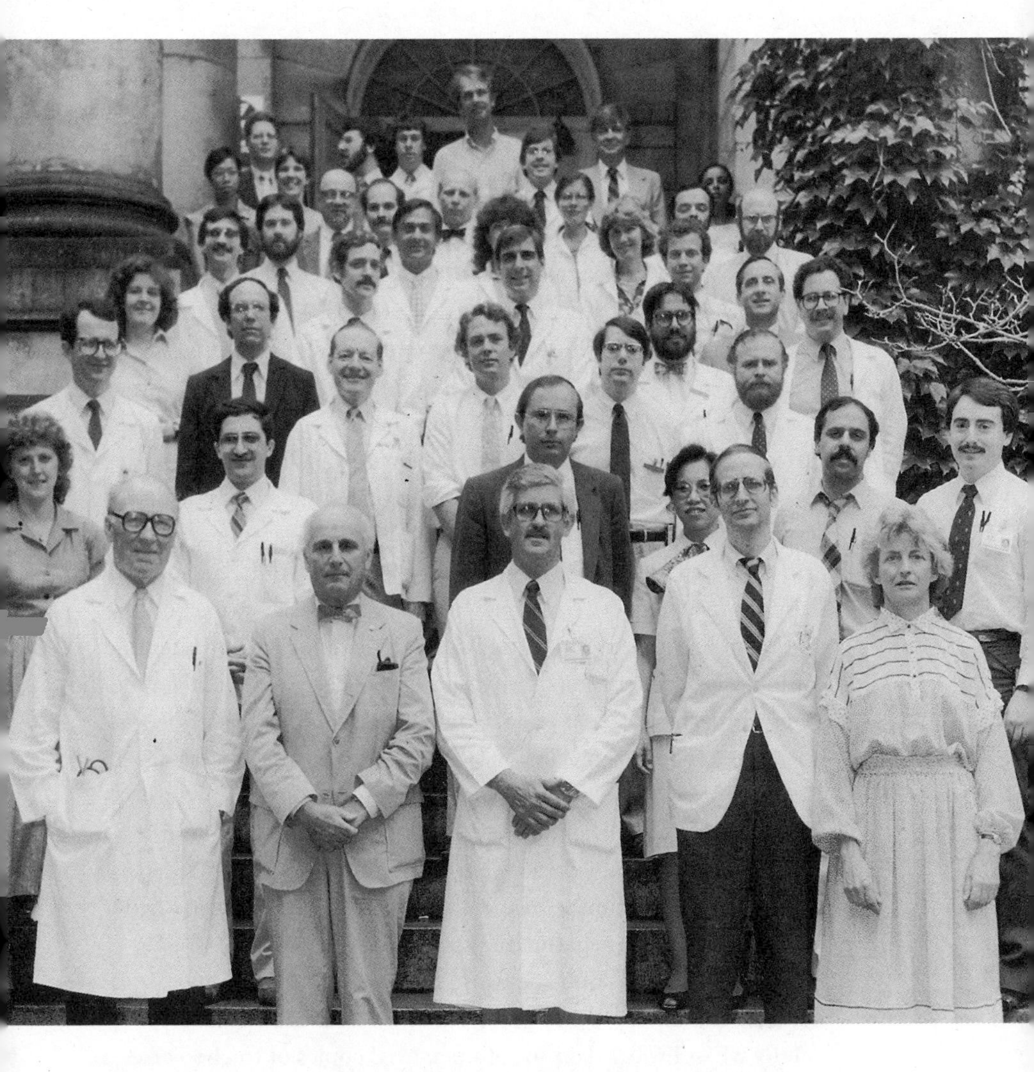

internal medicine. I was surprised by the prospect of joining this elite editorial board. I had used the much smaller fourth edition of HPIM in medical school and had been invited to write a chapter for the book while at McGill. I vividly remember receiving a letter from George Thorn, physician-in-chief at the Brigham and Women's Hospital (BWH) in 1976 asking me to consider a clinically relevant chapter on the clinical disorders of the hypothalamus and pituitary. I had been thrilled by that invitation, which I thought might have been triggered by my review of GH regulation published in the *New England Journal of Medicine* in 1973. George's letter (typed by his own hand, or so it seemed to me) was gracious and kindly asked me "to consider whether [I] might wish to contribute to HPIM." I did, and I wrote what I considered to be a quite satisfactory chapter on the disorders of hypothalamic-pituitary regulation for the ninth edition.

My meeting with Kurt was soon followed by meetings with the other editors: Robert Petersdorf, chief of medicine at the University of Washington in Seattle, who stopped by while visiting Boston during a trip to the East Coast; and Eugene Braunwald, George Thorn's successor as chief of medicine at the Brigham and Women's Hospital. Apparently, my ideas and experience were considered sufficient for the task, and I was invited to join Ray Adams as a co-editor of the tenth edition, which appeared in 1980. I learned enormously from the experience. I was impressed with Ray Adams's beautifully flowing sentences—my own writing talents being late in blooming. But I believe I did add a new perspective on the neurosciences as they were becoming relevant to neurology and internal medicine. Of considerable value was the fact that through my earlier research I had gained entry into the national endocrinology community. Over the next fifteen years, I was privileged to work with one of the best in that field, Jean Wilson of the University of Texas, Southwestern Medical School in Dallas. Together with Gil Daniels, my colleague in endocrinology at the MGH, we produced an enlarged, more definitive chapter on the disorders of hypothalamic regulation of the pituitary gland, including pituitary tumors.

As I traveled around the world, I marveled at the impact HPIM had on the concepts and practices of internal medicine, especially when I was asked to sign personal copies of the book for students and faculty. It sometimes seemed that in China and India at least, my editorship of the book carried more significance than my professorship at Harvard.

## The Alberta Heritage Foundation for Medical Research



I was barely ensconced in my new position at the Massachusetts General Hospital and Harvard Medical School when the phone rang one September morning in 1979. It was Dr. Lionel McLeod, dean of the University of Calgary's Faculty of Medicine. Lionel had been the hero behind my emerging academic interests as a student at the University of Alberta and honorary (faculty) class president of our graduating class in 1962.

Dr. McLeod had a request. Would I agree to host a visit by Alberta's Premier Peter Lougheed? Lionel explained that deep interest was growing on the part of the provincial government to establish an endowment fund for biomedical research and that the premier was looking into the details of how it might be organized.

The visit to the MGH was arranged on October 5, 1979. I met the premier in my office and arranged meetings with him and Charlie Sanders, head of the MGH, and a few other leading researchers.

In a letter to Lionel dated October 25, 1979, I expressed how enjoyable my meeting with the premier was, as well as my interest in the evolving plans and strategy of the Heritage Fund for Medical Research: "I must confess my astonishment at the degree of interest, knowledge and general information that was apparent on the part of the Premier. It is clear that he considers this endeavor to be a part of the 'heritage' that he will leave to the province and that he wants to do it right." I also noted to Lionel that I felt the premier's proposal was a "sound one" and that I felt "there is a genuine effort on his part to hold the whole endeavor at arm's length from government to depoliticize it and to allow academic freedom." I did caution, however, that "a major concern for all of you will be how to implement the first few years of a program which provides such massive amounts of money at a time when the necessary excellence and eventual development of a critical mass can only be accomplished over a period of several years."

The Alberta Heritage Foundation for Medical Research (AHFMR) was established formally in 1983 and became perhaps the single most important development in the growth of the biomedical reputation at Alberta universities. The funds were applied to a broad range of activities for training, recruitment, fostering faculty development and assuring permanent support for an outstanding group of faculty recruited from all over the world over the next twenty-five years.

I was delighted to accept an invitation to serve on the scientific advisory committee from Lionel McLeod, who went from

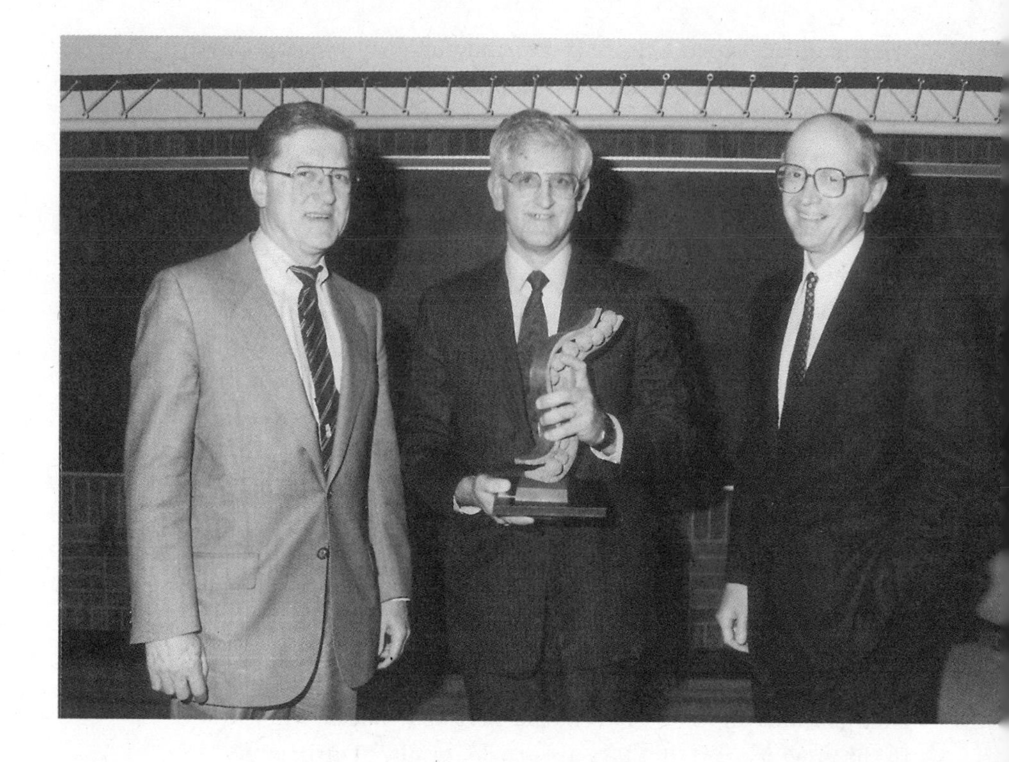

Receiving the Faculty of Medicine, University of Alberta 75th Anniversary Research Prize, 1988. From left: Lionel McLeod, president of the Alberta Heritage Foundation for Medical Research, the author and Dean Douglas Wilson of the Faculty of Medicine.

his position of dean of one of the two medical schools to be the first president of the foundation. I served on the committee from 1982 to 1989. I participated in one international review in 1994 and chaired a second one in 2004.

There is no disagreement among leaders of Canadian and US medical schools that the foundation enabled biomedical research in Alberta to establish an international reputation, placing Alberta's among the top research universities in Canada. As I reflected in a letter to the AHFMR leadership in 2004:

*Back in 1962 when I wanted to pursue medical research, I had to go elsewhere. The establishment of* AHFMR *completely transformed the landscape for scientific research in Alberta. It revolutionized the opportunities for Alberta to recruit outstanding scientists from around the world, to establish world-class research centers with the equipment and tools required to do specialized research, and resulted in the two main universities becoming recognized internationally for their research contributions. Without* AHFMR, *it is unlikely any of this would have happened.*

In March 2010 the Alberta government under Premier Ed Stelmach revoked the agreement that had established the AHFMR as a stand-alone endowment with independent governance to place it under a new consolidated entity called Alberta Innovates–Health Solutions. On a visit to Calgary in December 2010, I requested a meeting with former Premier Peter Loughheed. He greeted me affably to his comfortable corner office on the forty-fifth floor of the downtown Bankers Hall East tower. I asked him about his reaction to the demise of the AHFMR as he had envisioned it when established in 1983. He recalled the breakfast meeting with Deputy Premier Doug Horner at Calgary's Palliser Hotel in December 2008, when he was abruptly informed that the change had taken place and it was a "done deal."

"I was extremely distressed," he said. "I found it inexplicable and out of sync with the usual modus operandi. I could not understand why they did it."

## A Year as General Director

It was July 1981, the beginning of the new academic year and the beginning of my term as chair of the General Executive Committee (GEC) by vote of the chiefs of the hospital. I had been taken by surprise when asked to serve in that role so soon after my arrival at the MGH, and I realized that I was now christened into the internal politics of the hospital.

The GEC had an ancient history within the structure of the MGH's governance. It served as the quasi-public venue for most of the major discussions about the hospital's strategic planning and related matters. Everyone knew, of course, that the real discussions were not held in this forum but rather behind the scenes, where the chief of medicine (Alex Leaf and later John Potts) together with W. Gerald Austen, the powerful chief of the Department of Surgery, consulted with the trustees of the hospital and the general director. The trustees, a small group of eleven men and one woman, were known for their deep loyalty and careful succession planning. They met every second Friday of the month at 9 a.m. and were always fully informed about, and deeply involved in, any major issue relating to or concerning the affairs of the hospital.

With almost no exception, the GEC met every Wednesday morning from 8:00 to 10:00. The chiefs sat at the large oval table in the Trustees Room on the first floor of the White Building, immediately down the hall from the office of the general director. The meetings were efficient and usually concluded on time.

I have often wondered why the chief executive officer of the hospital was called the general director. The title was quite unique to the MGH and had a history that went back to the origins of the hospital in the early nineteenth century. I reckon that the minions who reported to the "general director" were considered deputies or soldiers to the general, who actually ran the hospital.

Charlie Sanders, a cardiologist who had grown up in Texas, was starting his ninth year as general director in July 1981. He had taken the helm after John Knowles vacated the position to become the president of the Rockefeller Foundation. Charlie was admired by nearly everyone and had a sufficiently distinguished career as a clinical academic to receive an appointment as professor of medicine at HMS. As he entered his ninth year at the helm, so did a particularly thorny issue that had emerged at the MGH two years earlier regarding the position the hospital should adopt about heart transplantation. The recommendation to proceed with this new technology on a limited basis had been put forward by Jerry Austen, the distinguished heart surgeon who had been chief of the surgery department for over a decade. I was aware that lengthy discussions had been held between Charlie and the board of trustees about how, if approved, to proceed with a technology whose efficacy remained highly controversial. In the end, the decision was made not to proceed with a large investment in space and staffing for this initiative. Jerry Austen was not pleased. Many in the hospital felt the issue affected the relationship between Charlie and Jerry; many also believe it was a key factor in Charlie's decision that came to light that summer.

Charlie called me to his office one Tuesday afternoon in early July before the regularly scheduled GEC meeting of the next morning. "Joe," he said, "I want to announce tomorrow morning that I'll be leaving the MGH." Although I swear infrequently, I vividly recall my response: "Oh, shit."

Charlie explained that he had already accepted a position as vice-president for research at Squibb Pharmaceuticals, a company based in Princeton, New Jersey, effective September 1, and would be leaving the MGH in about two weeks. He wanted me to introduce the topic toward the end of the regular business meeting at the conclusion of the GEC session the next day. I cannot overemphasize the impact of Charlie's decision on me, personally. I always felt he understood my aspirations for my department and was readily available to meet with potential staff members, particularly those in the basic sciences whom I had interviewed and hoped to recruit. Charlie, always optimistic, offered his help whenever I asked.

The GEC meeting started promptly at 8 a.m. with consideration of new faculty appointments by the staff, deliberations over the impending shortage of nursing staff, an update on the completion and occupancy of the new Wang Ambulatory Center (named for the Wang computer family) and so on. Toward the end of the meeting, I said I had a special announcement to make. With Charlie seated to my immediate right, I elaborated on our conversation of the previous afternoon and added that he would like to make a few comments. It was an emotional moment for Charlie. One felt the weight of his decision to leave an academic family to join a pharmaceutical firm. It escaped no one that resignation from important academic roles was usually given far in advance, allowing sufficient time for an orderly transition to another leader.[3]

The GEC broke from its regularly scheduled meetings in August, but the trustees, who had little more warning than the chiefs themselves, set about to identify a successor to head the hospital, almost certainly someone who could serve in an acting role while they formed a search committee and found a replacement. My first awareness of what might transpire came when I met with Sarge Cheever, who chaired the board of trustees. He reasoned that since I was chair of the GEC and enjoyed the confidence of the chiefs, I might consider stepping into the general director position for perhaps a year. My response was that I did not feel I could undertake additional responsibilities at such an early stage in the renaissance of the Department of Neurology. My own lab was doing well, although I already found it difficult to spend more than two mornings a week there. I was actively recruiting new faculty, and as principal investigator of the Huntington's Disease Center, sponsored by the National Institutes of Health beginning in 1980, I spent considerable time soothing the egos of the disparate community. I had no choice but to decline the offer.

Sarge and I met a week or so later, and he asked me to reconsider. It was a polite exchange, again ending with my insistence that it would not be possible for me to do my job as chief of neurology with the distraction of running a major hospital. A few days later, the phone rang in my office on the ninth floor of the Vincent–Burnham Building, also known as Kennedy 9. (The top floor of the building, called the Kennedy Wing, had been renovated and named for the famous Boston family who had contributed to the study of mental retardation through research efforts at the MGH and at the Eunice Kennedy Shriver Center, a few miles away in Waltham.[4])

The call was from John Lawrence, a trustee of the MGH, a former board chairman and an *éminence grise* in the best sense of that phrase, requesting in his raspy voice to meet with me on an urgent matter. John had been a formidable supporter of the MGH for more than four decades. He said he would come to my office; I couldn't help but wonder if he had ever been in that part of the hospital before.

"Joe," he said, "you have to do this for the sake of the hospital. Joe, people trust you, and you'll be able to return to your research quickly. It will only be for a short while, I'm certain. We have no other option that we are considering—you have to do it."

Of course, I said yes, and that fall, I found my life undergoing yet another swift transition.

My term as general director began in September 1981. The only immediate advantage of the position that I understood and appreciated at the time was the trustees' agreement to pay me a double salary—the first for my continuing role as chief of the neurology department, and the second for the job of hospital director. One year later, that stipend allowed us to purchase a contemporary house overlooking Meredith Bay on Lake

Winnipesauke in New Hampshire, a place we have cherished for the past quarter century. It served us quite remarkably as our steady domicile later, when we had migrated to San Francisco and were seeking refuge from that city's summer fog to enjoy the beautiful lake adventure during the dog days of August, or in which to spend the Christmas holidays with our growing family.

An immediate challenge on arriving in the general director's office was the urgent need to consummate an agreement with the German pharmaceutical giant, Hoechst, which had provided the resources and long-term commitment to recruit Howard Goodman from the University of California, San Francisco (UCSF), to the MGH. While at UCSF, Howard had achieved international celebrity status through his success in recombinant DNA technology. He had led the team that cloned human GH and also developed the potential for the commercialization of human proteins by placing their genes into *E. coli*, a bacterium particularly well suited for such manufacturing purposes. Hoechst had tried unsuccessfully to reach an agreement to support Howard at UCSF; the campus leadership at UCSF had been unable to convince the board of regents of the University of California that such an arrangement would be in the best interests of the university.

Howard was even more distressed than I at Charlie Sanders's imminent departure over the summer of 1981. The Hoechst agreement had been negotiated in the spring, just a few months before Charlie's announcement about leaving the MGH. Entrenched in the language of the agreement were conditions that depended heavily on Charlie's stature with the MGH community and his visibility within Boston. The German corporation was also convinced that the execution of some aspects of the negotiations needed Charlie's skillful denouement. Specifically, to house Howard's enterprise, the hospital had agreed to add four floors plus a floor for the requisite mechanical systems to an already-planned, six-floor research building. The space would be used to establish and recruit a faculty of between ten and fifteen, all of whom would be participating in the new powers of molecular biology to develop new therapies. At the basis of the extensive financial commitment to the MGH partnership was the recognition of the powerful potential of a new class of biological agents, which leaders at Hoechst felt could not be advanced as quickly in Germany because ethical concerns about the safety and ultimate use of recombinant DNA technology had been voiced there, and because of the perceived lack of scientific expertise in Germany to perform cutting-edge research in this still relatively new field.

The realities of the current situation became immediately apparent to me. The only site on campus for a new research building was on the Blossom Street side of the MGH campus, where the Resident Physician's House stood, a nondescript brick building with a small footprint built in the latter part of the nineteenth century. In the early part of the twentieth century, the house had served as the home of the general director of the MGH and following World War II as the on-site quarters for the hospital house staff. By 1981 it was used for a few offices for the staff and some conference rooms.

> Moving the Resident Physician's House to make room for the New Research Building, which in 1982 would be home to the Hoechst laboratories.

The agreement with Hoechst called for a groundbreaking ceremony by March 1982, just six months away. At first, it seemed simple to tear down the nineteenth-century building and begin construction of the new one. But it turned out to be much more complicated than that. The decision to clear the site was opposed by some residents in the neighborhood, who, led by mixed motives of preservation and the wish to deny further expansion of the MGH, suddenly came to appreciate the unlikely historical value of the red-brick structure. Neighborhood relations with a local developer and the residents on Beacon Hill had always been tenuous, and most expansion projects at the MGH were delayed for months or years by calls for public hearings, petitions to the Boston Redevelopment Authority (BRA) and Boston City Hall. The mayor of Boston at the time was Kevin White, whose support of the MGH often seemed duplicitous, even though he received his own medical care there.

Together with Ernie Haddad, the hospital's general counsel, we plotted the pros and cons of proceeding with the demolition of the residents' house or, of moving it to another location. The latter proposition was made unequivocally unattractive by estimates of the costs involved in the relocation. But as fall progressed, opposition to the demolition mounted, with City Hall sending signals of a protracted battle with the preservationists

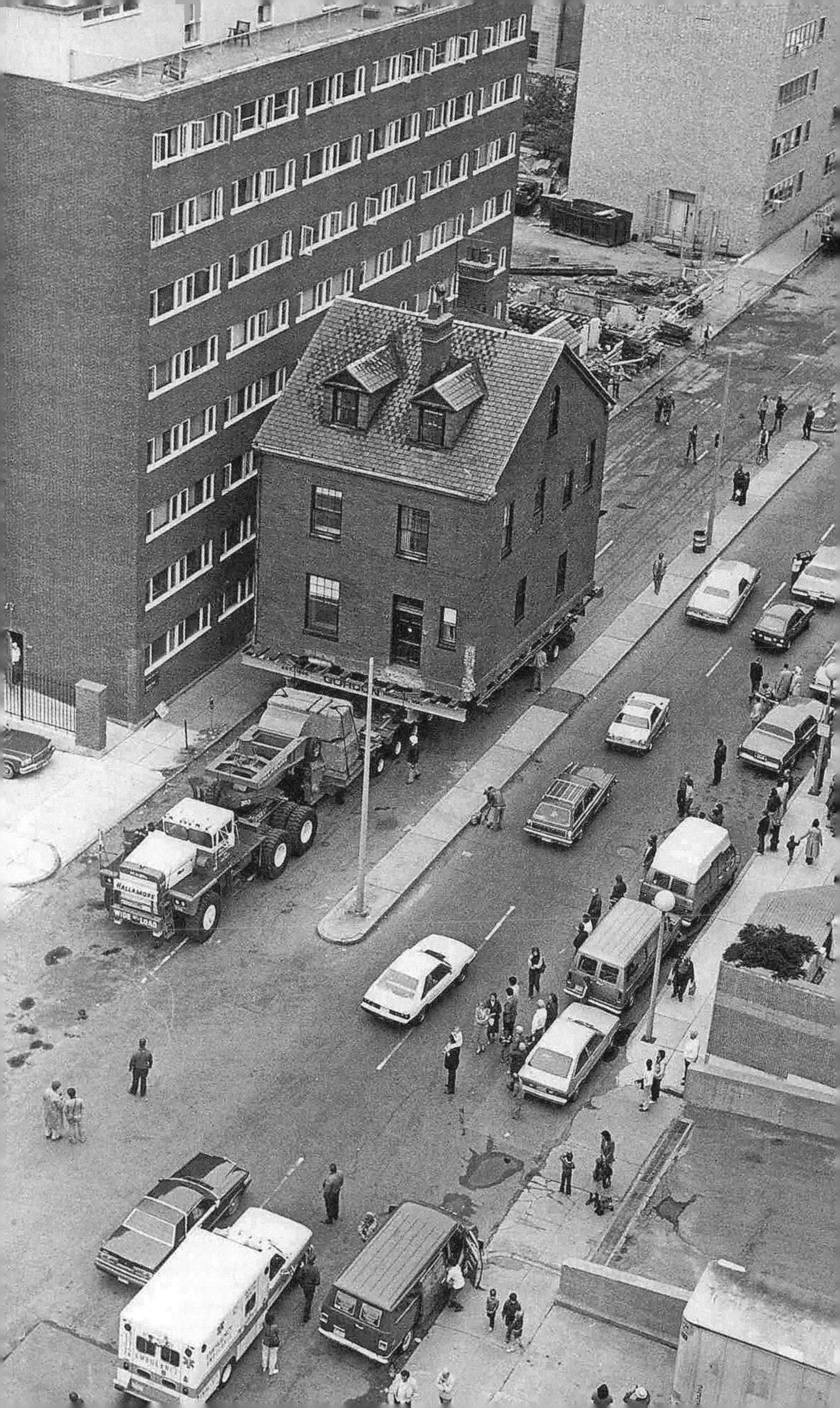
GORDON
HALLAMORE
WIDE LOAD

of Beacon Hill. Hoechst, for its part, threatened to withdraw support. We approached the board of trustees of the hospital with the estimated cost of relocation: nearly $500,000 and a potential site for its placement, directly off Cambridge Street, at the main entrance to the hospital.

Levels of anxiety increased as spring approached. The deadline for the agreement became imminent and trips to City Hall more frequent. In the end, we relented to neighborhood concerns and the hospital trustees reluctantly agreed to the relocation plan and approved the expenditure. On a dreary rainy Saturday morning, Rachel and I with a couple of our children, watched as the building moved from its century-old site to its new resting place—where it still sits—to the left of the main entrance of the MGH, as a museum of the hospital's artifacts. Howard Goodman was very grateful for my efforts, and our close friendship was sustained over the next two decades.

> Groundbreaking ceremony for construction of the Wellman Research Building (now the Thier Building), which would house the Department of Molecular Biology founded by Howard Goodman (far right) through support from the German pharmaceutical company, Hoechst.

Another development in the fall of 1981 associated with the Hoechst deal is engrained in my memory. It was an ordinary afternoon in the office when Kay Bander, a loyal and talented chief-of-staff who had worked tirelessly with Charlie Sanders during his tenure and who had agreed, to my delight, to stay on to assist "the new guy" in the office, called on the intercom to say a congressman from Washington wished to speak with the "head of the hospital." It was Representative Al Gore Jr., at that time, a youthful thirty-three-year-old member of Congress from Tennessee, calling about "this deal" with a German pharmaceutical company. It was 1982, just two years after the *Bayh–Dole Act* (or *University and Small Business Patent Procedures Act*) had been enacted by the US Congress, giving rights to research discoveries supported by the National Institutes of Health grants to the institution and investigators receiving the grants. The federal government was essentially relinquishing its rights to intellectual property to encourage the academic–industrial transfer of research discoveries and to facilitate translational research for new therapies for our patients.

Congressman Gore was very specific. He felt that the agreement with a foreign entity was "taking the cream off the top" of our research support and giving it to another country—hardly the purpose of the new legislation, he pointed out. I argued,

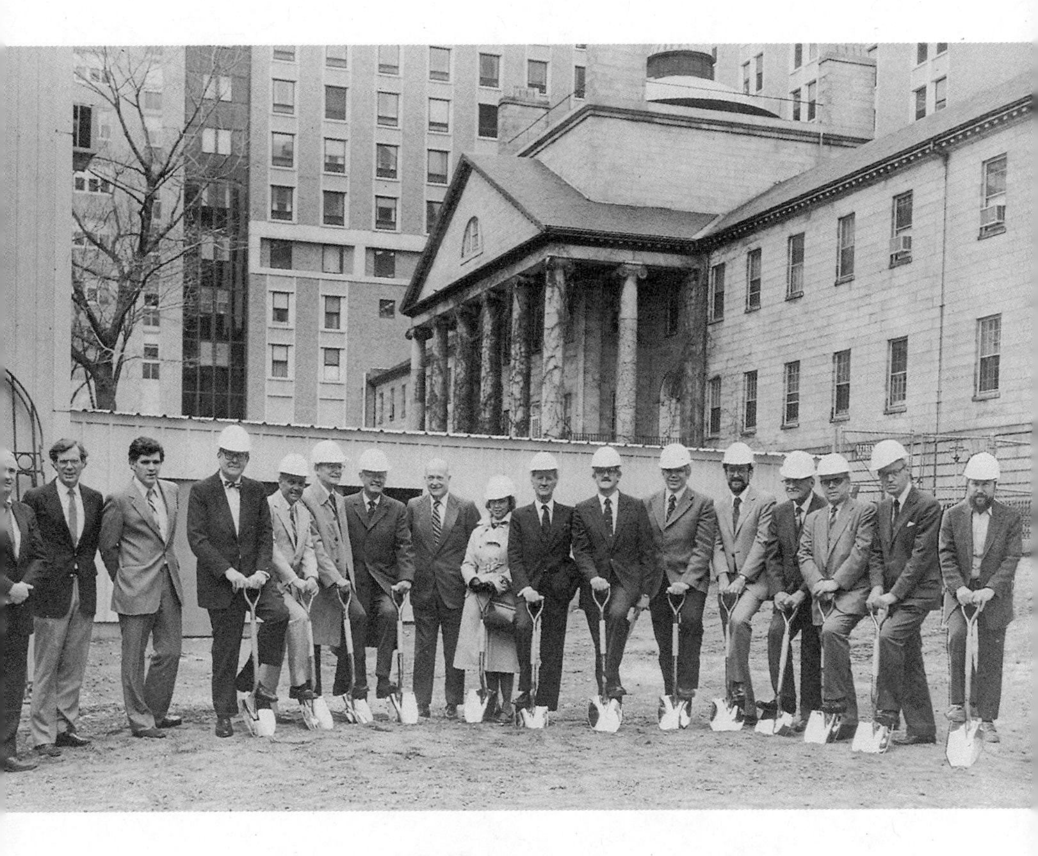

apparently persuasively, that the hospital maintained fundamental rights to any discovery resulting from the collaboration and would be certain to execute agreements for the development of promising therapies in the United States and not in a foreign country. I doubt that I fully appreciated how impossible it would be to assure such an outcome. Gore listened, indicated to me the possibility that I might expect to be called to congressional hearings and hung up. As I recall, the conversation lasted about thirty minutes; I never heard from him again. We did meet many years later, at a fundraising event in California, held in anticipation of his run for the presidency. The conversation I had with him many years before never came up.

A distinguishing feature of the agreement with Hoechst, which Howard Goodman had insisted on, was that the research laboratories were to be open and accessible to members of the MGH and HMS communities and that academic collaboration and publishing would be the same as with any other funded research. Howard's own appointment was in the HMS Department of Genetics, chaired by Phil Leder. Together, the two of them recruited, mentored and promoted a distinguished number of faculty in genetics.[5]

After all of the jags in the plans to establish this research facility, I was relieved in March 1982, when a group of sixteen people lined up for a photo to acknowledge our success in the groundbreaking for the new research building. As an interesting sideline to that event, Howard was unable to attend the groundbreaking ceremony due to a long-standing prior overseas commitment. A picture was taken of him later, shovel in hand, and superimposed on the "official" picture. Since this was before the days of sophisticated photo-enhancing software, one can clearly see that Howard doesn't look quite right in the picture.

It was a particularly rewarding day for me. The city had acquiesced, the Resident Physician's House had been relocated and Representative Al Gore had not called again. Howard was enthusiastic. He would patiently await construction, which moved forward quickly, and in the summer of 1985 he moved into a corner office on the ninth floor overlooking the hospital campus.

## Leaving the General Director's Chair

On May 12, 1982, after the successful recruitment of J. Robert Buchanan as general director, I was invited to share my impressions of a job I was about to leave. Following are the remarks I made to my audience:

*Mr. Lawrence, Dr. Cheever, ladies, and gentlemen. It is for me, an unusual and special privilege to report briefly to you this evening concerning the state of affairs of the Massachusetts General Hospital and to comment about my experiences as Interim General Director over the past nine months. With all due respect to William Shakespeare, I would like to describe for you the seven stages of an interim general director's life.*



### Stage 1: Exhilaration

*When I was approached by the board of trustees to serve as interim successor to Dr. Charles Sanders and, after some thought having accepted the responsibility, I entered a stage of exhilaration. I discovered that I was now the boss* *of the largest independent hospital complex in the world. The MGH is the second oldest hospital in the United States, founded in 1811, and is an institution that has served the community, New England, the rest of the United States and the world for many years. The MGH houses 1092 beds, has an annual budget in excess of $280,000,000 and employs more than 10,000 people, including full-time and part-time staff. It has a most remarkable record of major contributions to improvements in the quality of patient care, and to teaching the medical students of the Harvard Medical School and providing postgraduate training in all fields of clinical medicine. Its contributions to medical research are well known to all.*

*The initial stage of exhilaration lasted about a fortnight and was followed by:*

### *Stage 2: Panic!*

*There followed immediately a period of disrupted sleep and of nighttime problem solving; the phrase of "My God, what have I done?" was followed shortly thereafter by "My God, what have they done?" Part of my anxiety was precipitated by the recognition that the now famous Hoechst agreement, totaling more than $65,000,000, contained within the contract a clearly worded clause that ground had to be broken by April 1, 1982, for the initiation of construction for a new research building. Included in the contract was a clear statement that failure to accomplish this might result in cancellation of the contract and the return of the funds already received to the company. It became immediately apparent that a substantial part of the anticipated work of the new general director was now defined.*

### *Stage 3: Settling In*

*With the tremendous assistance of Larry Martin, who patiently provided a steep learning curve, I came to recognize in a new way the strengths and the vulnerabilities of this great institution and to discover the fiscal limitations that have been increasingly placed upon us by diminished external resources. With the patience and good advice of Kay Bander, I came to grips with the central issues of importance for the operation of the hospital. During this period of time I learned that the hospital has a major responsibility to improve certain aspects of its patient care opportunities, in particular those related to the construction of a new patient care facility and to the provision of improved and satisfactory patient care.*

## *Stage 4: "Oh, by the way..."*

*Within a short period of time I discovered that I had all kinds of new friends. And more than that, all manner of acquaintances became increasingly friendly. They were heard to say, "Joe, it is awfully good of you to do this—it is noble duty and we do appreciate it—oh, by the way—about that lab space I was promised." Or "What do you think about this new program?"—"Oh, by the way."*

*During this time I gained a particular affection for the Resident Physician's House. I learned that the small red-brick building located on Blossom Street, between the Edwards Research Building and Bartlett Hall, built in 1891, had an unusual degree of interest to the community and to certain members of the hospital staff. The plans initially were to destroy the building in order to make way for the new Wellman Research Building. It soon became apparent that such a plan was most unwise and that during the long process of obtaining permission from City Hall, from our neighbors on Beacon Hill and from our friends in Charles River Park to begin the construction, it would be best to make arrangements to move the house to another site. Hence you saw as you came into the ACC this evening, a hole at the front end of North Grove Street that will become the permanent location of the now famous little red schoolhouse.*

*The ACC opened on schedule in November, a tribute to Larry Martin and to Mr. Walsh, the general contractor. There are still a few squeaks in the new structure, but it has already demonstrated its worth to us all. It will be completed on time this June and more important, on budget.*

## Stage 5: Relief in Sight

*In January we learned of the appointment of Dr. Robert Buchanan. This appointment, greeted enthusiastically by all, made the function of the interim general director less difficult and introduced the beginning of the period of transition.*

## *Stage 6: Lame Duck Actor*

*At the beginning of my appointment I had declined to accept that title of acting director with the strong feeling that so far in my life I had not pretended to do anything, and I did not want now to make a pretention to run a hospital. The term interim general director had been carefully selected.*

*As any of you who are in acting know, there is nothing worse than a lame duck actor. At this point in the year, I found that the most important duties became those of holding the fort together and determining the important issues and decisions to be shared with the incoming director.*

### Stage 7: The Finish

*Much like the marathon runner approaching the twenty-sixth mile of the race, I feel now that the race has been a lot of hard work but fun, and I feel exhilarated and excited, once again. I am pleased to note that the Prudential Center is just around the corner and that Dr. Buchanan soon will arrive permanently.*

*I want also to express my appreciation to the chiefs of service who worked patiently with me during this time, to the hospital advisory committee, to Mary Macdonald and her staff, and to the many truly supportive people who shouldered the burden and the responsibility. And particularly, I thank those of you who chose not to bother me at all.*

*The opportunity to serve in this way has given me remarkable insights into the operations of the hospital, to its strengths and its weaknesses. I do not need to detail to you the sense of family and commitment, and the enduring knowledge of how a great history contributes to the worth and prestige of an institution, and how this affects those of us who work here. I would like to speak for a few minutes about the issues that I perceive to be important to the future of our success and the need for your continued support of our endeavors.*

*The research enterprises of the hospital are, in general, in good shape. We are concerned about the new reductions in federal budgets presently being proposed in terms of research funding, but, by and large, we feel that, if anyone survives, we will survive. The funding of the new Department of Molecular Biology under the able leadership of Dr. Goodman made possible by the Hoechst Company provides an important new addition to our research strength. The gift of Mr. and Mrs. Wellman to permit the building of a new research building secures our future in research.*

*On the other hand, our patient facilities, particularly those in the Baker and in the Vincent–Burnham Building, leave a great deal to be desired. We have patients crowded four to a room without appropriate bathroom facilities, who, although they continue to receive outstanding medical care, are not subjected to the most comfortable medical treatment possible, simply because of limitations in physical space. In order to keep pace with the demands of fine patient care, it is absolutely essential that we push quickly towards achieving the objectives of the capital campaign in order to improve these facilities. The trustees of the hospital are committed to this, the staff of the hospital is committed to this, and we call upon all of you to join in this important endeavor.*

*In conclusion, I want to relay to you the particular sense of achievement I felt at the time of the groundbreaking of the Wellman Research Building. This occurred on March 31 and I want to read to you the statement sent in a telegram by Mr. Arthur O. and Gullan M. Wellman at the time of the groundbreaking ceremony. Mr. Wellman said, "The best way for the people of the Massachusetts General Hospital to express their thanks to me and Mrs. Wellman would be by the use of my philosophy in the new research building, 'Make things happen; do it right; don't hurt anybody; be good to people.'" I think that epitomizes the philosophy of this great institution, and I encourage all of you to join us in the exciting years ahead.*

After a year in the general director's chair, I was pleased to gather up the knowledge I had gleaned in the position and move on. I was also keen to be able to spend more time in my laboratory.

## Research at the MGH: Hormones, Brain Peptides and Neurodegenerative Disorders—Alzheimer's Disease, ALS and Huntington's Disease

For two centuries, neurologists have fastidiously collected data on patients with disorders that affect the brain, the spinal cord, peripheral nerves and muscle. These disorders are commonly named after their discoverers: James Parkinson, a physician in London, who described the disease that bears his name in 1817; Jean-Martin Charcot and Pierre Marie in Paris and H.H. Tooth in England, who, in 1886, simultaneously described a condition affecting the nerves supplying muscles in the legs and arms, which came to be known as Charcot–Marie–Tooth disease; Freidreich, who had described an inherited ataxia; and Duchenne who wrote of an inherited muscle disease now called Duchenne muscular dystrophy.

In 1907 Alois Alzheimer, a German neuropsychiatrist, described clinical and brain changes of presenile dementia, now named for him. Although he did not recognize a familial form of the disease, it soon became evident that genetic transmission, although infrequent, was to be a major clue to the pathophysiology of the disorder. Of course, not all disease names derive from the person who discovered them: Lou Gehrig was a baseball player for the New York Yankees! He died of amyotrophic lateral sclerosis (ALS), a disease of the motor neurons that innervate the muscles throughout the body.

Each of these disorders is classified as neurodegenerative, meaning they are due to death of nerve cells in the nervous system. Onset is usually in adulthood, between thirty and sixty-five years; they are progressive and the symptoms of each one result from selective degeneration of nerve cells in the brain or spinal cord. Of growing interest to me was the emerging evidence that the disorders often occurred in families as genetic traits. With the development of new techniques for searching for genes that might be predisposed to them, the time seemed ripe to apply these to clinical studies in affected families.

Meanwhile, as mentioned previously, it had taken some time for me to create and recruit staff for my lab at the MGH South. The renovation of my laboratory was completed in the spring of 1979. Two technicians assisted me: Judy Audet, who had accompanied me in the move from Montreal, and Carol Milbury, whom I had hired in Boston. There were three post-doctoral fellows in the laboratory in the first year: Bill Millard, who had originally planned to join me in Montreal but was flexible given my transfer of activities to Boston; Paul Cooper, from the University of Western Ontario; and Otto Rorstad, who came from the University of Calgary, where he had graduated from medical school and completed a residency in internal medicine followed by a fellowship in endocrinology. Later in that same academic year, Steve Sagar, who had completed residency training at the MGH and spent a year in research at the Boston Children's Hospital with Robert Snodgrass, switched his activities to my laboratory. Judy transferred the radioimmunoassay technology for GH, and Otto developed a new radioreceptor assay for somatostatin.[6] Carol was an excellent animal surgeon. She worked with Bill Millard to perfect the jugular venous sampling technique. Bill had an interest in the role of the hypothalamic arcuate nucleus in the regulation of GH secretion.[7]

By early 1979 I had sensed a new opportunity for my laboratory and the department at the MGH. My team and I developed a collaboration with Ted Bird at McLean Hospital, which gave us access to human brain material being collected there as a resource for study by local researchers. We had access to the brains of patients who had died of Alzheimer's disease (AD) and Huntington's disease (HD) and set about assaying various levels of neuropeptides in these brains to determine whether there were any selective patterns of neuronal cell loss. By identifying glitches in the neuronal circuitry that these diseases caused, it might be possible to find new treatments. Such had been the case in PD where the dopamine cell population in the brain stem was shown to be selectively affected leading to the successful use of levodopa, a natural precursor of dopamine, in treating the symptoms of the disease.

Acetylcholine deficiency had been shown to be a reliable neurochemical feature of AD, and we documented an equally dramatic loss of somatostatin reactivity in AD brains. The findings in HD were particularly interesting. We demonstrated that somatostatin was selectively localized to a subset of neurons in the caudate nucleus and putamen, which were characterized microscopically as aspiny, or lacking the characteristic spiny processes that were the prominent synaptic connections found on the cells receiving input from the cerebral cortex: the spiny neurons. These spiny neurons were the main projection neurons out of the striatum. The neurons contained the neurotransmitters GABA and substance P (Susan Leeman's peptide).[8]

We were amazed to discover that the neuropathologic process that reduced the size of the neostriatum (consisting of the caudate nucleus and striatum) appeared to affect only the spiny neurons. These are the cells that receive a powerful input from the outer layers of the brain (cortex) that use the excitatory neurotransmitter glutamate, which might in a hyperactive state contribute to the cell death of these neurons. The somatostatin-containing neurons, on the other hand, were entirely spared. We showed that they stained selectively for an enzyme marker, NADPH-diaphorase, which became an excellent marker for the selectivity of the cellular loss in the basal ganglia in HD.[9] Much of this work was carried out by Neil Kowall and Robert Ferrante in a series of studies made possible through the establishment of the Huntington's Disease Center, as is described in chapter six of this book.

In the summer of 1981, I offered a position to John Growdon to leave Tufts Medical School and establish an Alzheimer's Disease Center at the MGH, applying for funding from the National Institute on Aging (NIA). I had served on the council of the NIA and was eager to participate in the emerging opportunity to study the disorder. John received funding for the center, one of the first in the NIA's national program, and led it with distinction for twenty-five years.[10]

Other serendipitous events would transform early genetic discoveries. One day, I received a call from Bob Horvitz—who I knew was at MIT working on *C. elegans* and who later received the Nobel Prize for his work—with a simple request. His father, who lived in Chicago, had been diagnosed with Lou Gehrig's disease, amyotrophic lateral sclerosis. The family requested a second opinion. I invited Bob's father to come to see me in Boston. He had distinctive features I thought diagnostic of ALS and suggested a referral to Robert H. Brown, a neurology colleague in the department who had been one of our distinguished chief residents. He was embarking on research to investigate diseases that affected the motor nervous system and had already developed the idea of tracking familial, or inherited, cases of ALS in search of genes that might be associated with the disorder.

Familial ALS occurs in about 10 per cent of cases and, in some families, is inherited in an autosomal dominant pattern, meaning that only one parent needs to pass the gene on for his or her child to get the disease. Linkage studies in these families, similar to those we used when studying HD, seemed a promising approach. But there was a major problem. As in many areas of medical research, the field was very competitive and the number of affected families small. Bob Brown confirmed the diagnosis in Mr. Horvitz and was deluged with pertinent questions from Bob Horvitz, who was reading everything written about the condition. Deep scientific curiosity led Horvitz to believe that the genetic approach was one way to advance knowledge about the disease. Together with Bob Brown, Bob Horvitz launched an initiative to collaborate with workers in other institutions with the goal of collecting a sufficient number of families effected by ALS to do linkage tracing.

The toughest person in the arena was Allen Roses of Duke University, who told Bob Horvitz that he had no interest in collaborating with "the Boston juggernaut." Horvitz argued effectively for collaboration, including making a visit to Durham, North Carolina, for a direct confrontation with Roses. It worked. They developed a very effective collaboration that resulted, five years later, in the identification of the first gene for familial ALS, a mutation in the enzyme superoxide dismutase, type 1 (SOD1). The disease in the studied families was caused by a single point mutation in an enzyme known to be important for detoxification of neuronal environments. Bob Brown and collaborators from around the world went on to define dozens of mutations in the gene and to identify other genes that cause ALS. This work led early on to the development of transgenic models for the disorder and for the search for effective treatments to slow the progress of the disease.[11]

During those days at the MGH, from 1983 to 1989, I was also privileged to be joined in my laboratory by M. Flint Beal, who worked on somatostatin assays and on models of brain disease linked to changes in neuropeptides.[12] Together with Neil Kowall and Bob Ferrante, we characterized the progress of Huntington's disease following the neurochemical signatures.[13] And, in 1989, I recruited Brad Hyman from the University of Iowa. Over the subsequent years, Brad brought extraordinary clarity to the anatomic distributions of plaques and tangles in AD and to new methods for the analysis of B-amyloid deposition in the brain, which is believed to play a key role in the disease. He became director of the Harvard Alzheimer's Disease Center following the retirement of John Growdon, who had led the effort so ably for twenty-five years.[14]

## Development of Child Neurology

As the larger organizational, programmatic and fiscal challenges of the department began to take form over the first several years of my tenure as chair, and after having completed a year as general director of the hospital, I divided my focus between my own lab and developing an academic program in child neurology. Adams had a longstanding interest in childhood development, and with support from the Kennedy family had established the Eunice Kennedy Shriver Center in nearby Waltham, Massachusetts, on the grounds of the Walter E. Fernald School for the mentally retarded.

After consultation widely with leaders in the field and an abortive effort to recruit Guy McKhann, a pediatric neurologist who had just stepped down as chair of the neurology department at Johns Hopkins, I approached Verne Caviness, a member of the MGH neurology family who had a long-standing interest in developmental neurobiology.

Verne was a gifted clinician and scientist. A graduate of Duke University and Harvard Medical School, he had also attended Oxford University where he gained a DPHIL in experimental pathology. Verne had established already an international reputation for his work on the development of the cerebral cortex and came recommended from those who knew of his intellectual prowess and experimental ingenuity.

When I approached Verne, he expressed surprise and then, with encouragement from colleagues and his wife, Madeline, he accepted my offer, agreeing to a position as vice-chair of the department.

Meanwhile, Adams agreed to accompany me to meet with members of the Kennedy clan to request additional support for our efforts in child neurology. We flew to Washington to visit Senator Edward Kennedy, his sister, Eunice, and her husband, Sargent Shriver. The meeting in McLean, Virginia, at Senator Kennedy's home was very productive, and the family agreed to establish a chair at HMS: the Joseph P. and Rose Kennedy Professorship in Child Neurology.

Verne accepted appointment to the chair, and for the next five years we worked seamlessly, Verne taking residence in the office next to mine. We had many long discussions over the years about the evolving field of molecular and cellular biology and the anticipated impact it would have on our appreciation of disorders affecting the nervous system. Verne has remained a steadfast friend throughout my years, and I was delighted on return to Boston from San Francisco some years later to accompany him on the wards as we shared teaching responsibility for our students and residents.

As the professorship in child neurology flourished and brought new research interests to the institution, I continued my work on ALS, AD, and, increasingly, Huntington's disease.

## Julieanne Dorn

In August 1980, soon after my lab had begun establishing efforts related to HD, I received a telephone call from David Dorn, a Denver-based oil executive whose family had established Forest Oil, one of the earliest of the American oil companies.

David asked me to see his wife, Julieanne, who was becoming progressively disabled with a condition that affected walking and coordination. Her memory was fine, but the family wanted to know whether her physical condition might be treatable. I invited David and Julieanne to Boston for a consultation that would be the beginning of a relationship with an extraordinary family whose friendship and support would become of great strategic importance as we moved forward with the Huntington's Disease Center's work.

Clinically, my examination indicated her condition to be most consistent with a diagnosis of HD, but the family history was not well documented. The CT scans confirmed focal basal ganglion atrophy also consistent with a diagnosis of HD. The family was concerned about the inheritability of her condition, and we set about doing everything possible to confirm the diagnosis and provide the family with an opportunity for genetic testing, should it become available, and to provide regular updates on the research of the center.

Thus was established one of the most cherished relationships a physician can possibly enjoy with a family, whose future became entwined with our work in ways that provided benefit to me and the department, and hopefully also to the family. David provided annual discretionary research support that allowed us to purchase equipment or other research tools difficult to fund through grants. I often told David that his support, which I could call upon from time to time, gave me a great sense of security and allowed us to move forward in our work in ways that could not have been achieved without him.

A few years later, in 1983, as Julieanne's condition continued to deteriorate, the family decided to honor her by funding a chair to support our research. After wide consultation and some reluctance on my part, it was agreed with the family and the dean that I would relinquish the distinguished Bullard Professorship. My preference had been to use the new funds to recruit another researcher to occupy the chair, but, in 1984, I was appointed to the new chair. It has now become the chair held by the chief of the Department of Neurology at the MGH, currently occupied by my greatly admired colleague, Anne Young, who succeeded me as chair in 1991. Julianne Dorn passed away in 1997.[15]

# SIX

# A Science Saga: The Search for the Huntington's Disease Gene

SOME MOMENTS NEVER FADE FROM MEMORY. August 5, 1983, was a Friday. It was muggy that evening, and I took the call in the bedroom. "Hi, Joe. It's Jim. We've got it!"

"It" was the linkage for the gene causing Huntington's disease to a DNA probe, G8. I was stunned. We had no clue where the probe was placed along the twenty-three chromosomes, and finding it meant that we had found the right chromosome and were closing in on the location of the abnormal gene itself. Amazingly, Jim had found the marker with the twelfth probe he tested.

"Are you sure?" I asked.

"It's linked in both families," Jim Gusella, who had joined my department a few years before, assured me. "The LOD score is over six!" The LOD (log of the odds) score is a statistical estimate used in genetics for the likelihood of an association between a DNA marker and a gene locus. A score of six means that there is only a one in a million chance that the association is accidental. Thus, the probability was very high that the marker we had found in Huntington's disease patients was very close to the gene.

## A Historical Perspective on Huntington's Disease

In the United States, George Huntington was the first to describe, in 1872, a disease that he, his father and his grandfather had observed in their medical practices on Long Island, New York. Named for them and their work on the disease, Huntington's disease (HD) has emerged as the prototypic autosomal dominant inherited disorder affecting the central nervous system. If a disease is autosomal dominant an individual only needs to get the abnormal gene from one parent in order to inherit the disorder. In simple terms, the child of an HD-affected parent has a 50/50 chance of inheriting the disorder

George Huntington was born in 1850 in East Hampton, New York. As recounted by Michael Hayden, Huntington was only eight years old when he first noticed patients in his father's care with inherited chorea.[1] At twenty-two, he described the deadly family trait in a three-page paper entitled "On Chorea," published in the *Medical and Surgical Reporter* in 1872.[2] Chorea, which takes its name from the Greek word for "dance," describes the involuntary jerking movements that patients develop early in their illness. Over time, they also experience intellectual decline. Huntington's succinct and compelling description of the disorder is graphic evidence that one does not need to publish a lot to be famous. It was the only paper he ever wrote! (This reminds me of the *New Yorker* cartoon featuring two elderly faculty members contemplating the announcement of a colleague's death on the bulletin board. One says to the other, "Poor old Ainsworth, published and published but perished all the same.")

Historical lore suggests that Huntington's disease arrived in North America early in the settlement of New England, possibly as early as 1630, when the John Winthrop fleet from East Anglia, England, arrived in Salem, Massachusetts. Indeed, it has been speculated, though without convincing proof, that some of the women tried during the infamous Salem Witch Trials might have suffered from HD.



## Genetic and Clinical Features of Huntington's Disease

Because HD is an autosomal dominant disorder, if a parent carries the mutated gene, each child has a one in two chance of getting the disease. Both men and women are equally at risk, and the gene penetrance—the probability that a person who has the mutated gene will actually get the disease—is 100 per cent. Having one copy of the mutated gene leads eventually to the disorder; although, in some cases, symptoms may be mild and not appear until the sixth or even eighth decade of life. When first diagnosed, almost all patients present with a family history; however, on very rare occasions, HD is found in an individual with no family history of the disease, most likely due to the appearance of a new mutation. The prevalence of the disorder is about ten per 100,000 persons in Caucasian populations, which extrapolates to a total of about 30,000 cases in the United States.[3]

The onset of HD is usually in the fourth to fifth decade of life. The average age at onset of chorea is thirty-seven years. In a study of 516 patients at the MGH, we found that the age of onset varied from early childhood to individuals presenting with symptoms in the sixth or seventh decade of life. With onset in midlife, most gene-carrying subjects have already borne children when their symptoms begin. Rarely, onset can be as early as two to three years. These "juvenile cases" are usually inherited from the father. When patients don't develop symptoms until seventy or eighty years of age, it is often because of maternal inheritance.

In addition to chorea, younger patients frequently suffer from rigidity or stiffness of muscles. Epilepsy can also occur in juvenile cases. Psychiatric symptoms of depression are frequent, leading to the risk of suicide. Personality changes, including paranoia or delusions, may appear ten to fifteen years before the movement disorder begins. The dementia that ensues, a prominent feature of the illness during the average life span of about seventeen or eighteen years, is distinct from the memory disorder of Alzheimer's disease. In HD, the cognitive disorder is characterized by abnormalities in judgment, difficulty in making decisions and generalized sluggishness of cognitive performance, attributes sometimes called "subcortical" dementia.

The brain changes occurring as the disease progresses are localized mostly in the basal ganglia, neuron-rich masses deep within the brain hemispheres. The basal ganglia include the caudate nucleus and the putamen (which together make up the neostriatum), brain regions that function to relay information from the motor cortex for coordination of movement. They also connect to the frontal lobes to play a role in judgment and cognition. In HD, the most intense loss of neurons occurs in the caudate nucleus and the putamen. These basal ganglia structures shrink in size, while the adjacent lateral ventricles expand, a change readily identifiable during life on an MRI or CT scan. The neurons that disappear leave no scar or indication of the cause of their death.

## The Quest for the Gene

Perhaps the most famous individual affected by HD was the folk singer Woody Guthrie, who for many years was labeled as an alcoholic and a miscreant until it was recognized that he suffered from an inherited disorder. After his death in 1967, his ex-wife Marjorie urged members of the US Congress to form a commission to study the medical causes and societal impact of the disease. A congressional imperative resulted in the funding for two HD research centers in the United States in 1980, one at the Massachusetts General Hospital in Boston and the other at Johns Hopkins University Medical Center in Baltimore. I was fortunate to head the MGH center for nine years, from 1980 to 1989.

Another individual crucial to the evolution of the two HD centers was Nancy Wexler. Nancy's mother had died of HD in 1978. The family, consisting of her sister, Alice, and their father, Milton, were devastated by the impact of the illness. Milton was determined to solve the riddle of the disorder, locate the gene and find a treatment. He formed the Hereditary Disease Foundation, which separated from the Committee to Combat Huntington's Disease, established by Marjorie Guthrie, over disagreements about how to make progress. Milton wanted to focus exclusively on cutting-edge genetic and brain research.

In 1979 Nancy, who had completed a PHD in psychology at the University of Michigan, was working for the National Institute of Neurological Disease and Stroke (NINDS), part of the National Institutes of Health. Her role was to be crucial to our eventual success in finding the HD gene. Nancy made her first trip to Lake Maracaibo in Venezuela in the fall of 1979 to initiate research on a large cohort of HD patients located there. Over the next several decades she organized field trips to establish family genealogical records of this Native South American population. Nancy became an impassioned zealot, driven by her own fear of carrying the gene for HD, and she now saw an opportunity to make a big impact. She convinced NINDS leaders to issue to the academic community a request for proposals (RFP) to study HD.

Alice Wexler wrote a stunningly revealing account of the family's participation in the search for the HD gene in her book *Mapping Fate: A Memoir of Family, Risk and Genetic Research*, published in 1995.[4] At the time of writing, neither sister had shown evidence of the illness.

## Planning for the Grant

In response to the RFP from the NINDS, we needed to put together a grant application, always a significant undertaking. I knew that the environment in Boston, with its rich history of neurobiology and molecular biology, was ripe for approaching the problem of HD, but I had no idea how the genetic studies might be accomplished. At the time, I knew little about HD, with the bulk of my experience being the few patients I had seen during neurological training, most of them in the final stages of their illness at Cuyahoga County Hospital outside Cleveland. In the Boston community, historical events had resulted in most HD patients being cared for at Boston University Medical Center and at the Boston Veterans Administration Hospital, where Professor Daniel Sax had followed many patients and their families. Interest in the neuropathology of HD at Harvard was developing at McLean Hospital under the influence of Dr. Alfred Pope, who had recruited Dr. Edward (Ted) Bird from Cambridge University in England to establish a Huntington's disease brain bank for study of the cytoarchitectural and neurochemical changes in patients who died at different ages, some from suicide, an all-too-common desperate outcome for patients, and something greatly feared by their families.

In the spring and summer of 1979, I organized several meetings of the key players—Dan Sax, Ted Bird and E. Peirson Richardson, chief of neuropathology at the MGH. Cooperation was favorably received, but no one had any idea of how to attack the genetics problem.

What transpired in August of 1979 illustrates the remarkable power of serendipity, or perhaps it is testimony to what Pasteur said, "Chance favors the prepared mind." I was preparing to leave my office at the MGH one Friday evening at about 6 p.m. when the phone rang. It was Kurt Isselbacher, chief of the gastroenterology division at the MGH, requesting that I see and consult on a young patient, the sixteen-year-old son of a friend of his, Alex Rich. Jody Rich, who was working that summer at the Woods Hole Marine Biological Institute on Cape Cod, had been struck in the eye by a baseball that afternoon. Over a period of an hour or so he had developed a headache, and the family wanted a neurologic evaluation.

I awaited their arrival about two hours later in my office. When Alex and Jody arrived, residual symptoms were minor and the examination normal. I reassured the two of them, not failing to mention that he ought to get in touch with me if any new symptoms developed.

Alex was a distinguished DNA scientist, having described a reverse turn of the DNA double helix that could be displayed under certain experimental circumstances. This phenomenon was referred to as left-handed DNA, or Z-DNA. I knew that the secret of our inherited characteristics must reside in our DNA and that an answer to the mystery of the HD gene would be found somewhere in the estimated six billion base pairs found in each of our cells. I told Alex about our evolving project and about HD. He said that he did not have much to offer from a scientific perspective but that he would think about my request for assistance with the genetic studies and call me back. A few days later, he suggested that I speak with David Housman, a professor of medical genetics at MIT.

I had the lead I needed, straight out of a patient-care experience! I contacted David and explained the circumstances and my hope that he would meet with me to discuss the problem. We got together soon thereafter in the conference room outside my office on Kennedy 9. At the time, I was reading *The Eighth Day of Creation*, the extraordinary account of the DNA story by H.F. Judson.[5] David was intrigued that I had been reading the book, which tells the story of the discovery of the double helix by James Watson, Francis Crick and Maurice Wilkins. Their discovery, published in *Nature* in 1953, led to the Nobel Prize in Physiology or Medicine in 1956 for all three.[6]

David brought me up to date on promising techniques under development in his and other laboratories. A crucial conference on genetic methods had been held in the spring of 1978 in Alta, Utah. The genetics group from the University of Utah, led by Mark Skolnick, had invited David Botstein from MIT and Ron Davis from Stanford as external advisors to review the work being carried out in Utah. As recounted by Robert Cook-Deegan in his elegant book *The Gene Wars*,[7] during that conference, a graduate student by the name of Kerry Kravitz discussed his work on hemochromatosis, a blood disorder, describing ways to map genetic relationships between the condition and a group of markers related to the immune system.

The notion of using genetic markers based on the structure of DNA became possible after the discovery of bacterial enzymes called restriction endonucleases that cut DNA into variably sized fragments based on the DNA sequence. For discovering and describing these enzymes, Daniel Nathans, Werner Arber and Hamilton Smith won a Nobel Prize in 1978. The fragments of DNA produced by the enzymes sometimes differed in size because of differences in the DNA sequence between individual people. These pieces of DNA were called restriction fragment length polymorphisms (RFLPS). They vary in size in different individuals, even when taken from an identical chromosomal region. Single base pair changes (polymorphisms) can arise as frequently as once every three hundred to five hundred base pairs in any individual. Scientists capitalized on this attribute by separating fragments according to their size by applying an electrical current (electrophoresis). Small DNA fragments move more quickly than large ones. The resulting separation on a gel medium is called a Southern blot (named for the English molecular biologist Edward Southern). This process results in each individual having a distinguishable DNA "fingerprint." RFLPS have since been replaced as a genetic tool following the complete sequencing of the human genome. Today, we can more precisely define the DNA sequences variations as single nucleotide polymorphisms or SNPs. Today panels of over one million SNPs are available to look for disease locations in the mapping process.

Early on, it was estimated that as few as 150 to three hundred RFLP markers spaced along the human chromosomes could be used as a map to register locations for placement of genetic markers or defective genes. David Botstein, Ronald Davis, Mark Skolnick and Ray White decided to communicate their ideas through a formal scientific forum. They collected their theoretical arguments into a paper published in *The American Journal of Human Genetics* in May 1980.[8] The notion of using RFLPs was a landmark and seminal discovery. It pointed to the potential strategy of using polymorphic DNA markers together with "linkage analysis" in families to search for the chromosomal site of unknown genes. Since then, linkage analysis, or linkage mapping, is typically the first step in the search for a disease gene. By comparing DNA polymorphisms in family members who are affected by a disease with those who aren't, it is possible to show "linkage" to the suspect DNA region or gene.

The paper by Botstein et al. would not appear until nearly eight months after David Housman and I had met at the MGH in August 1979. But long before this paper was published, the methodologies surrounding linkage mapping were in discussion in many labs, including that of Y.W. Kan and A.M. Dozy, who had been the first to show the utility of the technology in a clinical application at the University of California, San Francisco. They had reported in 1978 on the gene structure for beta-hemoglobin, the oxygen-carrying molecule of red blood cells. Beta-hemoglobin in a mutated form gives rise to a type of anemia called sickle cell anemia, so named because the red blood cells take on an elongated sickle shape instead of the normal round appearance. These red blood cells contain a mutation in the hemoglobin molecule. They break down as they attempt to force their way through small capillaries, and their shortened life spans lead to anemia. When they examined the gene for beta-hemoglobin with restriction enzymes and cut it into smaller pieces, Kan and Dozy noted that variations in the sizes of the pieces occurred due to single changes, or variations, in the base pair makeup of a region immediately upstream from the gene. They speculated that the technique would be useful among various races or individuals in assessing risk for a mutation of the gene for beta-hemoglobin.[9]

David Housman was thoroughly familiar with the concept. And, as luck would have it, he was also acquainted with the HD story, having already made the acquaintance of Nancy Wexler and having attended a few workshops sponsored by Nancy and her father through the Hereditary Disease Foundation. David told me that the approach would be a matter of collecting families with the disease trait and finding a marker close enough to be linked to the chromosomal site of the gene. In order to use the "strategy" of DNA polymorphisms, we would need families whose HD-affected members could be readily distinguished from those who were symptom free. Because of the onset in mid-life, one could make the reasonable conclusion that if individuals reached age sixty to eighty and were free of symptoms, they did not carry the gene.

David agreed to write the genetics portion of the grant application, and the whole proposal was submitted to the NIH in October 1979. The NIH received some sixteen grant applications for HD "Centers without Walls." Within the review structure of the NINDS, the application fell under the jurisdiction of Nancy Wexler herself, who had been assigned this portion of the NINDS portfolio. She worked closely with Katherine Bick, whose interest in neuroscience stemmed from her early research in psychology. Together, they were responsible for establishing the review process and the site visits that would be made to each of the institutions whose applications had been received.

The site visit to the MGH was scheduled for January 1980. We had proposed a total of six projects to study HD. Many were related to the collection of families in the New England area and to clinical and psychological studies. The application to the NIH described a "Center without Walls," and included four different institutions in Boston. The most important project in our proposal was the genetic studies, and I knew that a strong proposal in that area might separate us from the other applications submitted from around the country.

We practiced hard and carefully prior to the site visit with our group in Boston. We invited other geneticists to criticize our approach. I was very nervous. Nancy invited me to the Children's Inn on Longwood Avenue, where the site visit team was spending the night, for a nightcap and some last-minute advice concerning our application. She reviewed the strengths and weaknesses of our proposal and anticipated questions that the peer reviewers might ask, and also pondered appropriate responses. I knew she wanted our project to be funded, but we had to convince the scientists and neurologists gathered from around the country to review our project that it would be a good bet. We were requesting close to $4 million spread out over five years. In addition, although I was a neurologist, I had not been interested up to this point in the genetics of neurological disorders, and I had not written any clinical papers on HD. I would be on the spot with those members of the review committee who might be skeptical about my leadership. Nancy's help was key to our success. I left the Children's Inn that evening feeling reassured and comfortable with the preparations we had made for the site visit team.

The site visit exceeded our expectations, and two months later we were named as one of two centers funded for our planned work, with me as the principal investigator for this new project. The other center was to be at Johns Hopkins.

### Establishment of the Boston HD Center

The funding of our HD center began in July 1980. David Housman was pleased with the outcome—and worried. He did not personally have the time to devote to the project he had outlined in the application. What to do? David had an idea that would transform our approach and lead to a truly remarkable moment in the history of emerging neurogenetic research. He recommended that I meet with a young graduate student, James Gusella, who had grown up in Ottawa, Canada. Jim had obtained a BSC degree from the University of Ottawa and had gone to work with David, who was then at the University of Toronto, on a master's degree in medical biophysics, studying the control of red cell formation. Within a year, he moved with David to MIT and began PHD studies using techniques emerging in the new field of recombinant DNA technology.

Jim was completing his PHD thesis in David's laboratory on the genetic cloning of DNA from individual human chromosomes and was planning to begin a postdoctoral fellowship in the laboratory of Professor Leroy Hood at the California Institute of Technology. Jim's wife, Maria, a pediatrician, was establishing her own practice in Framingham, a suburb west of Boston, and was not keen on moving to California. David Housman suggested that I talk to Jim about leading the genetics project. I had already met Jim during the course of writing the grant. Our first conversation about him moving to the center was very productive, and he agreed to venture across the Charles River to the MGH to undertake what we all recognized was a very risky project—finding DNA markers that would link closely to the HD gene and provide a guidepost for the search for the abnormal gene itself.

Jim established a small laboratory in shared space on the third floor of the Edwards Research Building, one floor below where my colleagues and I were working on the brain regulation of the endocrine system. Jim's and my approaches and needs in research were vastly different; I was a physiologist and neurologist by training with no hands-on experience with DNA analysis. Jim had earned a PHD in somatic cell genetics and had no special knowledge of neurological disorders. Richard Erbe, head of the genetics unit in the pediatric department at the MGH, agreed to offer Jim space to initiate his lab and later to expand it. Jim set up the storage facilities to process blood samples from Michael Conneally of the HD Roster at Indiana University and from Nancy Wexler, who was cataloguing the family histories of HD patients from Venezuela along with Anne Young, a neurologist, who would be appointed my successor as chief of neurology at the MGH and who traveled to Venezuela each spring to examine the patients and their families. The blood samples were used to isolate and transform lymphocytes that became the source of the DNA for RFLP typing. The samples were placed into vats at –90°C until further analysis.

Meanwhile, I faced a dilemma with respect to Jim's appointment in a basic science department at Harvard Medical School, which I had promised him I would try to arrange to allow him access to graduate students and a more viable trajectory for

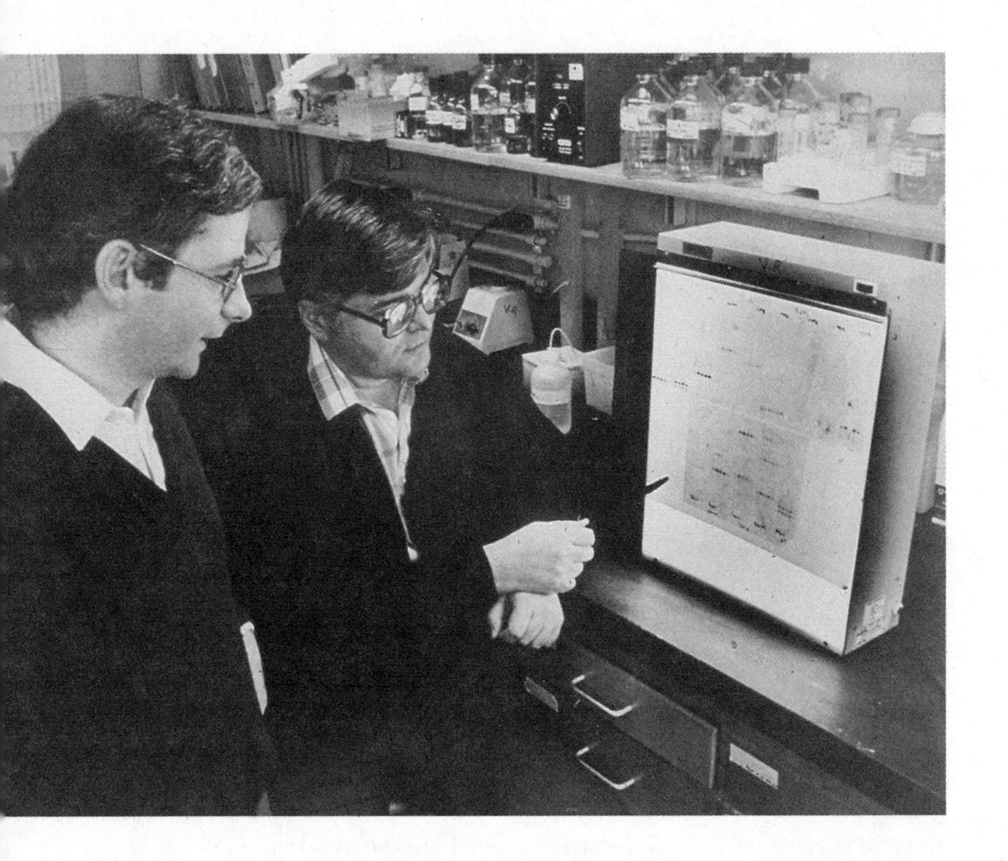

Jim Gusella (on the left) and Peter St. George-Hyslop at the computer, 1983.

academic promotion. The Department of Neurobiology, my first choice, was entirely refractory to any appointments in hospital departments affiliated with HMS. Furthermore the department saw little advantage to the appointment of an individual with interests in a very exploratory realm of science—searching for gene locations without any notion of what the gene might do.

I was very fortunate that Phil Leder, chair of the Department of Genetics at Harvard Medical School, who had just arrived from the NIH to head the new department, shared the vision of the importance of emerging technologies in human genetics. He offered Jim an appointment as an instructor and later promoted him to assistant professor. This turned out to be key in keeping Jim at the MGH. As he flourished, he received offers from many institutions to join basic science genetics departments. Phil not only made the initial appointment but also served as a mentor to Jim, meeting at least annually to review the progress of his work.

Eventually Jim was promoted to full professorship, and we were able to keep him in an expanding clinical department.

Research space was a serious problem at the MGH in those days. Jim used to attend the weekly meetings of our group, and I would often wonder, as he established his working approach to HD, how far removed he must feel from the luster of MIT. He would report to our combined research groups every month on the progress of his work. The first two years were exceedingly difficult for Jim as he began to appreciate the risk he was taking. The theory behind RFLPs was clear enough. But how many DNA markers would be needed to scan the whole genome? The theory described that markers placed ten million base pairs apart would be adequate. That meant three hundred spaced equally. Only a few markers were available at the time. Where would the rest of the markers come from? Jim concluded that the best he could do was to take whatever DNA markers he could locate from other laboratories working in the field of human genetics and test them one by one.

Blood samples from affected families had to be collected and their white blood cells separated and transformed into immortalized cell lines that could be frozen and stored for later analysis. Linkage studies in one large family located in Iowa would be done first. The pedigree of this family had been carefully collected and analyzed by Michael Conneally, an Irishman whose laboratory was located at Indiana University. Nancy was organizing the collection of samples from the Venezuelan pedigree, planning to use the information as a large reference family, not only to track HD but also to be used for other genetic studies that would use linkage analysis. By the third year of the project, DNA markers were being tested routinely. By the spring of 1983, a few runs had been made on individual family members of the Iowa pedigree. Incredible as it is, success began to emerge with the testing of the twelfth DNA marker. The marker was an anonymous piece of DNA (of unknown structure and function) that Jim's lab selected from a human genomic library developed by Tom Maniatis of Harvard University. Blood samples from a portion of the family from Lake Maracaibo were now arriving in Jim's lab. Both families showed positive linkage to the marker.

## Linkage in HD is Established

My first reaction to Jim's telephone call that August evening in 1983 was exhilaration. As the principal investigator of the Huntington's Disease Center Without Walls, I immediately recognized the extraordinary significance of the discovery: never before had a gene for an inherited disorder been located by gene "mapping" alone. It meant that the gene search had been narrowed by one thousand- to two thousand-fold. We had narrowed the search from three billion bases to a few million. The gene could be searched for in a much smaller haystack.

Almost as soon as the good news sank in, an afterthought followed. Although Jim had been working extremely hard, it seemed impossible that he could be so lucky. What if he were wrong? Even worse, what if he had made up the results? After all, this was a time when scientific misconduct was first being recognized and associated with the misplaced trust that was one of its enabling factors. As a member of the Harvard committee that investigated the work of John Darsee, then an assistant professor of medicine at the Brigham and Women's Hospital in Boston, and who was suspected for research fraud, I knew that questionable research reports could escape detection for some time. Darsee had, as it turned out, a long track record of dishonesty, likely beginning as an undergraduate and extending through his residency training at an Atlanta hospital affiliated with Emory University. One of the world's foremost cardiologists, Dr. Eugene Braunwald of Brigham and Women's, had been implicated in the process, not for any wrongdoing but for inadequate supervision of a research project in his laboratory. Those of us on the committee to investigate Darsee, chaired by Dr. Richard Ross, the dean of the Johns Hopkins University School of Medicine, underestimated the depths of Darsee's skulduggery. Our committee found no evidence that more than an event or two of research misconduct had occurred. We were later proven to be naïve for having been whitewashed by a very clever, very unprincipled man.

I had no reason to suspect that Jim was anything but a straight shooter; there was nothing in his character, temperament or past interactions with me or other mentors to suggest that this was even possible. However, given the importance of the findings, all possibilities, even the most unlikely ones, needed to be fully explored before the manuscript could be published. I arranged for Nancy Wexler and Jim to meet in the next few days to go over the data. Nancy flew in from Washington, and we met in my office. A few hours later, and after poring over the data and examining the results from both the US and Venezuela families, there seemed to be no room for doubt. There was indeed a linkage. We would assemble the data, make the appropriate figures and rush it forward for publication. We chose *Nature*, the best of the scientific journals, and submitted the manuscript in mid-October. It was accepted with only minor revisions and was scheduled to appear four weeks later, on November 15.[10]

## Announcing the News to the World

On entering the Ether Dome at the Massachusetts General Hospital, there is a momentary feeling of disorientation, of having entered an age long since gone. The dome covers a square-shaped observation room designed by the famous Boston architect Charles Bulfinch. From the exterior of the Bulfinch Building, the dome rises symmetrically atop the four stories of the old, original, Chelmsford granite landmark of the Massachusetts General Hospital, which opened in 1821. Bulfinch, who also designed the Massachusetts State House on nearby Beacon Street, planned the hospital facility for the poverty-stricken patients of Boston. The plan to form the hospital had been supported by the Brahmins of Boston, whose descendants still occupy premier slots on the MGH Board of Trustees. From inside the dome, the ceiling forms a half sphere high above the observation area, where the doctors of the MGH and the medical students of Harvard Medical School have since 1821 scrutinized patients and their medical problems. The Bulfinch Building can still be seen today from Cambridge Street in Boston, dwarfed though it now is by the surrounding oversized structures of the MGH complex.

The dome has not changed appreciably from its original design. A plaque on the wall immediately inside the northern entrance announces that the room is a national treasure, so designated by the US National Park Service. It cannot be renovated, relocated or torn down without federal approval, unlikely to be forthcoming. The Bulfinch Building was built directly on the bank of the Charles River to provide access to patients arriving by boat as well as by land. The rising tide came within a few feet of the base of the building. Surrounded now by the unsightliness of the newer buildings of the MGH, it looks like an ancient fortress resilient in its stance against the disorganized visions of later planners of academic medical centers. It was here in the dome in 1846 that the dentist-anesthesiologist Thomas Morton first used the volatile agent ether to lessen the consciousness and reduce the pain as surgeon John Collins Warren cut into a mass in the side of a patient's neck. (This was a momentous milestone, hence the name Ether Dome.) Ether allowed a patient to be rendered unconscious, be operated upon without moving away from the knife since the pain of the incision was masked, and awaken refreshed and without any memory of the event.

The dome is still used as a teaching arena. When I was chair of the department, every Thursday morning at 8 a.m. the neurosurgeons at the MGH met in the dome for clinical rounds to discuss their latest conquests. Neurology rounds started an hour later. The neurologists assembled to discuss the differential diagnoses and management of the extraordinary cases that are brought to the MGH, the court of last resort for patients with neurological disorders from all corners of the world. During rounds, the doctors sit in steeply layered rows of uncomfortable wooden seats, peering down into the central oval arena where the patients are introduced, examined and discussed. In the top row, there remain the original "bicycle seats" from where late arrivals could view the scene below, or where Harvard medical students, spending an obligatory month studying neurology at the MGH and hoping to avoid being questioned, would gather. In the right-hand corner at the front of the room is a closed glass-covered cupboard that houses the ancient Egyptian mummy of Padihershef, over 2,500 years old and probably a stonecutter from Thebes, Egypt, a gift made to the MGH in 1823. Soon after its arrival, the mummy had gone on a tour, with people paying to see him. In the end, he raised the equivalent of $1 million for the hospital. Now, he is sometimes absent from the closet on loan

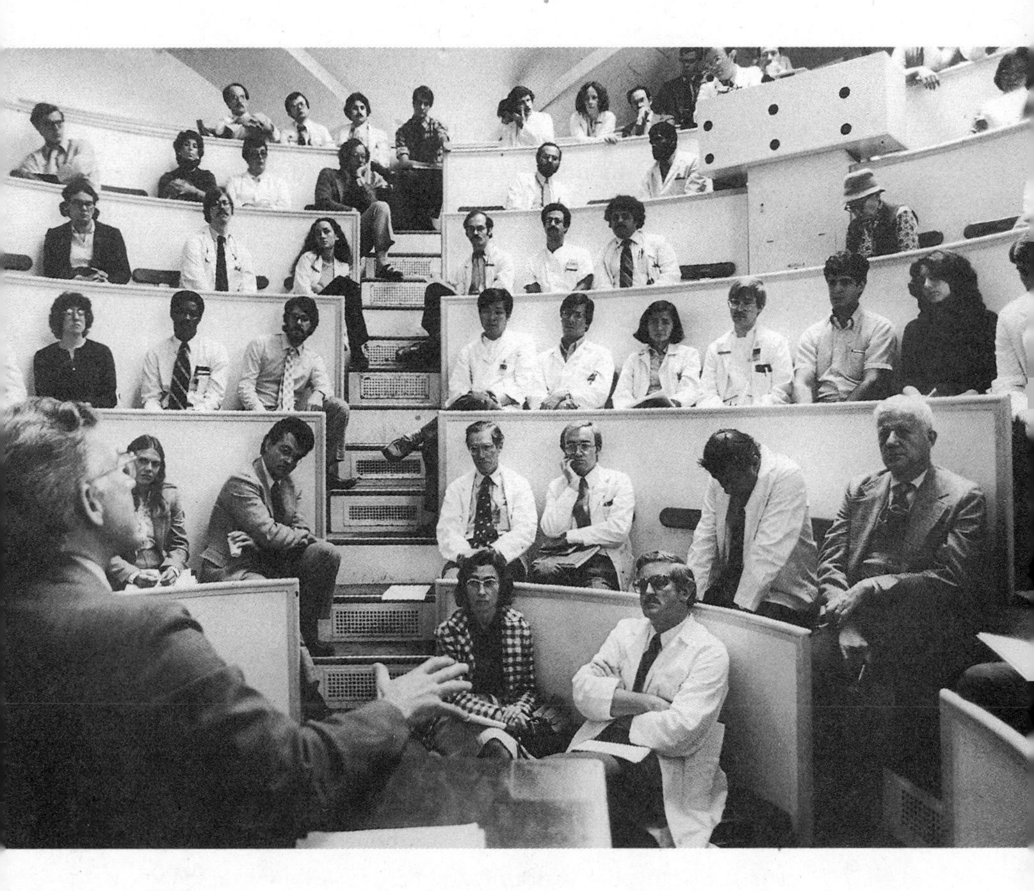

to local museums, but, in 1846, Padihershef witnessed the first application of anesthesia in the Ether Dome.

On the morning of November 9, 1983, a different kind of exhibit was scheduled in the dome—a press conference to announce to the world the discovery of the HD gene linked to chromosome number 4. The press conference had been convened on short notice after the general press became informed of the upcoming paper in *Nature* and had begun to call Jim's laboratory or the hospital's public affairs office for more details. The journal had agreed to the news session, although it would preempt, to some degree, the publication of the report the following week. The local television stations were to be in attendance, and a large contingent of the best reporters from the *Boston Globe,* the *New York Times, Time* magazine and the Associated Press was anticipated. The public affairs folk at the MGH had impressed upon Jim and me that it would be important for us to give an

Professor Fred Plum, chief of neurology at Cornell University Medical College, addressing neurology grand rounds in the Ether Dome, 1980.

accurate accounting of the discovery and that we should not give too much play to the significance of it. On the other hand, the hospital thrived on trumpeting discoveries like the one we were about to announce. There would undoubtedly be questions about using the test to diagnose the HD gene in young patients not yet symptomatic, and the really big concern: when will the gene itself be found, and when will we doctors be able to offer some treatment?

Martin Bander called Jim and me to his office the day before the press conference to put us through the paces of a mock interview. Martin was a short, dark-haired, dapper gentleman. He had been a science reporter for a number of newspapers prior to his arrival at the MGH, where he had worked for many years as the chief press liaison officer. He was a serious and relentless pursuer of the truth. He was stern in demeanor but soft underneath. He seemed particularly intense as we entered his office to answer a pretend series of questions. He was superb at making one feel the pressures of being under the gun, as he anticipated what questions would be asked.

We went through the ritual. "Jim, wouldn't you consider this discovery a lucky break?" Jim rankled at the question. He didn't want to be considered lucky. He wanted to be considered daring, adventuresome, hardworking and perhaps even obsessed with finding the HD gene—but not lucky. Serendipity is fine in science; it suggests the capacity to recognize the unexpected and to take quick brilliant advantage of it. But "lucky" implies a fishing expedition, looking for something without a carefully thought-out plan. Jim was "lucky," but he didn't want to admit it. He would say that he had been prepared to examine each of the DNA probes that became available to him, that he had a plan and that the plan had proven productive sooner than he might have anticipated. But there it was, and if he hadn't been looking, it couldn't have happened all by itself.

Then there was the crucial question, "How long do you think it will take to find the HD gene?" Jim responded, "In a few years." Bander pressed forward, "What will you do if the gene hasn't been found? Will you go on to something else? What if it takes longer than that?" We agreed that Jim would say that he hoped that the methods of localizing genes would permit him to find it in the next few years. Yes, he would pursue it to the end. It was not something that he could or would give up on.

The most difficult questions would be about presymptomatic testing, the issue of telling healthy subjects that they were destined to get a fatal disease for which there was no treatment. Would such a test be possible? Would it be offered? Would children be given the test if their parents wanted it done? Would it be possible to test an unborn fetus that was at risk? And, if the test were positive in the unborn child, would the physician recommend abortion? How long would it take to find a treatment for HD? I attempted to answer the clinical questions, but it was clear that we were in for a difficult time. Not because the questions might be unfair but because they had never before been asked in circumstances where the possibilities could bring them so close to potential reality.

The press conference lasted nearly two hours. I gave a brief presentation on the clinical features of HD and of the pattern of inheritance. I emphasized that each child of an affected parent had a 50/50 chance of getting the disease, a point that is often missed. Even if a dozen siblings are spared the disease, the next still has a 50/50 chance. And, if five siblings in a row inherit the gene, the next in line has the same chance, a flip of the coin. Each time the gamete is formed from the egg and sperm, the chance is one in two that the HD gene may be transmitted.

Jim followed with a brief presentation about the potential of molecular biology and how with the use of polymorphic DNA markers, or RFLPS, he had traced the presence of the gene through two families. He pointed out that the gene for HD had been narrowed to a span of DNA about five to ten million base pairs in length out of the total of three billion base pairs.

Nancy Wexler told of her tribulations as a person who was at risk for HD. She told of the experience of learning that her mother had the disease and discovering that it was not transmitted only through fathers to their sons, something once believed to be true. And she told of the challenge that she and others in her position now faced. Would she take the test if it became available? She wasn't sure.

Of the many reporters who attended, Larry Altman of the *New York Times* was the most skeptical about the results. Had the findings been confirmed by others? What was the statistical likelihood of finding a marker close enough to provide linkage and to have it happen on the twelfth throw of the dice?

I felt a bit foolish. And I was nervous. It had been so unexpected. If the results were true, it signaled a new era in the possibilities of using modern genetic methods to find the genes for each of the inherited neurological disorders. Any family with a disease that followed Mendelian inheritance could be tracked down in the same manner. But how could I be sure that it was true? One reporter asked if we thought we, as scientists, had gone too far. Where would the manipulation of genetic studies take us next? Another questioned the risk for the individual who tested positive if insurance companies were to discover the test results. Would the physician give such information to the insurance company when asked?

My reactions to the event were mixed. The attention given to our results was gratifying. We were on the front pages of all the national newspapers the very next morning. But what if the results didn't hold up? And how would we deal with the patients we were following in our clinic in Boston, who would now want to be tested? In the next few weeks, Jim arranged to share the DNA probe with other research centers around the world that wanted to confirm and extend his findings. He also fielded requests from clinical centers that wanted to use the probe for predictive genetic testing. Such a test would be based on linkage, and one had to have at least three members of a family in order to do the test: one who was old enough to be unaffected, one affected with the symptoms and the asymptomatic subject who wanted to predict the future. Individual patients without well-documented family members with the disorder would have to await the discovery of the gene itself.

However, while we shared the probe for research, we declined initially to provide it for clinical testing. The reason was that an important scientific question would have to be answered to understand the test's overall validity. Was HD due to a single mutation at the same site on chromosome 4 in all families? Or did some families have a mutation somewhere else on the chromosome or on another chromosome? If so, patients with symptoms identical to HD would fail to show linkage to the chromosome 4 location. Was the disease heterogeneous with other chromosomal locations? The G8 probe, now also labeled as D4S10, had already been sent to Peter Harper in Wales, to the HD center at Johns Hopkins and to Michael Hayden at the University of British Columbia in Canada.

While the research was being done to answer these critical questions, we began to make plans for how testing patients would be carried out. In earlier surveys from our own patients and from other centers, there had been a striking degree of concordance in response to the question, "Would you take the test if it becomes available?" Approximately two-thirds of the respondents answered in the affirmative. If available, they would want to know the results. Why? To plan for their future or to be able to make informed deliberations on whether or not they would want to have children. Others wanted to know just so they could settle the issue in their own minds. A reason frequently given by those who said they would not want to know was: why learn of a fate that has no treatment? Others said they would feel guilty if they had a negative test when others in their family were already suffering from the disease. Still others declined for religious reasons.

A few years later, Nancy approached Jim about doing the test. There had been tissue saved after her mother died, and her father was still living. Would Jim do the test? He came for my advice. I had no difficulty in responding. Although Nancy knew as much as any of us about the disease and the test, she should not enter into any special arrangements with a scientist like Jim. We were busily engaged in developing the criteria for presymptomatic testing, which would involve pretesting for psychological state, counseling about genetics and careful attention to the administration of informed consent. She should not be treated any differently.

## Could We Have Been Wrong?

A few months after the press conference I received a call from Martin Bander. He urged me to come to his office for a chat. He related that he had never, in more than twenty years of work in public affairs, had a news story that received such wide attention. I was still a young man; I had been at the Massachusetts General Hospital now for about five years, one of which had been spent as general director of the hospital. I knew Martin very well. He was a consummate professional, and I was pleased to take his compliment. The neurology department was thriving, and our venture into human genetics was being widely noticed. But Martin soon came to the point. He, too, had been troubled by the success. Was I absolutely certain that the results were valid? Had I reviewed the data very carefully? I assured him that I had but that I had not seen all of the primary data, only the DNA blots that Jim had shown us and the connections to each family member.

I left his office deeply concerned: Could there be a problem? Did he know something he wasn't sharing with me? There was no reason to suspect anyone. Yet the results did seem too good to be true. There was no way to share my concern with Jim. He would react strongly against any insinuation of less than the most stringent application of scientific pursuit. I came to appreciate that Bander was simply doing his job.

We eagerly awaited the results from Vancouver, Johns Hopkins and Wales, which soon began to appear, confirming our linkage. In the space of a few months the LOD score, the statistical log of probability odds that the data are significantly linked, had climbed to over ten and no false-negatives (an incorrect finding that indicated someone didn't have HD when symptoms proved that they did) had appeared. What was particularly striking was the fact that all families tested were positively linked. We appeared to be dealing with a single gene disorder, worldwide in occurrence, and probably spread throughout the world from a European, perhaps of British origin.

The fact that there was no treatment for HD wasn't the only downside to the discovery. As the principal investigator of the center's grant, as a collaborator with Jim providing equipment from my lab, and keeping close contact with his work, it was assumed and never contested that I should be an author on the paper. In the culture of science, the student, the postdoc or the junior professor who carries out most of the actual work appears as the first author, and the most senior leader of the group, in this case myself, as the principal investigator and director of the HD center, would appear as the last author. There were fourteen authors in all. Jim was quite appropriately the first author. I was, I thought appropriately, the last author. The others included Nancy, several doctors who had helped Nancy examine the patients in Venezuela (Anne Young, Ira Shoulson) and Mike Conneally and some members of his group from Indiana. None of the patients who I was following in Boston were included in the first results. I thought little about it and was delighted to be a member of the team. Only later did I learn that certain other senior professors at Harvard had found my participation objectionable. Perhaps they were right, but it was the most important work I had ever been associated with, and I felt that I had made a heavy intellectual investment and not just played a departmental role in the work. Still others explained away the long list of authors on the paper as yet another example of the less-scientific work of clinical research, as compared to basic science research.

## The Long Search for the HD Gene

This remarkable and early success was the first evidence to show conclusively that polymorphic DNA markers could be used to find the general region of a gene in an autosomal dominant disorder, where no clue existed about the function or nature of the gene or protein it produced. Although this early linkage was fortuitous, it took a full decade of intense work to finally identify the specific nature of the gene defect.

To understand the dilemma that faced Jim Gusella and other investigators as they searched for the elusive HD gene, let us recall that DNA polymorphisms are useful in linkage studies in families because they define a difference between regions of the genome. A polymorphism is useful in marking a DNA region in an affected family member that is different from that present on the normal chromosome that does not contain the defective gene. This technique of using RFLPs and linkage analysis has since proven to be extraordinarily powerful in identifying gene loci for more than five hundred diseases.

The process also has some severe limitations. In the case of HD, the first marker, D4S10, was linked to the extreme tip of chromosome 4 in a region labeled 4p16.3. Unfortunately, linkage can only accomplish so much. It was soon appreciated that the probe could be as far as four to five million base pairs away from the HD gene. The gene was confirmed to fall between the D4S10 marker and the chromosome tip (telomere), and dozens of additional DNA polymorphic probes were identified and a genetic map of the region developed. Then the search began to narrow the region that contained the gene and to search for so-called candidate genes. Very few identified genes existed in the region. As each candidate gene was identified, it had to be examined base pair by base pair to look for mutations that might be associated with HD. It is important to appreciate the difficulty that this represented. It was possible by linkage alone to narrow the search to about one to three million base pairs. Since there are about thirty genes per million base pairs, the region under study for HD could theoretically be the home of one hundred to two hundred genes.

A formidable task lay ahead. Jim Gusella's group led an international collaboration. A variety of techniques were used in the scientific search for the little straw in the remaining haystack. Human chromosomes were introduced into rodent (usually hamster) cells in a technique called somatic cell hybridization. Over time, most human chromosomes are lost leaving a hamster cell that has incorporated human DNA representing all or part of the remaining human chromosomes. Using the technique that Jim had developed in his PHD work, one could then search through fragments to find subregions of 4p16.3 that contained the HD gene. DNA from the region was also cloned—making genetically identical copies, which is standard operating procedure, enabling one to study the DNA more easily. Eventually, several genes were found and examined, and ten years later in 1993, one, called IT15 (for interesting transcript number 15), was shown to be the long-sought-after culprit.[11]

Within IT15, near the early part of the transcribed region (5' end of the gene), was found a trinucleotide (triplet) repeat containing the base sequence CAG, which is present normally in up to 34 repeats. The repeat was expanded in patients with HD. In studies from three centers with large populations of HD patients, it was shown that the average number of CAG repeats in normal individuals is approximately 19, with a range of 12 to 34. In confirmed cases of HD, they were invariably expanded beyond 37. A few patients were found with an intermediate number of 34 to 37, most of whom were asymptomatic. In a few instances, children born to parents, particularly men with this intermediate, or "premutation," range were subsequently found to have expansions into the symptomatic range, greater than 37, with development of HD symptoms. Increased expansions in repeats tended to occur more often in inheritance from an HD-affected father through errors of DNA replication in the sperm, and the triplet repeats rarely, if ever, expanded as much in the mother during egg formation. The aberration in sperm accounted for the inheritance of the juvenile form of the disease from the father.

HD was the third disorder in which such triplet repeats have been shown to be associated with neurologic diseases. The first was fragile X syndrome, the most common cause of mental retardation in males. Another, myotonic dystrophy, a disorder in which muscles develop abnormal sustained contractions (myotonia), was the second disorder to show expanded triplet repeats.

Where did the HD gene discovery lead? The gene was shown to encode a novel protein of unique structure but unknown function. It was called huntingtin, and is present in all cells of the body, including the brain and peripheral tissues, such as the liver, kidneys and pancreas. No abnormalities in the expression of the gene were shown to be associated with the selective neuronal loss in the HD neostriatum. Indeed, it was soon found that both the abnormal gene on the HD chromosome and the normal gene are transcribed into messenger RNA and produce two proteins, one of which is larger than the other because of the expanded CAG region that encodes for glutamine. Cell death cannot be accounted for simply by a deficiency in the protein or by an abnormality in its content within cells. At present, it seems likely that the secret to neuronal death in HD resides in the protein itself. CAG in the genetic code reads out glutamine, one of the twenty amino acids that are found in all of the proteins of the cell's regulatory functions. An examination of these normal proteins shows that none contain stretches of glutamine in excess of thirty-eight. This remarkable observation correlates well with the critical range for expansions that cause HD. Studies in brain cells indicate that huntingtin is found in the cytoplasm and nucleus of nerve cells. It is also present in the axon and in synaptic terminals. By 2011 the speculation was that the protein, because of its abnormal length, may be metabolized abnormally, resulting in neuronal toxicity that accumulates over decades and eventually leads to the selective cell death characteristic of HD.

Subsequent studies revealed that a fragment of the elongated huntingtin protein accumulates as intranuclear aggregates in the cells affected in the neostriatum. At first it seemed likely that this accounted for the cell damage and premature death of these neurons, but later studies suggested that the inclusions are efforts by the cell to sequester the toxic protein away as insoluble aggregates, as a mechanism of protection from adverse effects of the elongated protein. Further studies have shown that the abnormal huntingtin or its fragments may interfere with mitochondrial function or the regulation of other genes. The work on huntingtin within the MGH department was greatly facilitated by the expertise of Marcy MacDonald and Marian DiFiglia.

Nine other diseases in which a similar pattern of CAG repeats occurs have now been identified. In each, there is selective neuronal loss in a region of the brain important for a particular function. In some of the disorders the manifestations are ataxia—difficulty in walking and difficulty with performing smooth muscle motions. In others there is abnormality associated with muscle tone producing rigidity or epilepsy. In each case, it appears that the gene expresses the protein, and the abnormal length of the glutamine repeat in some way leads to selective neuronal cell death.

## Presymptomatic Testing

Presymptomatic testing or diagnosis of HD was not possible before 1983. It all changed with the discovery of the gene location and the availability of RFLP analysis. DNA polymorphisms linked to the disease allowed predictions to be made as to whether family members harbored the abnormality and the likelihood of becoming afflicted with the disease. We reported the first findings on genetic testing in the *New England Journal of Medicine* in 1986.[12] Several conclusions could be drawn from our data. First, the prediction of disease could be changed by testing from 50/50 to about 95/5. But only about half of the families who inquired about the validity of the test had sufficient family members to do a satisfactory linkage test. We were surprised that when the test was first offered, fewer than 20 per cent of individuals at risk actually requested it. In retrospect, this may not be surprising in view of the fact that no treatment exists.

The test's precision increased greatly with the discovery of the gene. All that is required is a sample of blood or a scraping from inside the mouth containing a sufficient number of cells to provide a DNA sample that can be amplified to analyze for the HD gene mutation. By 2011 the sensitivity of the test exceeded 99 per cent. Presymptomatic testing for HD has raised many ethical issues that have been widely discussed: Who should be tested? Who should know the results of the test? Who will pay for the test? Should anyone be told they will get a fatal disease when there is no effective treatment? What percentage of informativeness is sufficient? And most important, particularly in the US, how can a positive test be kept confidential, since knowledge of it threatens an individual's insurability?

The discovery of the HD gene mutation led to the widespread commercial availability of genetic testing and eliminated all complexity and uncertainty inherent in the linkage test. Ethical issues related to HD testing remain to be considered in each case. Most individuals considering HD presymptomatic testing have experienced the full tragedy of the illness in a parent, sibling or other relative, as well as its impact on the social, financial and behavioral well-being of the family. The psychological consequences of a positive—or negative—presymptomatic diagnosis of HD may be profound. The numerous potential consequences of an HD gene diagnosis should be explored in every patient prior to testing, enabling each at-risk individual to make an informed and voluntary decision regarding the risks and benefits of the test.

Most centers report that a significant proportion of those who initially enter testing programs, after carefully considering the pros and cons of living with the knowledge that they have an HD gene "positive" diagnosis, decide not to proceed with testing. This underscores the need for careful individual counseling before sending blood for genetic testing. It is often the anxiety associated with living at risk and the opportunity to rid oneself and one's offspring of the dreaded illness that brings people to genetic testing centers. However, the test has an equal probability of producing the opposite result, enhancing the psychological stresses that motivate the decision to seek testing. A cogent rationale for testing exists when the individual believes the benefits of early positive HD gene diagnosis (personal, family planning, professional reasons, etc.) outweigh the profound negative aspects of knowing that he or she will suffer the dreaded familial illness.

In 1994 the World Federation of Neurology Research Group on Huntington's Chorea provided formal guidelines for administering the test for HD. These include: (1) counseling of the highest standards to inform the individual about HD and the personal implications of genetic testing, as well as providing post-testing support; (2) absence of coercion by family members, employers, insurers and others; (3) consideration of the possible impact of a test result on a relative who is not being tested; (4) exclusion of the HD genetic test from any routine blood investigation without informed consent of the individual; (5) confidentiality of test results; (6) exclusion of minors; (7) prenatal testing only if the parent has already been tested; (8) delay in testing individuals with a serious psychiatric condition (especially depression carrying the risk of suicide) and the institutionalization of proper psychiatric services.

Recommendations for HD testing processes now include: (1) pretest counseling of the risk, options and benefits of testing; (2) a neurologic examination to identify and treat those individuals who already have disability due to HD or another neurologic/psychiatric disorder; (3) psychological/psychiatric screening for clinical depression, suicidality and emotional dyscontrol; and (4) post-test follow-up counseling to support the individual tested and his/her family members.





The variability between the actual repeat length and age of adult onset of HD is so great that the repeat length itself lacks clinical value for predicting age of onset or severity. Many recommend that test results be reported as either positive or negative, or indeterminate if repeat length is between thirty-three and thirty-eight. Genetic testing of individuals with early symptoms of HD can provide definitive confirmation in a cost-effective manner.

## Treatment

There is no effective treatment for the neuronal degeneration in HD. The physician faces the challenging task of assisting patients to live as fully as possible with their neurologic limitations and their anxiety about the future. Genetic counseling of at-risk individuals is now more important with the advent of presymptomatic testing.

Early in the illness, patients' are primarily disabled by their reactions to the diagnosis, manifested as sadness and irritability, and some cognitive deficits. Depression and anxiety states are common, but psychologic counseling and either tricyclic antidepressants or benzodiazepines can help. Another symptom, a sleep disorder with frequent restless movements, may cause sleep deprivation. Clonazepam at bedtime is often beneficial. If chorea is disabling, tetrabenazine, haloperidol, or clonazepam may help improve function. Most patients are less impaired if medicated at low doses rather than medicated to suppress chorea. We have found that the motor dysfunction in HD is exacerbated by weight loss and, occasionally, dramatic improvement occurs if patients are placed on very high-calorie diets that enable weight gain. In 2008 an old drug, tetrabenazine, was approved in the US for HD patients because its use demonstrated modest effects in delaying the symptoms of the disease.

Patients and family members must be warned about the loss of driving skills, which is an inevitable consequence of HD. Myriad social, interpersonal, financial and medical problems plague those with disabling HD, so patients should have a team consisting of a social worker, psychological counselor and neurologist. The lack of appropriate long-term-care facilities for patients with late-stage illness or HD patients with psychiatric manifestations is a source of much anxiety on the part of patients, family and medical staff. Patients with serious emotional dyscontrol present difficult management problems. In our experience, phenothiazines have some limited effectiveness in controlling destructive behavior. Relaxation therapy and trials of lithium, tegretol, valproate, or beta-adrenergic blockers may be helpful.

## Future Efforts

The goals of future research in HD have been crystallized by the discovery of the HD mutation, and work is underway to learn: (1) the biologic function of the normal huntingtin protein, (2) the biologic function of the huntingtin protein containing an expanded CAG trinucleotide repeat, (3) the effect of the HD mutation in a transgenic mouse, and (4) the rules that underlie the instability of the mutation during transmission from parent to child. Most believe that the autosomal dominant HD mutation causes the huntingtin protein with its expanded stretch of polyglutamines to take on a new destructive function. Characterization of the biologic effect of the mutation may lead to ideas for therapy. In this regard, the transgenic mouse model of HD has been extremely useful in understanding the illness and for testing of potential therapies.

## The Evolution of Neurogenetics at the MGH

The neurogenetics group thrived under Jim's leadership. In my view, he is one of the most distinguished investigators I've known, and his motivation grew to tackle difficult problems presented in the search for genes for other neurodegenerative disorders. Soon after his laboratory was up and running, Jim hired Rudy Tanzi as a technician. Rudy, twenty-one years old, was fresh out of college at the University of Rochester with a degree in history and microbiology, and had formed, during the summer after graduation, a rock band called Fantasy. Referring some time later to that period of his life, he characterized himself as "living life as a bushy-haired, scruffy musician and playing keyboard once again with musicians from my high school days." Tanzi was a facile scientist familiar with the technology of restriction fragment polymorphisms. The opportunity to join Jim's efforts seemed just right for both of them, and he proved to be a critical force in the emerging efforts in HD. He later entered the graduate program in neuroscience at Harvard, a program that I helped establish with Torsten Weisel, chair of the Department of Neurobiology, as a vehicle to allow access for faculty in clinical departments to graduate students and to allow the emerging interests that many students were developing in pursuing clinical research problems. After completing his PHD, Rudy established his own laboratory to pursue work in Alzheimer's disease and by 2011 he was the Joseph and Rose Kennedy Professor of Neurology at the MGH and director of the MGH Genetics and Aging Unit. Other key individuals in the advancing work on Huntington's disease were Marcy MacDonald and Marian DiFiglia, both professors of neurology at the MGH.

Jim quickly expanded his laboratory efforts to work on other problems and became a magnet for young trainees in neurology, from Boston and around the world, who wanted to enter this new discipline. Postdocs arrived from Canada, two noteworthy ones being Peter St. George-Hyslop, who arrived after completing neurology training at the University of Toronto to work on identifying genes for AD, and Guy Rouleau, who came from Montreal and would find the gene for neurofibromatosis type 2. The promise of neurogenetics became apparent to some of our finest neurological residents. Robert H. Brown, who had a medical degree from HMS after completing a DPHIL with Denis Noble at Oxford, pursued genes for familial periodic paralysis. He later found the first genetic abnormality in ALS (Lou Gehrig's disease) with the cloning of the SOD1 gene.

Besides the work in Huntington's disease that finally identified the HD gene, members of the MGH group included Xandra Breakfield, who isolated the gene for torsion dystonia, and Susan Slaugenhaupt, who found the gene for familial dysautonomia.

By 2011 Jim Gusella was leading the interdepartmental, interdisciplinary Center for Human Genetic Research at the MGH, focused on the ongoing revolution in human genetics. The center concentrates hospital-wide efforts in genetic variation, investigating a variety of diseases (both neurological and beyond).

## What is to be Learned from All of This?

The work on the elucidation of the genetic basis of HD speaks to the essence of what medical science is. The story of HD epitomizes the conception and birth of a staggering and history-changing breakthrough. The background elements important to this story include: the compelling need represented by the clinical tragedy demonstrated by HD, the imperative coming from advocacy groups through Congress, and the means realized by funding from the US Congress through the NIH. A vision for a means toward finding the genetic basis of HD coalesced with knowledge of an emerging technical possibility and inspiration provided by David Housman. Of course, the inspired grasp of benefit–risk balance and the historical destiny of a great department (of neurology) in a great institution (the Massachusetts General Hospital) with exceptional leadership instincts and an informed sense of the clinical possibility of discovery didn't hurt! And, at the height of the story, there was the grand payoff for a big gamble on a young investigator, Jim Gusella, and a first-pitch swing that "put one out of the park," which might be called "luck," but still a quality of luck that would have had no meaning without the history of all the elements outlined in this chapter. Finally, running through the HD story from its beginning to the present moment, of course, are the ethical issues raised by genetic testing and the imperative we clinical scientists feel in pressing forward to find new treatments for our patients.

# SEVEN

# *From Bethesda to San Francisco*

AFTER A FULL DECADE AT THE MGH it seemed appropriate to undertake a serious period of study in molecular biology to strengthen my research portfolio. I sensed that my research work by this time had become somewhat prosaic, not grounded in the emerging powers of cellular and molecular neurobiology, and my laboratory lacked the capacity to clone genes. My observations of the growing importance of genomics in attacking the clinical problems we faced in neurology convinced me to take this step.

## Sabbatical at the NIH and an Opportunity on the West Coast

In the fall of 1987, I was awarded a Fogarty International Fellowship for a research sabbatical at the National Institutes of Health to work with Michael Brownstein. Michael, Dorothy Krieger and I had collaborated at several symposia and had edited a couple of books on the emerging importance of brain neuropeptides that functioned as neurotransmitters or neuromodulators. Dorothy, an endocrinologist at Mount Sinai School of Medicine in New York, and I had written an extensive review on the subject for the *New England Journal of Medicine.*[1]

While on sabbatical, I worked hard in Mike's laboratory to master the fundamentals of the use of DNA restriction enzymes and production of DNA gels. But I found the effort more frustrating than productive, verging, quite frankly, on humiliation as I watched young college and graduate students in the laboratory show far greater facility with these techniques than I. Tutorials with Mike helped, but I found myself more intrigued by associating with other Fogarty scholars in the Stone House up the hill from Mike's lab, which served as the Fogarty International Center. Among other advantages to the center were free lessons in computer technology and office applications.

I had the opportunity to engage frequently with Julius Axelrod, whose work on the biochemistry of neurotransmitters in the catecholamine pathway had led to his being awarded the Nobel Prize in Physiology or Medicine in 1970. He had been a mentor to Solomon Snider, professor and founder of the Department of Neuroscience at Johns Hopkins University. Every day, Julie (as he was affectionately called) appeared at his laboratory down the hall from Mike's to carry out the latest of his experiments. He and Sol Snider were both known for being prolific in neuroscience. It was said that Julie came in with a new idea Monday morning, carried out the critical experiments and had another paper to submit to a periodical by Friday.

As I think back to that 1988–1989 sabbatical year, I realize that it was the introduction to WordPerfect, e-mail and simple computer programming that made the year most beneficial for me. I admit this only as a critique of my own capabilities and not as a reflection of Mike's efforts or the fertile environment of his laboratory.

As the sabbatical year advanced, I was looking forward to a variety of projects, including the completion of the extensive remodeling of "Building 149" in the Charlestown Navy Yard. Together with John Potts, who was then chairman of the Department of Medicine, I had been a strong supporter of a grand-scale plan to relocate major basic science components of the MGH from the crowded inadequate laboratories of the main campus on Fruit Street to the ten floors of the old navy arsenal in Charlestown. Although the site was twenty minutes away across downtown Boston and on the other side of the Charles River, it was the only site available for rapid development into a substantial, sustainable, research campus.

I negotiated for the sixth floor to provide space for our expanding neuroscience activities. We were able to convince Larry Martin, the associate general director (and no relation to me), of our group's evolving needs. We were assigned approximately 60,000 gross square feet and planned to move the laboratories of Jim Gusella, Marian DeFiglia and Bob Brown to the new site. We were joined by David Corey, whom I had recruited from Yale, together with his spouse, Xandra Breakfield, and Robert Martuza, a junior member in neurosurgery who was working on the genetic profiles of malignant gliomas.[2] The emerging portfolio of investigators also included a new research group in neuropeptides consisting of Steve Hyman,[3] Steve Fink[4] and Michael Comb, who had worked with Howard Goodman and was setting up an independent laboratory.[5]

The expansion in neuroscience at the MGH was certainly something to look forward to. My new office at the MGH was an imposing corner suite overlooking the Boston Harbor, but I never moved into that space or worked in the beautiful new laboratories rapidly emerging at the old navy warehouse. Indeed, by August 1988, as I began to sense my growing frustration with laboratory work, an unexpected series of events unfolded and ultimately set my career on a different trajectory. It all began with a call from L. Hollingsworth (Holly) Smith Jr. from the University of California, San Francisco. Holly explained that a committee chaired by him had convened to begin the search for a dean of the medical school to succeed Rudi Schmid, and that he was calling to explore my interest in visiting UCSF for an interview.

Holly Smith was a legendary figure in the national fabric of internal medicine. While a student at Harvard Medical School he had worked with George Thorn, then the physician-in-chief at the Peter Bent Brigham Hospital, which in 1976 would merge with the Boston Lying-in Hospital and the Robert Breck Brigham Hospital to form the Brigham and Women's Hospital. Holly had graduated from Harvard Medical School in 1948 and was accepted for internship and residency in internal medicine at the MGH. After two years of military service during the Korean War, Holly returned to Harvard, where he was admitted to the distinguished Society of Fellows. He continued work at the MGH and met and married Margaret Avery. They honeymooned in Sweden, where he undertook a sabbatical year at the Karolinska Institute. Holly later returned to the MGH as chief resident and before long was asked by Walter Bauer, the remarkable chief of medicine at the MGH, to head the endocrine division. Walter Bauer was a legend at the MGH and noted for his prescience in appointing promising young people to distinguished posts. In his memoir, Holly, who had expected to continue on in research, recounts a dramatic encounter, "Walter Bauer called me into his office and said in effect, 'I am going to make you chief of the Endocrine Unit. I believe that you can make it in academic medicine and therefore I'm going to support you fully for the next five years.' Then he leaned forward and said (I remember the exact words), 'If you don't make it, I'm going to kick your ass out of here.'"[6]

Holly's new position had opened when Fuller Albright, an endocrinologist, suffered permanent brain damage following unsuccessful surgical treatment for Parkinson's disease, leaving him totally incapacitated for the remainder of his life. Holly led the unit with great distinction, nurturing the careers of Daniel Federman, who would later become chair of the Department of Medicine at Stanford and then dean for medical education at Harvard Medical School, and Mitch Rabkin, who went on to head the Beth Israel Hospital in Boston.

After a sabbatical at Oxford in 1963–1964, Holly made a dramatic exit from the Boston scene, never to return. It was a stroke of imagination and courage. He accepted the position to head the Department of Medicine at the University of California, San Francisco, where he led a major academic expansion taking UCSF to academic heights widely admired and respected. I had met Holly once during the search for Alex Leaf's successor as chair of the Department of Medicine at the MGH, but at that time he had been too entrenched in San Francisco to give serious consideration to a return to Boston. Now, we were to meet again, this time to discuss my career.

## A Visit to San Francisco

Holly Smith convinced me to visit San Francisco in October to meet with the search committee. My visit was "light and lively." I had no serious interest in the job—I loved neurology and felt we had the strongest group at the MGH of anywhere in the world. New recruitments were now moving along very well, our residency training program was thriving and we had trained an expanding cadre of outstanding people who were populating leadership positions all over the country.

Much to my surprise, I enjoyed the two-day visit to UCSF. I found the members of the search committee representing the diversity of the UCSF community from the nursing, pharmacy and dental schools to be an outstanding group. With my visit over, I returned to Boston and immediately left for the annual meeting of the Society for Neuroscience in Toronto. I had just arrived in Toronto when I received a call from Holly asking me how I felt about the visit to UCSF. In his legendary role as a "ruthless recruiter," he told me of the great impact my visit had had there and that although he was not able to offer anything definitive yet, he was almost certain that when the search committee held its next meeting they would recommend that I consider the job as their preferred candidate. Flattery was a great strategy—and I fell for it, only to realize that I had a serious problem on my hands.

## San Francisco, Here We Come

The issue of a move to San Francisco complicated Rachel's and my life in a number of ways, and it certainly managed to create discontent during the remainder of the sabbatical at NIH. The next call from UCSF was from the chancellor of the campus, Dr. Julie (which he preferred to Julius) Krevans, a hematologist who had trained at New York University and then rose through the ranks at Johns Hopkins as professor of medicine and dean of medical education. He had come to UCSF in 1971 to serve as dean of the medical school, and a decade later he succeeded Dr. Phil Lee as chancellor. Julie had now entered the recruitment process to encourage me to return for a second visit in January 1989.

Rachel sent clear messages that she was not interested in another move. She had sought career advice about entering social work in Boston and intended to pursue other activities close to her interests. She had been active working in the library at Belmont High School until my sabbatical, and she looked forward to a change when we returned to Boston after my sabbatical. Despite her misgivings and the growing attraction of the developing neuroscience group at Charlestown, I allowed my personal ambition to drive me onward, and I agreed to another visit. By this time, the pressure was escalating from the UCSF side and Bill Kerr, CEO of the hospital, and Haile Debas, chair of the Department of Surgery, had become particularly persuasive.

Haile had a remarkable personal story. Born in Eritrea, educated in medicine at McGill University and trained in surgery at the University of British Columbia, he had enjoyed a productive academic career following postdoctoral training in gastrointestinal surgery and research at UCLA. After Haile's brief stint at the University of Washington, Rudy Schmid had recruited him to UCSF to chair the Department of Surgery. He had been there about eighteen months when I first met him in 1988. In that short time he had established himself as the most forward-thinking chair in the school, and his influence was to be critical to my decision to go to UCSF as dean.

I began a process of rationalization that proved decisive in the months ahead. It went like this: I had succeeded in developing a new strategic vision for the department at the MGH, focusing on emerging opportunities in neuroscience and genetics. I was now being offered a more expansive landscape. My own research had reached a plateau, and my plans for introducing new techniques and approaches to my own laboratory work seemed more remote. I increasingly found that my advice to the best students and residents was to extend their research experience in the best labs in the Boston area. Chris Walsh, for instance, went to work with Connie Cepko in the basic science departments at Harvard Medical School; Bob Brown began collaborating with Bob Horwitz at MIT and Tom Maniatis from Harvard's Faculty of Arts and Science. And finally, we had a family tie breakpoint. Neil was finishing high school and planning to enter college at the University of Rochester, my alma mater. Doug was ensconced in the pre-med program at McGill, and Melanie had selected Brown over Harvard College, ostensibly to get farther from home. She had then applied to medical schools, with acceptances to both Harvard and Stanford, and had chosen the latter. Her preference for Stanford signaled a healthy desire to be away from any influence I might have had over her acceptance at Harvard (I had none), or my surveillance of her progress at HMS (which I knew wouldn't happen). So with Neil going to college, Doug in Montreal, Melanie in Palo Alto and Brad recently married to Karen Lenington and living near Boston, our attachments to Boston looked negotiable. We had not been blessed with any grandchildren at that point.

None of these rationalizations resolved Rachel's hesitation about another move. I appreciate now, in retrospect, how selfish my ambitions were and how I offered explanations that were largely self-serving.

The second visit in January and subsequent negotiations led to the requirement of an affirmative answer on my part by mid-February. Rachel and I traveled to Miami in February for a meeting at the Howard Hughes Medical Institute and extended our visit to spend a few days driving up the Atlantic coast of Florida to Palm Beach. My mind was made up and Rachel seemed reluctant but flexible. As we approached the Breakers in Palm Beach, I decided to find a phone, call Julie Krevans and indicate my continuing interest in the position as dean of the medical school at UCSF, pending further discussion of details of available assets and resources that would be committed by the school. I said I was available immediately for a third visit. Then I called Bob Buchanan, head of the MGH, with the news that I was in serious negotiations. Bob, in turn, informed Dean Dan Tosteson, and pretty soon I began to receive calls from colleagues at Harvard urging me to return to Boston at the end of my sabbatical. Particularly memorable was a call from Gene Braunwald, a co-editor of *Harrison's Principles of Internal Medicine,* reminding me that giving up an active role in neurology might jeopardize my position as an editor. That was a serious concern because the substantial royalties from the textbook had provided for the bulk of the tuition needs of our four children, thanks to which they would graduate from college with minimal debt.

Before accepting the position as dean, I spoke with Jean Wilson, a co-editor of HPIM and a person whom I admired greatly. From his perch at Southwestern Medical School in Dallas, Jean had a perspective of UCSF that was different from the one I could get from contacts on the East Coast. He was very specific. He felt that UCSF was one of the top two or three research and clinical care medical schools in the country, surpassing in some areas the work at Harvard. He encouraged me to take the position if I really wanted to be a dean. I realized that if the HPIM editorship rules were applied, I might lose my role there—but, fortunately, this didn't happen.

Julie Krevans and I reached an agreement a few weeks later. I took advantage of a visit that Rudi Schmid, the outgoing dean, made to Bethesda in April and got a detailed account of the challenges and opportunities facing UCSF. The most notable issue that emerged was the serious lack of research space for any further expansion.

Rachel and I set about considering the details of the move to be undertaken over the summer and fall after the conclusion of my sabbatical in May. I took on my responsibilities at UCSF in July, and we moved in October, just in time for the devastating Loma Prieta earthquake, rating 7.3 on the Richter scale, on October 17, 1989, during the opening ceremony of the World Series at precisely 5:07 p.m. Pacific Standard Time. Mike Bishop, a professor of microbiology and immunology at UCSF and a recent recipient of the Nobel Prize for his work with Harold Varmus, was particularly disappointed. As a loyal Giants fan he had been scheduled to throw out the first pitch on that day. That never happened, of course, as the city mobilized to face challenges it had not seen since the earthquake of 1906.

The night the earthquake took place Rachel was in Ohio, and I was in Washington, DC, to honor Herb Boyer, professor of biochemistry at UCSF who, with Stanley Cohen, professor of biochemistry at Stanford University, had first shown the practical experiments demonstrating the feasibility of recombinant DNA, and was to receive the Medal of Science at the White House that night from President George H.W. Bush. When I returned to my hotel after the ceremony to watch the World Series, I was greeted by a televised firestorm of burning houses and collapsed bridges. I will never forget the feelings that overcame me. *Why have we done this?* I kept asking myself over and over. Then I called Rachel. Her comment was, "I could have told you this was not a good idea."

Sleep was next to impossible that night. I woke up in the middle of the night in a panic. I found myself obsessed with the possibility of a sustained power failure at the UCSF campus. I knew how many research experiments and samples were customarily kept frozen at low temperatures and cringed at the disaster that could befall the research community if results from experiments were lost. Finally, at about 2 a.m. Eastern Standard Time, I called San Francisco. I was told the hospital had emergency power. I hadn't worried about that. I was also told that the power to the school and campus did remain off for about twelve hours, but fortunately not enough to cause any damage, much to my relief.

I returned to Boston to pick up our car then drove to Ohio to meet Rachel, and together we continued on to San Francisco, concerned about what we might find when we arrived there. As it turned out, the damage caused by the quake had been somewhat exaggerated that first evening. By the time we arrived a week later, the city was up and running at full speed except for the collapsed section of the upper deck of the Bay Bridge, which would not be repaired for many months to come.

## UCSF: A Brief History

A bit of history about UCSF might help describe my sentiments about joining a "frontier" medical school. It had, I learned, a very interesting history. A South Carolina surgeon by the name of Hugh H. Toland had arrived in California in 1852 on the heels of the California Gold Rush. The UCSF *Alumni Bulletin* in the fall of 2008 describes his adventure:

*After a few discouraging months as a miner, he sold his claim and headed to the coast to establish a surgical practice in booming San Francisco. Toland located his office near the waterfront at Montgomery and Merchant streets and within months became the city's foremost surgeon, managing what was reportedly the largest practice on the West Coast. In 1864, he decided to establish a medical school in San Francisco and purchased land for that purpose in North Beach, at Stockton and Francisco streets, opposite the*

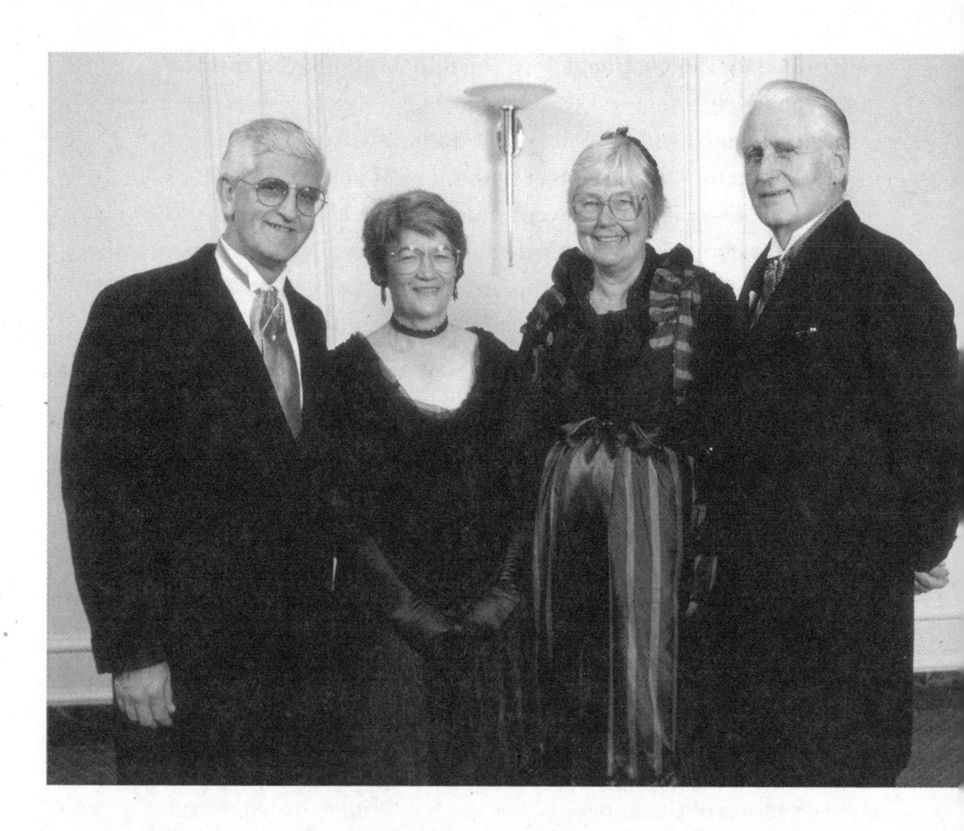

UCSF Foundation fundraising event, 1990. From left: the author, Rachel Martin, Margaret Smith and Holly Smith. The event recalled the 1869 founding of Toland Medical College, the forerunner of UCSF.





*San Francisco City and County Hospital. By 1870, Toland Medical College had a class of 30 students and had already granted diplomas to 45 graduates. Toland sought to affiliate his medical school with the University of California, which was not yet two years old. In March 1873, the trustees deeded the Toland Medical College to the UC Regents, establishing the Medical Department of the University of California. In 1874, it became a coed campus for medical education.*[7]

UCSF grew in stature as a clinical and educational institution during the early years of the twentieth century and would become the oldest medical school in continuous operation west of the Mississippi. Following the relocation of the Stanford University School of Medicine from San Francisco to Palo Alto, UCSF became the only medical school in the city. And, following the successful recruitment of a number of key faculty members in the two decades following World War II, it emerged in international ascendancy from a backwater clinical school to a preeminent research university. By the last two decades of the twentieth century it was recognized as one of the world's leading biomedical, clinical and research centers, with strong schools of medicine, pharmacy, nursing and dentistry.

Among the important developments that led to the ascendancy of UCSF was the recruitment of outstanding leaders in the clinical departments and in basic science. In addition to Holly Smith, who chaired the Department of Medicine, there was Marv Slesinger—a Harvard Medical School classmate of Holly's who had come to head the VA service—and Rudi Schmid—a world-renowned hepatologist who was recruited to the Department of Medicine and later served as dean of the school from 1982 to 1989. Other departments flourished under new leadership. J. Englebert Dunphy headed surgery, Robert Fishman came from Columbia to head the neurology department and Charlie Wilson headed neurosurgery. Equally stunning recruitments were made in the basic science departments and the Department of Physiology, to which Fran Ganong brought enormous prestige.[8] Other distinguished appointments included Alex Margulis as chair of radiology and Mel Grumbach as chair of pediatrics.

An even earlier period in the renaissance in research at UCSF began with the Cardiovascular Research Institute, founded in the 1950s and headed by Julius Comroe. Not long after, William Rutter arrived to chair the biochemistry department, and then in the late 1960s and the 1970s came Mike Bishop, Harold Varmus, Bruce Alberts and Marc Kirschner. Their arrivals were powerful harbingers of the growing importance of basic cell biology, genetics and biochemistry, which grew through the largesse of expanding federal research and support from the NIH.

## A Crisis of Space at UCSF

Life as a dean, though on occasion exceedingly frustrating, would prove gratifying on the whole. The school was in considerable flux. Several department chairs were dysfunctional or nearing retirement. I was expected to move expeditiously by appointing search committees and leading the appointment of the next generation of leaders, hopefully as successful as the last. The basic science departments had felt strong support from Dean Rudi Schmid, but the clinical departments considered their status under siege. They had not been able to identify new research space for more than a decade, and communications between the basic science chairs and the clinical departments were at a minimum. New recruitments were being made in the basic science departments into space provided by the dental school, but the clinical departments were having a difficult time recruiting.

UCSF's school of pharmacy, the top ranked of such schools in the country, was in even more dire shape than the clinical departments. The faculty had finally agreed to relocate to a recently vacated insurance office building at Laurel Heights, about two miles away from the main campus. At its new location in Laurel Heights, the school of pharmacy would expand by 100,000 square feet, vacating approximately 40,000 square feet on the site of the main facilities of UCSF Medical Center and the Children's Hospital, located in a neighborhood called Parnassus Heights. When I arrived on campus, it was estimated that construction would be completed in two to three years. But serious problems needed to be resolved before the school could move. The university had purchased the Laurel Heights property without fully disclosing its intention to transform it into a wet laboratory for basic biomedical and pharmaceutical research.

I had been assured by Chancellor Krevans and by my friend Holly Smith that all legal issues were now behind us and that we were free to proceed with the detailed plans for renovation. Community activists, however, thought otherwise. Opposition to the renovation was strong and growing. As Bruce Spaulding, vice-chancellor of UCSF during this period, related to me in retrospect in August 2009, the debacle had its origins in the agreement that the regents had made with the community in the 1970s to restrict growth on the Parnassus campus to a total of 3,554,000 square feet:

*The event that pushed the neighbors over the edge was the construction of the school of dentistry building. The campus as it expanded to the west, took over private housing and closed 4th Avenue, south of Parnassus. This was perceived as arrogant and insensitive, the basic dilemma being that our highly dense, high-rise campus was in the middle of an almost exclusively residential neighborhood. The Mount Sutro Defense Committee was formed, and the legislature threatened to hold up the entire University of California budget if the regents did not impose a building moratorium.*

This agreement to a space limitation was succeeded in 1982 by a long-range development plan (LRDP), which was required as part of a periodic university-wide mechanism for public comment and approval for all campus developments across the system. California had extremely strict environmental laws under a 1970 statute known as the *California Environmental Quality Act* (CEQA). Spaulding explained to me: "This law requires an exhaustive environmental impact report (EIR) for any building project greater than 30,000 square feet. One of the standards for review of projects is that the project must be consistent with the LRDP for each of the 10 UC campuses."

The board of regents, whose membership included the governor and other political appointees who mirrored the current political makeup of the state, met, on average, ten times per year and were always in the public eye. Each meeting included public sessions attended by advocates and opponents of the university. As a consequence of this very public endeavor, the regents adopted an extremely prescriptive format for campus LRDPs. Each had to be approved by the full board and have a full environmental impact report prepared for the proposed actions. A weak or ill-advised LRDP could hamstring a campus for over a decade.

The 1982 LRDP had such an impact. It confirmed the space limitation, accepting the moratorium on expansion at the Parnassus site and adopted a philosophy of "scattering to the four winds." It proposed expansion into other sites and failed to acknowledge that the genius of UCSF's success lay in the close proximity of the "best and brightest" at the Parnassus campus. The premise that emerged was expansion to sites all over the City of San Francisco and northern San Mateo County. "The flaw in this approach," Spaulding told me, "was that faculty and staff in these disparate sites felt isolated as second-class citizens and as individuals who were no longer able to participate in daily interaction with their colleagues and co-workers at the main campus." A series of acquisitions followed, the most notorious of which was the purchase of the Laurel Heights campus, a

362,000-square-foot office building that sat, like the Parnassus campus, squarely in the midst of an influential middle-class neighborhood.

Many felt that the university had paid too much for Laurel Heights—a total of $55 million—without due diligence to the controversies that would emerge. The neighbors firmly held to the belief that Chancellor Krevans had made a promise that the building would be used for administrative purposes only. "Hence," Spaulding notes, "one of the four lawsuits to stop UCSF's utilization of the building was nicknamed the 'Julie Lies' lawsuit by the press, and it sought to hold Julie to his 'promise.'"

Spaulding recalls:

*Accusations came from the faculty that campus leadership was stubborn and timid. Stubborn because it pursued the litigation at a cost that ran up to $200,000 per month at the height of the fight. Timid because the campus left the building fallow for fear that the litigation, which stretched on for almost ten years, would result in a permanent injunction for the development of laboratory space in the building.*

The plan for Laurel Heights was not realized. With each passing month, new avenues of legal opposition were mounted by community activists, and by the third year of my deanship a dark pessimism had settled over the campus. There were desperate moves to find alternative solutions, and there was great fear of an exodus of the best faculty to other opportunities propelled by space constraints.

## Intellectual Growth and Collaboration

Despite the unfolding saga, to which I shall return below, much was accomplished during the first three years of my deanship. Sixteen new department chairs were recruited in three years. Among them was Floyd Rector, a distinguished nephrologist, who took over the chair of medicine from the ineffective Richard Root, who, after five years of failed leadership, had become seriously depressed and dysfunctional.[9] Other early recruitments included David Bradford to head orthopedics, Ron Arenson in radiology, Larry Shapiro to head pediatrics and, much to my delight, Steve Hauser to succeed Bob Fishman as chair of neurology.

Steve had been a senior neurology resident at the MGH during my first year there as chief, and we had worked together seamlessly on the ward service that winter when I was the attending neurologist. He joined Howard Weiner at the Brigham and Women's Hospital to work on new treatments for multiple sclerosis and then spent three years in basic immunology at the Institut Pasteur in Paris. On his return to Boston, I had arranged a modest laboratory for him at the MGH, where he quickly excelled in his work, getting substantial funding and developing a rigorous research program.

I had first offered the chief of neurology position at UCSF to Robert Barchi at the University of Pennsylvania, but negotiations had foundered, and I was very pleased when the search committee followed my recommendation to approach Steve. In the end, Steve proved to be an extraordinarily effective clinical leader, not only in his own department but across the entire school. Over the next fifteen years he was president of the American Neurological Association, succeeded me as editor of the neurology section of HPIM and was subsequently appointed editor-in-chief of the *Annals of Neurology*, succeeding Richard Johnson of Johns Hopkins University.

Early on during my years as dean, I established monthly luncheon meetings with all the department chairs—basic and clinical—and invited Bill Kerr, head of the hospital, to join us. In the reporting relationships, Bill reported to the chancellor as did I, and I felt it important to include him in our academic meetings whenever his schedule permitted. We scheduled department reviews and received a report from one of them each month. Attendance was high, and I sensed a growing camaraderie among the chairs.

The UCSF School of Medicine had a strong clinical and research presence at the San Francisco Veteran's Administration Hospital (SFVAMC) and at the San Francisco General Hospital (SFGH), the latter serving the indigent population of the county. The chairs of the clinical departments were at the Parnassus campus, and vice-chairs of great stature and distinction were placed at the other two sites. Marv Slesinger served as chief at the SFVAMC for many years but was retired when I came to the university. At the SFGH, Merle Sande, a renowned expert in infectious diseases enjoyed engaging the competition at Parnassus with a confrontational style we all admired.

Neuroscience was thriving at UCSF. Zach Hall, who had served on the faculty in the Department of Neurobiology at HMS in the 1970s, was appointed chair of the Department of Physiology, succeeding Fran Ganong, who had been chair for over two decades. Fran was a dear friend during my days in neuroendocrine research at McGill and at the MGH. He sponsored me for the Bowditch Research Lecture of the American Physiological Society when he was president of the group. When Zach replaced Fran he began recruiting, and Mike Stryker, Steve Lisberger, Michael Merzenich and later Alison Doupe came together to form a group in systems neurobiology. I urged them to formulate a plan to renovate space for a center in the sixteen-story research tower and to seek support from the Keck Foundation in Los Angeles. I took the proposal to the program director at the Keck and represented our strengths in neuroscience to their board of directors. We were awarded a substantial sum to form the Keck Center for Integrative Neuroscience, which remains a strong entity on the Parnassus campus.

Other major appointments to basic science positions during those first three years of my deanship included Ira Herskowitz to chair biochemistry and Elizabeth Blackburn—well known for her discovery of the enzyme telomerase, which acts to lengthen the ends of chromosomes—to chair the Department of Microbiology and Immunology. Liz was reluctant to take on this assignment, but I twisted her arm firmly, and she became a terrific addition to our leadership group.

While all the new recruits were filing in, I established a new Dean's Seminar Series that was well attended by graduate students and both basic science and clinical faculty. The seminars dealt with emerging clinical problems that showed great promise of improved therapies from recent research. A patient was usually presented in grand rounds fashion, followed by in-depth reviews of the clinical enigma and the relevant ongoing research.

One month each year I joined the staff at the SFGH, where the neurology department was led initially by Roger Simon and later by Richard Price, a brother of my friend Don Price of Johns Hopkins, to make daily rounds with the residents and students to examine and discuss neurological problems. I enjoyed these sessions immensely and was able to maintain my expertise in the clinical field through these bedside occasions and through my continuing editorship of *Harrison's Principles of Internal Medicine.*

## The Gladstone Institute and HIV-AIDS Research Initiatives at the SFGH

Founded in 1980, The Gladstone Institute was located at the San Francisco General Hospital and grew in stature during my tenure into a formidable organization. Robert Mahley served as its president and worked closely with the board of trustees, which included founding members Richard Brawerman, Richard Jones and David Orgel, who would later be succeeded by Al Dorman. The institute's initial focus was cardiovascular disease, Bob Mahley's area of research. Although independent, all the members of the institute held UCSF faculty appointments, and their recruitment and promotion standards were equivalent to those in UCSF's other strong science and clinical departments.

Among the other distinguished research and clinical activities at the SFGH was the effort led by Merle Sande, chair of medicine at the hospital, focusing on the HIV-AIDS epidemic that at the time was shattering the lives of so many individuals in San Francisco and beyond. Holly Smith, as my associate dean, led lengthy discussions with the Gladstone trustees about expanding the focus of the institute to include HIV-AIDS. In the early 1990s, the institute outlined a program in virology and HIV-AIDS with the recruitment of Warner Greene from Duke University. Holly had known Warner as a productive Howard Hughes Medical Institute (HHMI) investigator. Holly served for many years on the medical advisory board of HHMI, which accounted in part for the great success of appointing HHMI investigators at UCSF.

To accomplish the dramatic expansion of The Gladstone Institute's research portfolio, a new footprint for research laboratories was required. Our solution was to seek approval from the city to construct two floors of research space on top of the building that housed the Department of Pathology at the SFGH. The request was approved, and the new institute, the Gladstone Institute of Virology and Immunology, opened in this new space to great fanfare in 1993.

A decade later, after my return to Harvard Medical School the institute expanded further with the development of a third institute—the Gladstone Institute of Neurological Disease, under the leadership of Lennart Mucke, who had been a resident in neurology with me at the MGH in the 1980s. Lennart had first come to the MGH as a medical student from Germany. I had been so impressed with his intelligence and good-natured ambition that we had offered him a residency slot following internship at the Cleveland Clinic. He was subsequently appointed chief resident and I had urged him to pursue an academic career. He had gone on to the Scripps Clinic to work with Michael Oldstone, and then to UCSF. Some years later, shortly after I had left UCSF to return to Harvard, and in recognition of his accomplishments, Lennart was appointed the Joseph B. Martin Distinguished Professor of Neuroscience at UCSF, which made me very proud indeed!

> The author and wife Rachel in San Francisco on the occasion of daughter Melanie's wedding to Jeffrey Fowler, 1991. Back row, from left: Neil D. Martin, Douglas R. Martin, Jeffrey Fowler, Melanie Martin, Karen (Lenington) Martin, and J. Bradley Martin.

The Gladstone Institute would go on to totally outstrip the available space at the SFGH, and in 2004 it relocated to a five-story new research building adjacent to the UCSF campus at Mission Bay.

## Life in San Francisco

What of our family life? During the first six months in San Francisco Rachel and I lived in a university-owned, two-bedroom apartment about two miles from the main campus while we acquainted ourselves with the different communities in the city. Eventually, we purchased a home on Clayton Street at the end of Parnassus Avenue in the area referred to as Ashbury Heights, a few blocks away from the rough and tumble area of Haight Street, so scarred by the events of the 1960s. We were within walking distance of the medical school. The house was newly renovated and served us well for the next three and a half years.



Rachel became actively involved with me in the social duties of the dean's office. We became an effective fundraising team, working closely with the UCSF Foundation formed by Julie

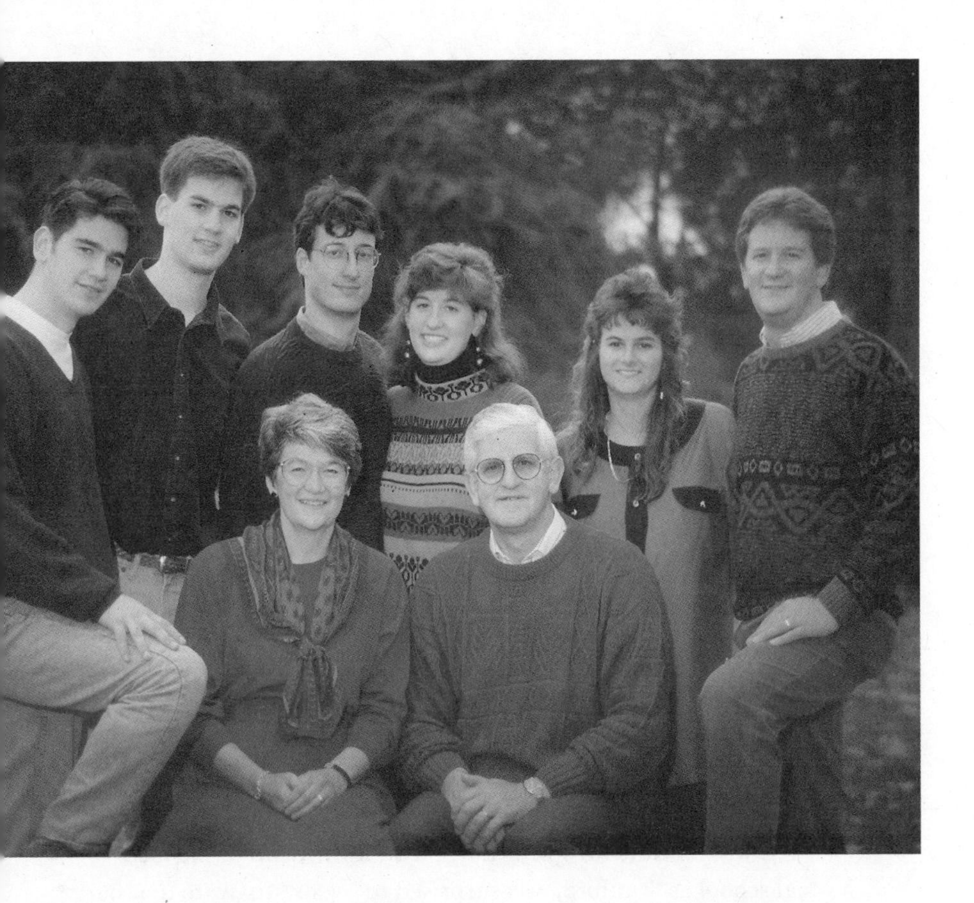

Krevans as a private vehicle to engender support from the community, to encourage our positive presence in the city and to assist in developing the resources needed to upgrade campus facilities.

In June 1992, it was time to attend Melanie's graduation from the Stanford University School of Medicine. She was completing the five-year Scholars in Medicine Program and had matched to the Stanford-affiliated program in primary care / internal medicine at Valley Medical Center in San Jose. At this point Melanie was newly married to Jeff Fowler, whom she had met at a barbecue outside the temporary housing where they both lived. Jeff came to Stanford University as a graduate student in chemical engineering from rural England, southwest of London. His undergraduate work had been at Imperial College in London. He had completed a master's degree in engineering at Washington University in St. Louis before moving on to Palo Alto.

Jeff and Melanie announced their engagement in the summer of 1991 and were married in San Francisco on New Year's Eve that year, six months before her graduation. We were delighted that they chose to be married by the pastor of the First Mennonite Church of San Francisco, Joyce Wyse.

In April, just before Melanie's graduation, Rachel developed progressively more disabling back pain and radiating pain in the right leg, extending to the tip of the great toe. I recall walking with her from our Clayton Street home down the hill to Golden Gate Park. She was disabled with pain on each forward movement of the leg, necessitating short uneven steps. As the symptoms progressed, weakness in upward movement of the right ankle and in extension of the big toe led to consultation with Bob Fishman in neurology, who advised conservative watchful waiting. But with further progression and an MRI scan that revealed a disk fragment within the spinal canal in the L5, S1 space, Charlie Wilson chose to operate, opening the spinal canal (laminectory) followed by removal of the ruptured disk. Surgery was scheduled eight days before Melanie's graduation in late May, and Rachel, stoic through it all, insisted on attending the outdoor ceremony.

It was a beautiful spring day. David Korn, dean of the medical school at Stanford, was surprised to see us, unaware that our daughter had spent five years in his school. Rachel took along a wheelchair but left it in the car as she walked the distance to the football stadium for the formal graduation proceedings and back to the main campus for the follow-up brunch. I heard no complaints from her, and the day ended with great satisfaction all around.

We treasured the friendships that developed during those years on the West Coast. Our social events with Haile and Kim Debas and with Bill and Janet Kerr at their homes or at ours allowed the pressures of our work to defuse and made us even more effective and efficient when we worked together. I also had a close working relationship with Bruce Spaulding that turned into a wonderful personal friendship Rachel and I enjoyed with Bruce and his wife, Dianne. We discussed the many challenges facing UCSF. These discussions became critical to the eventual deliberations at UCSF, leading to the identity and adoption of a site for the second campus at Mission Bay.

Rachel and I joined a book club with Bob and Mary Fishman and Bob and Evie Jaffe. Bob had been chair of the Department of Obstetrics and Gynecology and was an internationally recognized expert on gonadotropin hormones. We were joined by two families of Wallersteins, not related: Bob (a psychoanalytic psychiatrist) and his wife, Judy, a children's psychologist, and Ralph (a distinguished professor of medicine) and Betty. Nancy and Sidney Unobsky and, for a while, the famous venture capitalist John Doerr and his wife, were active in the group. The events were held in rotation among our homes and introduced some of the best discussions about literature (among other things) we ever had.

Holly and Margaret were our close friends and often invited us to their home in Kentfield or to their magnificent country home near the coast in Inverness. We also saw Rudi and Sonya Schmid at these parties.

We learned to love opera, shared ballet tickets with the Schmids and with Mike and Kathryn Bishop, and admired the emerging effective leadership of Michael Tilson Thomas, conductor of the San Francisco Symphony.

The weekends also saw me on campus, but sometimes not in my office! In 1990 I began a regular Sunday morning biking routine. I drove from our home to the bike cage on the street below the Parnassus campus and ventured out on an eighteen-mile ride through Golden Gate Park to the ocean, along the shoreline around Lake Merced, back to Golden Gate Park along Sunset Boulevard to ascend back to the UCSF campus. It was a ride that could be made during the four seasons of the year and yielded some of my fondest recollections of the beauty and uniqueness of our San Francisco experience.

## "Laurel Depths"

By 1992, despite the growth of our programs and collaboration, frustration was mounting over UCSF's failure to resolve space constraints. By the beginning of the third year of my deanship

I was tiring of explaining the failure to reach an agreement over the Laurel Heights issue to the chairs and faculty. Chancellor Krevans was a noble and well-meaning man, but strategic planning was not his forte. Any plans for campus expansion would require resubmission of a new LRDP. Julie Krevans began that process in 1990, but by 1992, it seemed to me that we were proceeding in fits and starts. I reached a level of impatience not ordinarily in my nature and wrote a scathing letter to the chancellor. Although I never did send the letter it read, in part:

*March 10, 1992:*
*I am writing to express my extreme dismay regarding the events of the past few months.*

*We have spent innumerable hours deliberating the "short term" space needs of UCSF. We undertook this "crisis planning" under the assumption that the outgoing President of the University of California a) had a major commitment to the future of UCSF, and b) wanted to be of assistance to us before he left office....*

*When I assumed the position of Dean at UCSF I came with the hope that the Laurel Heights debacle was nearing an end....As we proceed into the next academic year it is apparent that we have made no advance on the space crunch on Parnassus....*

*Julie, we are on the brink of disaster. I can identify ten to fifteen young people whose laboratories are one-third to one-half of the size of those they can occupy at other institutions. We have a very short time window in which to demonstrate to these people that they should stay here....*

Then in the final paragraph I added:

*I believe our crisis has been heightened by the ineffectual planning of the past three months. I would urge you to demonstrate your commitment to finding a way through this morass. We do not have very long.*

My letter made explicit the ineffectiveness of the leadership on the UCSF campus to engage University of California President David Gardner with force about the seriousness of our plight. Nine months later, when Krevans announced his intention to retire, the resolution of the Laurel Heights debacle, dubbed "Laurel Depths" by Holly, seemed as distant as ever, while opposition from community activists continued to grow and spread.

It was regrettable that in place of being recognized by the San Francisco community as a jewel for clinical excellence and research prowess, UCSF was instead plagued by comments about its contribution to radioactive wastes (causing cancer) and support for animal research (cruelty unjustified). These "dangers" made the development of laboratories in a bedroom community surrounding Laurel Heights quite indefensible. This, despite the fact that the *US News & World Report* rankings, as doubtful as their credibility might be, consistently ranked both the medical school and the hospital among the country's top ten, while in total annual NIH support, UCSF was regularly placed in the top two or three in the country. In addition, it was the largest regional employer after the City of San Francisco.

Despite the problems we were having with space, and my worries about the "Laurel Depths," we continued to be successful not only in recruiting able new leadership but also in picking off the best young faculty applicants from around the country. The strong cohesion of the interdepartmental collaborative programs provided powerful incentives for the brightest and best of the emerging generation of new investigators in developmental biology, genetics, structural biology and neuroscience to join the school. We continued to attract the top tier of graduate students, as well as medical students, competing favorably with other top schools such as Harvard, Stanford, Yale and Columbia. I remember one poignant moment as Cori Bargmann and Marc Tessier-Lavigne sat together in my office, Cori coming from a postdoc with Bob Horwitz at MIT and Marc from Tom Jessell's lab at Columbia. They had both turned down offers from many other institutions to join our campus, largely inspired by the cooperative culture of UCSF, especially notable for its welcome of junior faculty and its reputation to support, mentor and promote junior investigators.[10]

## Chancellor

When Julie Krevans announced that he was retiring as chancellor in the summer of 1992 and a search for his successor began,

I wavered between having no personal interest in the position to eventually accepting the invitation of University of California President Jack Peltason to take the job beginning July 1, 1993. I approached Haile Debas and we made a deal. If I took on the challenges of the chancellor position, he would agree to stand as a candidate for the dean's job. After four years as dean, I found myself faced with yet another career move, this one requiring quite a different set of skills from those of an academic leader. I was now in charge of a large campus with a fantastic hospital, four wonderful schools and an incomplete LRDP.

As I began my work as chancellor, two incredible opportunities emerged that my colleagues and I pursued over the next couple of years: emerging discussions with President Gerhard Casper and his colleagues at Stanford about the possible merger of the clinical activities of our two schools, and the search for a campus site to relocate our basic science laboratories.

## Merger Talks between UCSF and Stanford

Gerhard and I had first met in October 1994, at a California Business and Higher Education Forum in Palm Springs. After a particularly sobering presentation on the challenges facing academic health centers brought about by anticipated cutbacks in Medicare reimbursements, we found ourselves together on a walk between sessions, musing about how it could be different. We talked about the duplication of expert tertiary care services, expensive redundant activities and the ongoing need to purchase or upgrade expensive equipment; each of these factors, of course, make it very difficult to break even in the business of medical care delivery. We agreed to convene a small group of our leaders, principally the deans of our medical schools and the heads of our hospitals to discuss the matter.

The notion of greater cooperation between our schools had actually surfaced two years earlier when I met with Dean David Korn, a pathologist who had been the dean during my daughter Melanie's tenure as a medical student. The two of us had met for lunch in a restaurant in Burlingame, midway between our campuses, to think about collaborative efforts in research and education. These discussions, however, had never progressed further while I was dean.

The Stanford and UCSF discussion was carried on by a group that met regularly at the president's house on the Stanford campus over the late fall and early winter. By the spring of 1996, we were ready to share our thoughts with the department chairs of our respective institutions.

I had a terrific team at UCSF. Bill Kerr was CEO of the hospital, Haile Debas was dean of the school of medicine and the three of us worked seamlessly to advance our vision for UCSF. Haile had just recruited Lee Goldman from the Brigham and Women's Hospital in Boston to be chief of medicine at UCSF. Bill and Haile both joined in the Stanford discussions with open minds to explore the feasibility of greater cooperation.

The Stanford participants were Peter Van Etten, CEO of the Stanford medical enterprise, and replacing David Korn was Eugene Bauer, the new dean. Victor Dzau, a cardiologist, was chairman of medicine at Stanford. I had known Victor from his days at the Brigham and Women's Hospital in Boston, where we had collaborated on some endocrine research related to cardiovascular regulation.

The meeting with the chairs raised more issues of skepticism than promises of collegial interaction, but Gerhard and I pressed on, planning to present our thoughts to our respective administration boards in late spring. The task ahead was easier for Gerhard because the private board of Stanford University met without requirements for public disclosure. I, on the other hand, faced the more arduous task of having to prepare the regents of the University of California to consider a public–private merger of our clinical enterprise.

To gain another perspective on the matter, I proposed the idea of an outside committee to review the implications of a clinical merger to the regents, which they accepted. The committee consisted of Warren Hellman, an investment banker in San Francisco; Sam Thier, head of the MGH and former president of the Institute of Medicine in Washington; and Richard Rosenberg, an executive at the headquarters of the Bank of America. Their deliberations, carried out with dispatch, lent renewed credibility to the enterprise. They reasoned that the fundamental changes in the marketplace placed competitive enterprises such as ours at a disadvantage and that a merger would facilitate the next era of clinical development and forge a partnership without equal anywhere on the West Coast.

By June, however, the UCSF regents were sharply divided over the idea. The leader of the opposition camp was Frank Clark, a corporate lawyer who lived in Los Angeles and who pictured himself as the regents' watchdog over all matters relating to the five hospitals of the UC system. In Los Angeles, he was often a hostile observer of the UCLA hospital activities led by Chancellor Charles Young and Dean Gerald Levy, and was viewed by some as a vigilante.

Frank required special private auditions before any important event went to the full board of regents. So Bill Kerr, Haile and I made the visit to his estate in Los Angeles to argue the pros and cons of a hookup with Stanford. He listened politely as we presented our perspective, and we came out of the meeting convinced that we had made the case. We were wrong! The June meeting of the board of regents was a disaster. Frank went vocal at a public session of the meeting declaring his opposition to the idea, specifically noting that the Stanford Hospital was not in the same league as UCSF, that we would sacrifice quality of care through this proffered alignment and that he would do everything he could to prevent it. His views were widely disseminated in the Bay Area media, where he accused me and my colleagues of cooking the documents and of not fully sharing all the financial and programmatic downsides with the board. Some of his allegations were particularly painful. In a word, he publicly called us deceivers and liars. I personally felt I had been pistol-whipped and publicly humiliated.

We were not sure of how we should proceed. Regent meetings over the summer were less frequent. Bill, Haile and I agreed with our Stanford colleagues to stand down from any further definitive discussions while we considered the options and the strategy to take. The events were not conducive to putting aside an emerging opportunity that I would soon learn about regarding the position of dean at Harvard Medical School. I looked

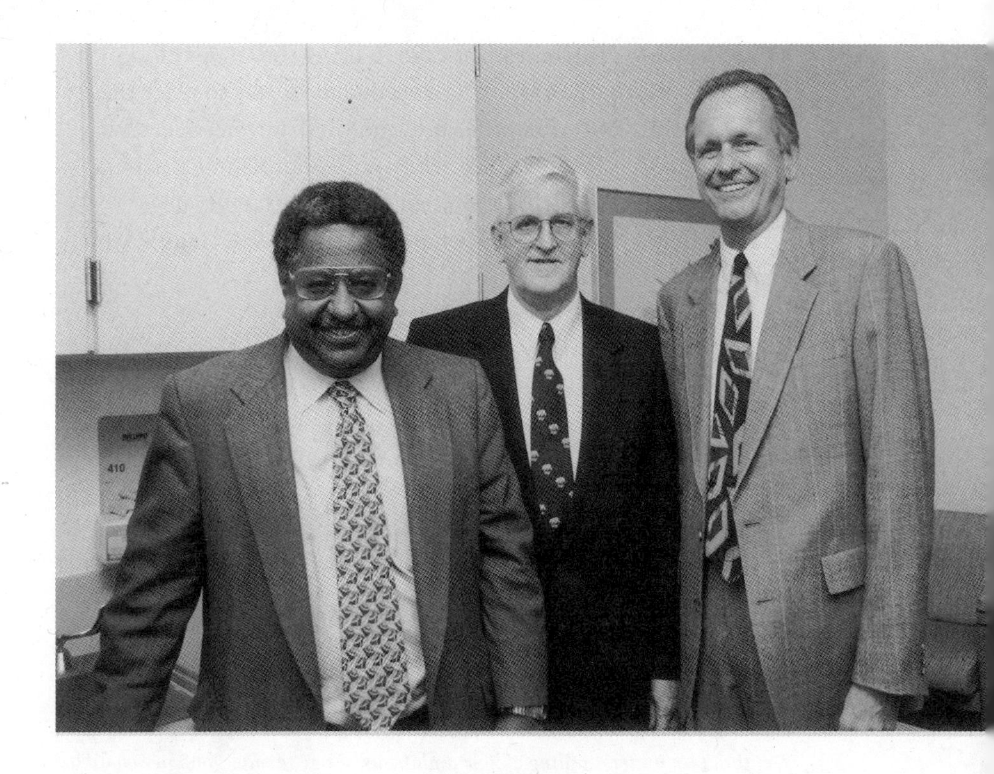


forward to getting away that summer to New Hampshire to clear my mind and contemplate my options for the future

The author with colleagues Dean Haile Debas (left) and Hospital Director William Kerr (right) at UCSF, 1995.

By the early fall, the dust from the media storm had settled and merger talks were re-established. The regents agreed to the formalities of the arrangement. Frank Clark persisted in opposition but was outvoted by other members of the regents. But I was becoming distracted by this time because I was actively engaged in talks to return to Harvard, as dean of the medical school.

When I returned to Harvard in the summer of 1997, it was with the full confidence in the leadership of the two universities, both at the trustee (Stanford) and regent (University of California) level and of the senior administrative staff in both hospital settings. I expected the approved merger to move forward with growing pains, no doubt, but ultimately for the benefit of everyone—students, staff, faculty, and, of course, the patients. How wrong I was.

The first signs of trouble arose after the appointment of Peter Van Etten from Stanford as CEO of the new enterprise, leaving

UCSF's Bill Kerr at a disadvantage to bring the troops along from the northern campus. The second error was to place the administrative staff in office buildings halfway between the two campuses, near Candlestick Park in South San Francisco, where ownership of the combined entities by faculty never fully emerged. I shared my perspective with Steve Hauser, who responded:

*You did not mention the decision by Bill Kerr not to assume the role of CEO, after it was assumed by all that he would take this on. Bill's notification to us that he would not take on this role was a major blow to the confidence of faculty at both institutions.*

Steve then went on to say:

*As the merger evolved in its early months, another problem was a failure to project a consistent vision in terms of the ultimate organizational relationship between the institutions, or the range of possibilities that would be reasonable to consider. It was difficult to plan coordinated clinical services without an understanding of how ambitious our academic synergies could be or should be.*

In short, the plan unraveled in a painful way over the next two years despite all efforts by community leaders such as Warren Hellman and Regent Howard Leach, on the UCSF side, and trustees like Isaac Stein on the Stanford side. After my move back to Boston in 1997, I was succeeded by Haile Debas, who served as chancellor for a year before the appointment of J. Michael Bishop. I kept in touch with all of them, doing what I could to encourage my colleagues Haile Debas and Bill Kerr to press on. The failure was the result of several emerging contentious issues that are skillfully outlined in detail by John A. Kastor in his book *Mergers of Teaching Hospitals in Boston, New York, and Northern California.*[11] Significant among these concerns was a growing reluctance by the department chairs to fully execute the details that would integrate clinical services, which had been such a powerful initial motivation for the merger. The exception was in pediatrics, where Larry Shapiro, chair of pediatrics at UCSF, and Harvey Cohen from Stanford sought arrangements that were clearly of benefit to the faculty and patients. Another reason for the failure was a growing perception that the UCSF infrastructure in information technology lagged behind modernization already partially executed at Stanford. This raised concerns that a siphoning of funds might result from the south campus to the north.

In the end, it came apart with great sadness on my part and not without some persistent concern that had I stayed the outcome might have been different, although I seriously doubt that such would have been the case.

I had an opportunity to reflect on the circumstances in a chat with Bill Kerr. His feels that the "principal reason for the failure was trying to bring together two very different cultures—in San Francisco a public university with a strong commitment to offering services to all comers, versus a private hospital (Stanford) that depended on the 'carriage' trade. Furthermore, there were disparities in the salaries of the clinical faculty—Stanford paying more—and when this became evident to UCSF faculty members, demands surfaced for equity."

Bill was very pensive when he added, "Then there was the nurse's strike at the Packard Children's Hospital at Stanford. When Peter [Van Etten (the head of the Stanford Health System)] capitulated, the effect on UCSF, with the California Nurses Association, was instantaneous. All of our nursing costs escalated almost overnight."

Bill feels that the effort collapsed when the Stanford faculty revolted supported by their dean, Eugene Bauer, despite strong encouragement on the part of Gerhard Casper to make it work. The result was that it came apart despite continuing efforts by business leaders from the regents and the UCSF family who tried to keep it on track. By 1999 the parties had negotiated an exodus from the agreement that left many wounded by the whole episode.

"I still believe it was the right thing to do," Bill told me.

## The Continued Search for a New Research Location

The relocation of research activities and the speedy alleviation of the stranglehold of space constraints that had been imposed on the Parnassus campus by the 1976 agreement was an issue

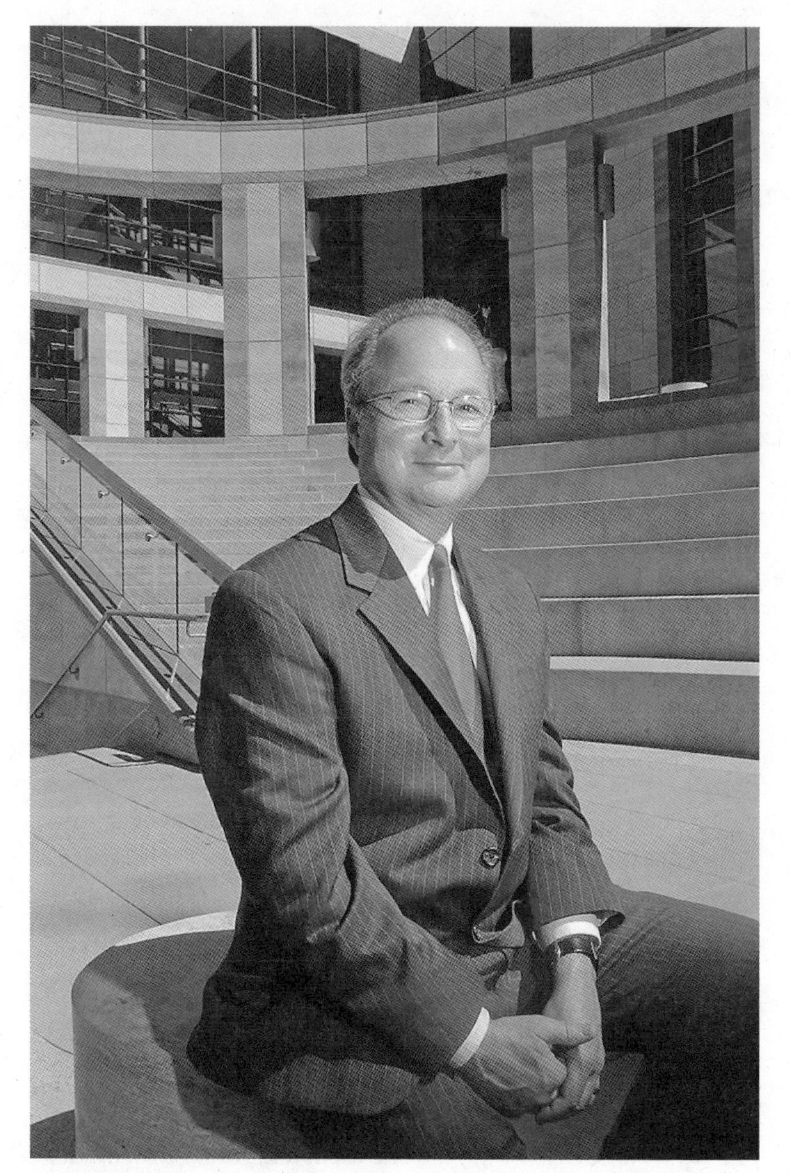
Bruce Spaulding.

that dominated the years I was at UCSF, and it was the second major issue I faced as chancellor of UCSF. By 1993, as I began my tenure as campus leader, many of the senior faculty and my own associate deans pressed for a solution to the research space impasse, urging expansion on the tightly packed Parnassus site. The challenge to doing so was not insignificant.

The 1976 agreement, reached between Julie Krevans as dean and Phil Lee as chancellor on the one hand, and the neighborhood on the other, had already been breached in the 1980s with the construction of small projects. By 1990 that limit had been exceeded by several hundred thousand square feet, although such calculations depended on the exact methods used to measure existing structures, some of which were nearly a century old, highly inefficient and subject to earthquake damage. The completion of a new library in 1992, a justifiable pride of Chancellor Krevans, sealed the issue for the community activists, who demanded the removal of the old University Hall to deactivate space to abide by the space ceiling agreement. Completion of the new library provided space for renovation of the old library into a much-needed medical education center and some laboratories. The laboratories provided space for the recruitment of Stephen Hauser as chair of the neurology department.

As I assumed the chancellorship, the advice given by Vice-chancellor Bruce Spaulding, with which I quickly agreed, was that there was grave danger to the entire LRDP process if there remained even the façade of a possibility that the regents' agreement of 1976 would be abrogated. I concluded that it was unwise to do so, recognizing the long-term damage of engaging in such a contentious issue to the campus, while still in litigation over the Laurel Heights home for the school of pharmacy. Such additional litigation would stall every avenue of strategic initiative. My response was to declare, openly and unequivocally, that no effort would ever be made during my administration to break the covenant made by the regents.

But this decision required moving toward a new solution, and community support would be needed to achieve this goal. The strategy Spaulding and I took was to meet directly with the local community activists, among whom were prominent lawyers and other professionals who lived in the Parnassus Heights area, to make the case that we understood their concerns about any increase in density at the main campus. At the same time, we asked them to appreciate the value UCSF brought to the city as a whole, to listen to our dilemma and be advocates while we tried to convince city authorities of UCSF's need for a new home within the city limits or close by. We argued that if the university was to remain competitive in the world of expanding basic and clinical research, education and patient care, new space and perhaps a new campus was essential. We initiated the process by meeting in the chancellor's office with a small cadre of four or five of the most influential leaders in the community. Bruce Spaulding spoke of the space crisis we faced and of the need for successful strategic planning required by the LRDP.

We hoped for an open comprehensive analysis, in partnership with the community activists, of the many sites currently housing university activities. These sites included the San Francisco General Hospital, the VA hospital and other sites that had to be rented as a result of the space crunch. To accomplish this, we needed to create a viable plan for the Laurel Heights campus (see Map 5). Taking each of these factors into consideration, we needed a community advisory group (CAG) with a membership of thirty to forty, structured to represent local communities all over the city. These meetings, I hoped, would give a new sense of transparency and openness that would serve everyone's needs.

Bruce went about restructuring the CAG to meet these objectives and would meet with them on a monthly basis for the next three years as we developed the environmental impact report (EIR) that met with court approval, making possible a new plan for Laurel Heights. As part of the plan, we agreed to use Laurel Heights for a new campus to house a Center for Social and Behavioral Sciences, led by Professor Nancy Adler. The successful completion of the LRDP, approved by the regents in 1997, was made possible by the symbolic act of honoring past agreements and a call for collaborative engagement with the community without foregone conclusions. The school of pharmacy remained cramped in its former quarters.

So by the summer of 1995, Vice-chancellor Bruce Spaulding and I had some important fact-finding to do. Expansion was essential, or UCSF's fabled biomedical research community would be in jeopardy through attrition, through either the loss of key faculty or failure to recruit promising young people. But we were required to do any analysis that we felt necessary within the structure of the LRDP now already underway.

Following lessons I'd learned from Dean Rudi Schmid, who had preceded me in the dean's office, we took advantage of two important initiatives. The first was to work collaboratively with the school of dentistry, led by Dean John Greene, to continue to search jointly for outstanding biomedical scientists to occupy dental school space and to strengthen research there with space otherwise unavailable to the school of medicine. The second was to recruit brilliant young investigators through the power of the UCSF community structure, to whichever department had an open position and a state-funded FTE (full-time equivalent, or full-time position).

Michael Bishop, who with colleague Harold Varmus had shared the Nobel Prize in 1989 for their discovery of oncogenes, had a profound impact on the UCSF science community with the establishment of the Program in Biological Sciences (PIBS). Membership in the PIBS was a status symbol given only to the best basic scientists in either the preclinical or clinical departments. PIBS became a powerful example of collegial interaction that served us well during recruitments as well as a landmark of success in graduate PHD education, attracting the best and the brightest from across the US. Junior faculty members of great distinction were recruited by these promises of collaboration within UCSF to the departments of anatomy and pharmacology with appointments that would not have fit well with the traditional slots in comparable departments around the country.

At the same time, during this period there were several major losses from the basic science community. Marc Kirschner had gone to HMS to start a new Department of Cell Biology, a merger of the departments of anatomy and physiology. Harold Varmus went to direct the NIH, and Zach Hall soon followed to head the National Institute of Neurological Disorders and Stroke. Finally, Bruce Alberts became president of the National Academy of Sciences, a position he would hold for two six-year terms.



## Initiating the Search for a New Campus



In our search for a new campus, Vice-chancellor Bruce Spaulding and I began what became for me a tremendously profitable learning experience. Bruce had come from Fresno, California, where he worked as a county administrator after a prior posting as the county manager in Las Vegas. He joked that if he could deal with the Las Vegas mafia, he was up to dealing with the neighborhood cliques in San Francisco and schmoozing with San Francisco Mayor Willie Brown. Bruce had been recruited by Julie Krevans and would prove to be a terrific colleague during the extensive search for a new campus location. Preferences for location varied among the faculty, in part based on where they lived—in the City of San Francisco, north in Marin County, across the Bay Bridge in Oakland, or in adjacent suburban regions. Others on the faculty wanted to take over the derelict buildings of the Letterman Army Research Laboratory in the Presidio, a concrete fortress of a research building then over forty years old that was to be vacated imminently and shut down (see Map 5).

The Presidio lab was Holly Smith's first choice, and I received him quite regularly in the chancellor's office when he presented detailed plans of how to secure the site. There was also pressure from Congresswoman Nancy Pelosi who saw our location in the Presidio as a viable use of the vacated army facility. I was suspicious of its location adjacent to a wealthy San Francisco neighborhood and foresaw more problems than opportunities in taking on another community resistance group over UCSF's spread in the city. The facility was in many ways a military bunker built in concrete with very few windows and little flexibility for renovation. I foresaw enormous expense in upgrading the facility to house modern molecular techniques. I rejected this option and we moved on.

The results of the search Bruce and I conducted came down to three options. The first was a large space of vacant land adjacent to Route 101 immediately south of the city in the suburb of Brisbane, exactly halfway between UCSF and the San Francisco International Airport, an area known for its windy and foggy character. It was across the highway from Candlestick Park where the baseball Giants played in the spring, summer and fall, and where the football 49ers shared space in the fall. It was also not far from the headquarters of the biotech company Genentech.

The plot of land had been purchased by Mr. Yu-How Chen, a Taiwanese billionaire businessman who intended to build multiple high-rise apartment complexes similar in dimension to those he had so successfully built in Taipei. Mr. Chen, or Chairman Chen, as he preferred to be addressed, was an affable man, and Bruce and I spent many hours, even days, negotiating with him. In 1995 we traveled to Taipei and met with him in his imposing office headquarters, which housed his Tuntex Corporation. We visited Kaohsiung, in the southern region of Taiwan, to see the emerging highest skyscraper then under construction anywhere in Southeast Asia.

Referring to the Chairman's land, Bruce reminisced that it was:

*Approximately 15 acres in San Francisco, at Executive Park zoned for office, biotech and housing. He also had 526 acres on the other side of Route 101, slightly to the south. These holdings were in the City of Brisbane....The General Plan for the City of Brisbane, developed in 2000, called for a "mixed use development with residential, office, biotech, a golf course, entertainment, retail and hotels."...Our talks with the Chairman and our MOU [memorandum of understanding] were about 89 acres on the Brisbane site. His donation was the 89 acres in Brisbane.*

Chairman Chen envisioned the UCSF basic science campus we proposed to build as the anchor tenant for his development of a major residential business complex spaced over more than 200 acres. A major downside was the fact that the site was a landfill that had included treated garbage, and the problems of toxic materials could not be ruled out. We foresaw great difficulty in getting the regents of the University of California to approve, even tentatively, any site that might carry such liabilities. Mr. Chen was so eager to make a deal that he seemed prepared to underwrite any clean-up required, however, so we kept the option on the table.

We used the Chen offer as a leading asset as we advanced our exploration to consider other potential sites for an expanded UCSF presence. We signed a memorandum of understanding in which Chen agreed to the donation of land. We used this as a trump card in setting up a "contest" between a location in

Brisbane and another in Harbor Bay in Alameda County, which were two viable options outside of San Francisco.

The second potential solution was to build the campus across the bay in Alameda. The site was a tract of land adjacent to a naval base on a portion of the island of Alameda called Harbor Bay. If we chose to relocate there, we would need to provide a ferry service to connect faculty and students to the San Francisco location of the Parnassus campus. The property was owned by Ron Cowan, a wealthy developer whose mansion graced the very top of the peak of Tiburon to the north in Marin County. The site was available immediately. We explored the ferry option, looked at the fiscal viability of providing shuttle service and took the twenty-minute ride across the bay in a boat Mr. Cowan brought along for the occasion. The sales pitch from Mr. Cowan had us interested for several months, but the driving distance across the Bay Bridge for those living in San Francisco or north in Marin County seemed unacceptable. The notion of a ferry commute soon became unrealistic when we analyzed the traffic required to make it a financial success. Alameda was not a routine point of landing for ferries from the ferry building north of the Bay Bridge in San Francisco. To create a new landing south of the bridge seemed highly impractical and created other issues, with respect to parking, for example.

We moved on to the third choice, which would eventually emerge as the preferred solution to our relocation woes. The area located south of the Bay Bridge in San Francisco was a vast urban wasteland of an old railway yard (see Map 5). It was called Mission Bay for historical reasons, having once been the mouth of Mission Creek before the extensive reclamation of land in the area by landfill, coming mostly from the rubble of the great earthquake of 1906. The entire area of over three hundred acres was owned by the Catellus Corporation, a southern California commercial development company. They were eager to explore a link to UCSF and proposed a sale of up to thirty acres to the university for about $5 million an acre, amounting to a total sale value of about $150 million. We knew that number was untenable, not only because of our limited resources but also because the university did not generally favor private land deals.

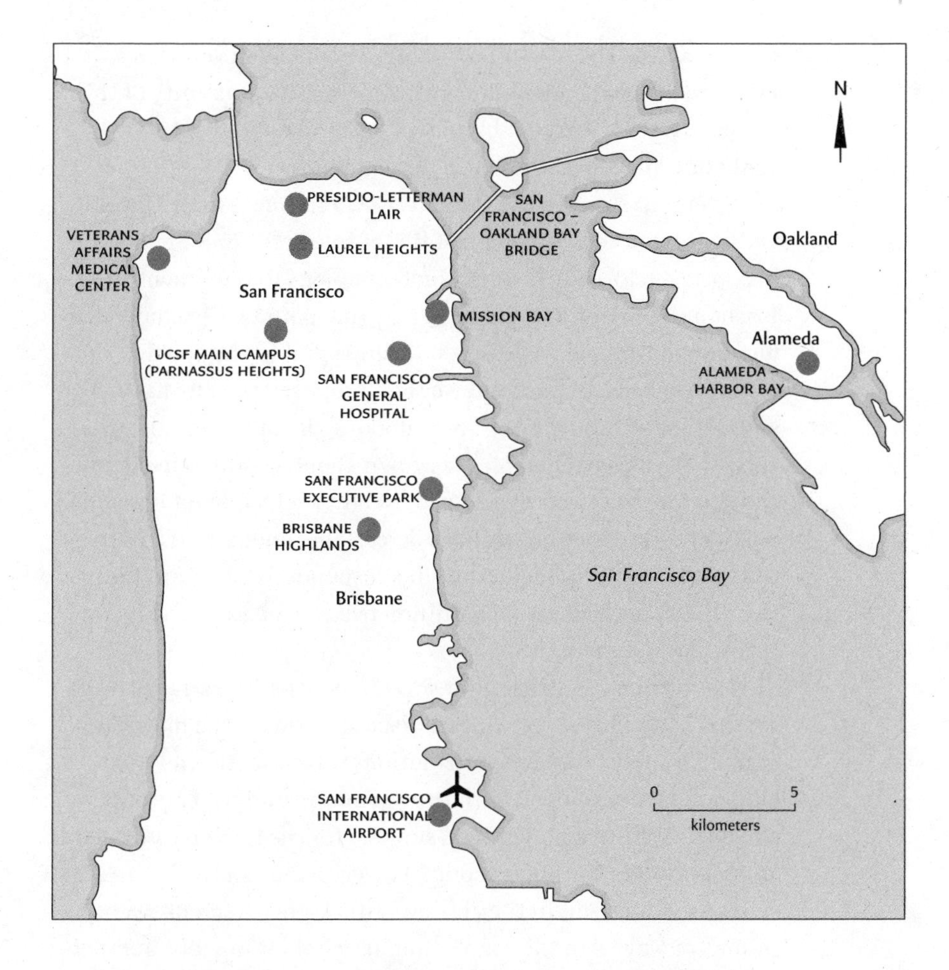


Map 5: UCSF and vicinity: the search for a new campus.

The Catellus project we were interested in was in its earliest stages of planning. Catellus itself was undergoing a transition in leadership with the appointment of Nelson Rising, who seemed to be more flexible in our discussions than his predecessor, who I never met, was. We met with Nelson, and over the course of several meetings suggested a proposal: the university space would be the anchor tenant for a mixed development site that would eventually include housing, commercial entities, shops and restaurants. This development, we reasoned, could hopefully encourage development of a San Francisco–based biotechnology industry. He showed great interest in our proposal. Up to this time, despite the great success stories of companies like Genentech, located in South San Francisco, and Chiron, located across the bay in Emeryville, there had never been a San Francisco–based biotechnology business. The proximity of the university, with its great history of entrepreneurial activities, could become a nidus for such development.

We emphasized to the Catellus Corporation, and to Mayor Willie Brown, that we had an offer of free land from Mr. Chen in a location already favoring biotechnology development in Brisbane, south of San Francisco. At this point, we excluded the location in Alameda as essentially unworkable and too distant from the main campus, and we then proposed the outrageous suggestion of asking Catellus to make a gift of land to the university. We approached Mayor Brown about a commitment from the city for street access and urban rights, which *in toto* provided a plot of forty-three contiguous acres, large enough for a potential campus development. Catellus responded that the value of their land approached $200 million because of its potential for future development.

Negotiations continued for several months. To gain approval for this approach we continued discussions with the mayor to gain his support for city contributions. The effective relationships we had developed with the community advisory group served us well. We had gained support for the university's need to expand to maintain its competitive position in the biomedical sciences. A location in the city, even if it were fifteen or twenty minutes away from the main campus, would bring jobs and new industries. The location would also facilitate interactions across the Bay Bridge with UC Berkeley, where UCSF had a major collaborative graduate program in bioengineering. We felt that the site would encourage biotechnology and medical device companies to locate and interact with the UCSF and UC Berkeley research communities. We took several precautions in our evaluation of the site, including depth-core testing the entire area to find the cleanest site for the potential new campus.

A formal agreement was reached in December of 1996, with the final agreement put into writing on January 16, 1997. We finalized plans to publicly announce the agreement, which specifically included the plans to develop UCSF at the Mission site. The gift of the land was booked at $166 million, the largest gift ever recorded at UCSF. The Catellus Corporation agreed to donate thirty acres of land to the university. The city, taking into account the need for city streets under any commercial or residential development plan, agreed to cede space calculated at approximately thirteen acres for the development of green space on the new campus.

The outcome of the discussions led to the formation of the Bay Area Life Sciences Alliance (BALSA), with strong leadership support from key individuals like William J. Rutter, who had founded Chiron while a member of the faculty of UCSF, and of businessmen like Donald Fisher, chairman of Gap clothing stores, and Warren Hellman, a wealthy investor from San Francisco. Bill Rutter headed the group. Warren, as previously noted, had served as one of three outside members who had strongly supported the merger of UCSF and Stanford and would continue to work to bring the effort to a final outcome after I had returned to Boston. The financial and political support we received from these visionary leaders was invaluable. Other notables from the city included Bob Burke, Sandy Robertson, Gerson Bakar and Rudi Nothenberg. Robertson was CEO of an investment banking concern, and Rudi was a former key person in the mayor's office, whose support gave great credibility to our efforts with Mayor Willie Brown. BALSA members provided strategic wisdom, funded the $2 million master plan and also paid for the site tests that we performed.

In 2011 Bruce Spaulding recalled the inner workings of the deliberations with the Catellus Corporation, as well as Bob Burke's key role in the negotiations:

*The way negotiations worked with Catellus/Nelson Rising, was that we had negotiating sessions on Wednesday afternoons. Robin Jones, a representative of the office of the president, and I handled these until Bob Burke volunteered to join us. For the last six months, Bob participated with passion and vigor as a volunteer. To Nelson, he represented all the powerful folks on the BALSA board and UCSF's Foundation leadership. The negotiating sessions required preparation, and there was a period of time when Bob was spending between twenty and twenty-five hours a week between the actual sessions and getting ready for them.*

The proposal experienced easy sailing through the often tough-minded board of regents with the support of all the parties involved, and by the spring of 1997 the strategic plan was approved, and the course set into motion to create the Mission Bay Campus of the University of California in San Francisco. When I resigned in June 1997 to return to Harvard, my successor as chancellor, Haile Debas, ably led the next phase of planning until J. Michael Bishop was appointed chancellor in July 1998.

The lessons learned from this adventure were many. First and foremost was the importance of establishing a CAG whose members came to appreciate the needs of the university. The novel arrangements with a major developer willing to take on a risky adventure with a not-for-profit entity and a mayor ready to help his friends on the campus, were all factors that played in the final outcome.

## Looking Back

Nobel Prizes bracketed my tenure at UCSF. Mike Bishop and Harold Varmus received the award for their work on oncogenes in October 1989. When the Monday morning announcement came, I was in Boston preparing for our move. I missed the celebration but spoke with Mike and Harold on the phone. Ten years later, after I had just returned to Harvard, my friend and colleague neurologist Stanley Prusiner received the prize for his work on prions, infectious proteins that cause spongioform encephalopathy like that found in mad cow disease (bovine spongioform encephalopathy) and in Jakob-Creutzfeldt disease. I was sad to have missed the champagne that flowed early that morning in San Francisco. Perhaps if I had stayed on, I might have been invited to the Stockholm celebrations.

Rachel and I often reflect on the partnership we enjoyed as we jointly undertook the responsibilities of the office of chancellor. I cannot express adequately the tremendous value Rachel gave to our professional experiences. She provided gracious hospitality to hundreds at our social events and gave me wise counsel and support in the successful fundraising required to complete UCSF's first capital campaign, an amount that exceeded $500 million.

Outside the sphere of work, we were privileged to enjoy the luxury of living in the chancellor's residence those four years. The incredible house designed by an American architect, George Rockrise, had the feel of a Frank Lloyd Wright creation. (The architect, whom we had the privilege to meet, did not appreciate my reference to the similarity—professional sensitivity, no doubt.) It was constructed in 1964 and had been the home of four chancellors before us. We enjoyed the ambience very much. It was perched on the side of Mt. Sutro, which ascends steeply above the Parnassus campus in the midst of seventeen acres of pine and eucalyptus forest, with a 180-degree view northward. The view encompasses a small piece of the Pacific Ocean and the Golden Gate Bridge, sweeping across San Francisco Bay to Oakland and the Bay Bridge. The vantage provided spectacular views of the features of a wonderful city: the fog rolling in regularly in the afternoon, the city lights incandescent in the moonlight, the hum of the city from the balcony, as well as a vista of birds, including red-tailed hawks, crows and, on occasion, eagles.

We loved living there and spent many happy evenings with our family and with friends and university acquaintances. We were blessed to have had several years with close proximity to Melanie and her new family. While we were in San Francisco, Melanie and Jeff welcomed a son, Gareth, at Stanford University Hospital on August 28, 1995. There was more joy when Brad and Karen and Josh and Courtney moved to Sunnyvale, an hour's drive away, as Brad was transferred there by his company, Analog Devices. They were there for two delightful years and then moved back to Boston in 1997, the same year Rachel and I did. In 1997 Melanie and Jeff welcomed Charlotte to the world in their new home in Basel, Switzerland, where Jeff had been transferred in his job with the pharmaceutical company, Novartis.

If San Francisco had been such a success, why did we choose to move back to Boston? Although the experience at UCSF proved amicable and in the end likely the right thing to do, it did limit Rachel's emerging opportunities for further study and engagement in an area of her own interest. Reflecting back now on our time in San Francisco, I cannot break away from the gnawing sense of guilt over the personal sacrifice that Rachel made for me when we moved there. I hope our shared experiences in the wonderful community of San Francisco assuage to some degree the trouble I caused for her.

The return to Boston, to a job I swore I'd never be interested in, was driven by a combination of factors. First there was dissatisfaction over the public duties inherent in a position as leader of a major research campus, with little opportunity for direct contact with students and close participation in academic planning of the research mission. Second, to our surprise, our children had all returned to the East Coast, three to Boston and Melanie and Jeff, who after two years in Switzerland were to move to North Carolina. With a job offer on the table, grandchildren present and arriving, and Rachel interested in moving back east, we chose to do so.

My letter of November 1996, announcing my resignation to University President Richard Atkinson, was not an easy one to write and followed a difficult period of contemplation. My decision to resign was taken principally, I explained to the president, because of my desire to return to a more intimate connection with the science and practice of medicine, which I had difficulty sustaining in my role as chancellor. And, I wrote:

*Timing is never perfect in the making of life's decisions. We are, after lengthy deliberations, poised to embark on one of the most important and influential mergers in the history of academic medicine. It was deeply gratifying to me to read the conclusions of the Hellman Committee's review regarding the UCSF-Stanford merger. Their findings confirm my own convictions regarding the importance of this action...*

*In many ways, my decision comes at a timely moment:*

- *We have just completed the first capital campaign for UCSF, raising more than a half billion dollars. Annual contributions to the campus have exceeded $100 million in each of the last three years.*
- *We have completed the work on our long-range development plan, and I believe that the regents will be very pleased with the recommendations that we will bring to them for approval in January.*
- *Relations with our neighbors in San Francisco have improved dramatically over the past few years. This can be attributed, I believe, to extensive consultation with the community in the LRDP planning and in deciding*

*wisely not to resurrect the controversial question about changing the ceiling on space at the Parnassus campus.*

- *An exciting plan has been developed for the use of Laurel Heights, including the development there of a Center for Social, Behavioral and Health Policy Studies. The plan received regental approval last year following extensive consultation to resolve a decade of community and legal controversy over the use of the facility.*
- *We are completing the building program and faculty recruitment to establish a National Cancer Institute designated Comprehensive Cancer Center at the UCSF–Mount Zion campus. Our cancer research building—the first new research building for UCSF in many years—will be dedicated in a few months.*

In the end, I continued, my decision had to be placed within the perspective of what I wanted to do with the rest of my academic life. Having served as dean and chancellor, I knew that as dean at HMS, I could share directly in the enormous gratification of participating fully in the academic life of the institution, and interact directly with individual students and faculty. But:

*I wish this decision could be as easy as following the advice of Yogi Berra—when you come to a fork in the road, take it! But clearly it is not. I will miss UCSF and all its wonderful people very much....*

# EIGHT

# *Return to Harvard Medical School*

SPRING IN SAN FRANCISCO is a rejuvenating experience, particularly for those of us who have only known Canadian and New England winters. The crocuses bloom in February, the azaleas in early March and the tulips of the Tulip Festival at the Queen Wilhelmina Dutch Windmill in Golden Gate Park are in full majestic bloom by late March.

## An Invitation from Neil Rudenstine

It was early April 1996 when I received a phone call from President Neil Rudenstine of Harvard University, inviting me to have dinner with him during his coming visit to San Francisco. He wanted my advice about the search he had recently begun for a successor to Dan Tosteson, dean at Harvard Medical School.

Tosteson, whose deanship was concluding after a remarkable twenty years, a record almost unique to medical school deanships in the late twentieth century in the United States, had agreed to stay on for an additional four years when invited to do so after Neil's appointment as president in July 1991. Dan

Tosteson's tenure was celebrated for the introduction of a new medical school curriculum in the 1980s, featuring small group tutorials focusing on clinical cases. Problem-based learning had been championed by other schools as early as the 1960s, for example at Case Western Reserve University, and in the 1970s at McMaster University in Hamilton, Ontario, but the imprimatur given to case-based tutorial teaching by Harvard served as a catalyst for the transformation of medical education worldwide. Despite the stellar achievements in the area of medical education, however, many faculty members at HMS thought that the last years of the Tosteson deanship suffered from deteriorating relationships among the hospitals affiliated with Harvard and felt that the dean's office often seemed disconnected from the daily activities of the faculty.

Neil Rudenstine had prepared for the search with great care. He had consulted widely within and without the university and had formed a large faculty advisory committee that included basic scientists and hospital-based faculty. When he called me in 1996, consultations had been underway for over a year. We met for dinner at the Ritz-Carlton Hotel on Stockton Street in San Francisco, where he was staying. It was my first encounter with this kind, gracious, Renaissance scholar. He inquired about my time in San Francisco, allowed that he understood there were some exciting activities going on there, and then we spent the rest of our time together discussing the challenges and opportunities at HMS, and the search for a new dean. I made some suggestions for potential candidates for the position, and as the evening wore on, we became comfortable with each other. But there was neither a hint of his interest in me as a candidate nor did I have an interest in the position.

I was reminded of a conversation with Rachel as we traveled to San Francisco seven years before, driving the 3,000 miles from Boston to the West Coast. As I reflected on the job ahead in San Francisco, I had commented that there was one aspect of the new job that already brought me great comfort. So unlike the situation in Boston and at Harvard and my experience at the Massachusetts General Hospital: at the University of California San Francisco we would own our own hospital!

I had always felt a trifle embarrassed when Dean Tosteson visited the MGH during one of our General Executive Committee meetings of the hospital department heads, held each Wednesday morning. He seemed estranged from the inner workings of the hospital as we knew it. His reports on HMS activities were perfunctory and largely irrelevant to our hospital community.

Tosteson tried to bridge the gap between the school and our world by inviting some of the chiefs to his office once a year with our hospital CEO—in my case Robert Buchanan—for a review of my department's activities, its opportunities and challenges. I appreciated his effort and felt that he was engaged and interested.

Even so, it was after one of Dean Tosteson's visits to the MGH that I commented to Rachel, "That is a job I would never take." How wrong I was!

Flash forward twelve years: Neil Rudenstine called again in July of 1996 to ask whether my family and I would be spending the month of August in New Hampshire. I had mentioned to him how much we treasured our vacation each summer in the Lake District in Meredith, and had indicated that we would be going there again. This was the first occasion where he asked whether I might personally be interested in the position of dean at HMS. The timing could not have been better: the accusations leveled at me by the regents in June of that year were still festering like a boil, and I felt enervated and depressed.

I agreed to meet with Neil's faculty advisory group at the Harvard president's house in Cambridge in mid-August. The group included basic science department chairs Phil Leder and Gerry Fischbach, both of whom were said to be interested in the job; Marc Kirschner, who had arrived five years earlier from UCSF to chair a new Department of Cell Biology; and Barbara McNeil, chair of the Department of Health Care Policy. I requested a private session with Gene Braunwald, who was stepping down as chief of medicine at the Brigham and Women's Hospital. I knew Gene quite well from our decade together as editors of *Harrison's Principles of Internal Medicine*, and wanted his frank view on the role of the dean at HMS. I asked him whether it was a doable job. He urged me to give it serious consideration.

By mid-October, Neil and I had reached an agreement and the news of my intention to return to Boston was announced at public gatherings in both San Francisco and Harvard in November, followed by an invitation to have lunch with members of the Harvard Corporation. In attendance at the lunch was the chairman of the Harvard Corporation, Robert Stone, who was familiar with HMS since his daughter, Jennifer, had graduated from there a few years earlier. He was a noted yachtsman, a winner and subsequent sponsor of the America's Cup—the foremost world yacht racing event—and a wonderfully empowering figure in the Harvard orbit. Also present were Ron Daniel, treasurer of the corporation and a leading partner of the consulting firm McKinsey & Co. in New York; Henry Rosovsky, who had served as dean of the Faculty of Arts and Sciences (FAS); Hanna Gray, just retired from the presidency of the University of Chicago; and Jamie Houghton, whose family ran Corning Glass in Ithaca, New York.[1] We covered many topics, among them the emerging power of molecular genetics and the possibility of new treatments for illnesses.

Then, quite abruptly, one member brought up the topic of the contentious mergers of the Harvard hospitals: What did I think about them? What did I intend to do to smooth the troubled waters? I remember citing a quote from the Bible (Romans 12:15) that I'd often used but later had to "look up" because I was uncertain of its origin. I suggested that I would enter the fray with the attitude that "I would rejoice with those who rejoice and I would weep with those who weep." Even now, I'm not sure what I meant exactly, but I know I expanded on the extraordinary qualities and international reputation of each of the hospitals and said that I looked forward to learning more about what each considered their strengths and weaknesses, and the challenges that lay ahead. I focused on how we might take actions to strengthen relationships between the medical school (and the university) and its affiliated hospitals.



## Returning to Harvard



Between November, when my transition to HMS was announced, and July 1997, when I actually began my term, I sought counsel from former and current academic and administrative colleagues at HMS about the salient issues facing the school. Visits to Boston and videoconferencing were frequent during those months and helped me establish a dialogue with my new partners in the dean's office and learn more of the internal dynamics of the school and the nature of the somewhat fractured relationships among the hospitals affiliated with the university. The round of meetings continued with colleagues in the affiliated hospitals, chairs of several major departments, not to mention with the chairs of each basic science department, whom I knew were going to present the biggest challenge for a new dean. I asked three questions of each of the chairs: What do you perceive are the strengths of HMS? What do you find to be the greatest weaknesses or limitations? What would you suggest we do about making HMS a better place? I listened to their experiences and took careful notes. Those notes were, and have been kept, confidential and never shared with anyone. But in the course of the next few years I would consult them from time to time, especially when I faced challenging issues within a given department.

## Transition Issues

Upon further review with Dean David Bray, executive dean for administration at HMS, and associates, I encountered several issues that would not await my arrival on July 1, 1997. I discovered, to my dismay, that the medical school had confronted the Harvard Corporation with a demand to disconnect the PHD program from the administrative control of the Faculty of Arts and Sciences in Cambridge. Dean Tosteson had encouraged the basic science chairs at the medical school to write directly to the corporation members, bypassing the usual route through the president. The action was driven by the disproportionately large number of graduate students in the biological sciences at HMS, amounting to three times the number of those at the college, as well as an outrage over the administrative fees assessed to HMS for services the school considered inefficient and unusually constraining. I listened to the arguments, spoke with the president and soon realized that this issue would not get resolved before I took over in July, or any time soon.

Another significant action was about to take place before my tenure began. Under the leadership of Marc Kirschner, whom I knew from our days at UCSF, and Stuart Schreiber, chair of the Department of Chemistry at the FAS, a proposal had surfaced to establish a new interfaculty initiative called the Institute of Chemistry and Cell Biology. The idea was to establish a high-throughput screening mechanism to examine potential drug targets using biological assays, taking advantage of Schreiber's extraordinary platforms of combinatorial chemistry. The medical school was prepared to underwrite the construction costs for a new laboratory and to provide approximately 10,000 square feet of valuable research space adjacent to Kirschner's Department of Cell Biology.

I reviewed the plan in the months before I arrived back in Boston, met with the key spokespersons and discussed the proposal with Dean Jeremy Knowles of the FAS. Jeremy indicated intellectual support but was not willing to contribute financially. He understood the scientific potential but was concerned about the use of space for this purpose. I was fully aware from discussions with Dean David Bray that there was virtually no space within the Quad buildings at Longwood for further program expansion and that the potentially available 30,000 square feet would be reduced by one-third should the plan go forward (space always seems to be a paramount issue in academic institutions).

I resisted initially, but in the end I surrendered to the idea. As I reflected on the successful outcome of the endeavor a few years later, I was very grateful I had done so. It was the first academic entity of its kind in the United States and a powerful vehicle that led to the development of new commercial enterprises. It also became a major building block for the subsequent establishment of a platform in chemical biology led by Schreiber at the Broad Institute, where he would eventually move his entire research operation.

Before actually beginning my tenure as dean, I also learned that efforts to update the medical school's information technology platform had been fragmented. To my surprise, there was no e-mail system that reached across the campus or extended to include the hospitals; interdepartmental communication of activities such as seminars and visiting speakers was almost nonexistent. The medical education curriculum was still almost entirely hard copy-based, and the preparation of teaching materials was disorganized and largely departmentally based. I was delighted that the recognition of these deficits had already led to the appointment of Daniel Moriarty, the new promising chief information officer at HMS. He would become a key advocate and intellectual leader as we pursued these improvements—one of my top priorities. He would later be succeeded by John Halamka, who served for eight years as my chief of information technology, introducing MyCourses, the web-based curriculum that enabled students to interact directly with their instructors in course planning and providing confidential online assessment of the quality of the teaching.

## Getting Started as Dean of HMS

During the first two months of my tenure I arranged to meet with each of the eighty or so basic science faculty whose laboratories were located on the HMS Quad. Investigators, both senior and junior, described for me the focus of their research as I sought to gain their perspectives on the school and what we might do together to improve it. In the dean's office, David Bray very ably and, I felt, with full transparency, undertook a systematic review of the opportunities and liabilities the school faced. Together with Jim Adelstein, who announced his intention to step down as academic dean in July, we went over the details of finances and the political landscape surrounding HMS. I was delighted to note during our planning sessions that in the winter prior to my arrival the medical school endowment exceeded $1 billion, a tribute to the fundraising skills of Dean Tosteson.

In general, I was pleased with what I found. I had not negotiated any specific requests about institutional support with Neil Rudenstine before accepting the job, trusting him to help me accomplish what I intended to do after I had developed a strategic plan. Already, however, I knew that the greatest challenge ahead was to re-establish effective working relationships with the hospitals affiliated with HMS.

## A Shifting Landscape

Everyone in the HMS circle acknowledged and was concerned about the persisting trauma that had resulted from the rather hasty efforts to merge the major teaching hospitals into a single or at least cooperative clinical enterprise. During his last two years as dean, Dan Tosteson had sought outside consultant advice, had convened hospital leaders and listened to their recommendations about how to proceed with a more definitive—and more collegial—set of cooperative arrangements for the complex clinical enterprise known as the Harvard Medical Center (HMC). A major consultative effort in this regard had been entrusted to Steve Ruma, a close friend of David Bray and Dan Tosteson, who had over many years consulted for the school.

When I began my tenure as dean, my perspective had changed about the hospitals: at one point, I didn't think the deanship was manageable because of the network of hospitals. Eight years later, as I stepped into the role of dean, in the midst of failed health care reform under the Clinton administration and the persistent budgeting challenges of a hospital-based enterprise, I could only comment, "Thank God, Harvard University and its medical school don't own any hospitals!"

By the mid-1990s, the failure of progress to develop new hospital affiliations led two of the hospitals, the MGH and Brigham and Women's Hospital, to proceed on their own. There had followed a remarkable, if not infamous, weekend consultation at an offsite location at Babson College with a small contingent of academic leaders, hospital CEOs, and board of trustee chairs. The leaders of the two hospitals announced a tentative union—Partners HealthCare—on the Monday morning following the retreat and to the extreme embarrassment of the dean; he first heard of the plan details on the pages of the *Boston Globe*. The reactions, immediate and largely hostile from many of the faculty and leaders of the other hospitals, ranged from disbelief to doubts about the likelihood of success. By the time Tosteson had called President Rudenstine that Monday morning, Hooks Burr, a member of the board of trustees at the MGH, had already been to see the president to fill him in on the events of the weekend.

The transformative impact of this nascent agreement on the affairs of the faculty and administration proved to be profound.

Largely as a reaction to the competitive edge they expected from the emerging Partners brand, the Beth Israel Hospital (BIH) and the New England Deaconess (NEDH) hospitals initiated talks. The communication of this "merger," described by many as essentially a takeover of the NEDH by the BIH, was initially devastating in its impact on the faculty and departments involved. The service chiefs were appointed almost entirely from the BIH contingent resulting in a major flight of surgeons and anesthesiologists to other Boston hospitals. The economic foundation of the institution collapsed and, as revenue losses reached into the tens of millions of dollars, endowments were used to rescue the operating budget, and in the next three to five years, senior management turned over several times. Children's Hospital chose to go it alone, not acquiescing to strong pressure from Partners CEO Sam Thier or efforts by the two boards to discuss potential benefits of a conjoined effort. For their part, the trustees and management of CH had as Fred Lovejoy, a professor at CH, described to me, "very little interest in being swallowed up" by the giant.

I was familiar with the panoply of critical issues created by these "mergers," having been briefed during my earlier meetings with the hospital CEOs. Of particular importance had been my meetings with Jack Connors, chairman of the board of Partners; Bill Boyan, chairman of the board of Children's Hospital; and Alan Rothenberg and Robert Meltzer, successive chairs of the dysfunctional Beth Israel Deaconess Medical Center (BIDMC). I listened at length, learned some of the graphic details of intertwining activities, and sought assurances from each board chair that the role and position of Harvard Medical School would be taken seriously in any future deliberations on hospital relationships, especially in terms of its impact on the school's missions of education and research.

In the last year of Dan Tosteson's deanship, a separate agreement had been reached with Mitch Rabkin, CEO of the new BIDMC, to form a new educational entity—the Harvard Medical School–Carl Shapiro Institute for Education and Research. Funds from the BIDMC and HMS were commingled to establish unilaterally a special agreement that had no counterpart or symmetry in any of the other teaching hospitals. To compound the conflict, Dan Tosteson had agreed to be appointed to the board of trustees of the BIDMC, a step that was perceived by many, especially Sam Thier, as totally inappropriate.

By June 1997, the HMS landscape had some deep potholes and frost heaves, and the chance of being derailed early in the course of my tenure seemed high. After some lengthy discussions with hospital board chairs and academic retreats to focus on common ground for HMS faculty and affiliates, I undertook a renewed effort to examine the feasibility of new inter-institutional alignments. I wanted to revisit the concept of the Harvard Medical Center that had frustrated Dan Tosteson in his final years as dean. Were there structural changes in governance and in strategic planning that could bring our clinical and research activities across the HMS complex into better alignment? Initially, our group of hospital representatives and deans were encouraged by recommendations from the Boston Consulting Group (BCG), led by David Matheson, a consummate insider to health care planning in the Boston region. I gathered the leaders together for several meetings, extended invitations to many department chairs and to key faculty. We hired a skilled negotiation team led by Eileen Shapiro, a graduate of the Harvard Business School, who had worked extensively in the techniques and strategies for negotiating difficult relationships.

Sam Thier was quite willing to meet and talk with Mitch Rabkin, whom he had known since their years together at the MGH. Mitch had served the BIH with distinction for over twenty-five years, and his efforts had received national acclaim, especially for their focus on patient-centered care and the strategic effort to elevate the role of the nurse in a team-care approach to patient needs. Joyce Clifford, the head of nursing during much of Mitch's leadership, was formally recognized inside the institution and across the country for developing new safety and satisfaction standards that became the envy of other hospital leaders in the Boston area and beyond.

The efforts continued to flounder. In the end, I realized the futility of wasting further effort on any grand schemes. But I remained troubled over our failure to grasp solutions that I felt would almost certainly be better for our patients. What benefit could possibly be derived from four competing heart transplant programs in Boston, two of them at Harvard hospitals. What about competing liver transplant programs where surgical experience was modest compared to other transplant programs around the country? The small number of patients treated at each of the centers was justified, based entirely on hype that they were each excellent programs. Even more problematic, I felt, was the competition between Boston Children's Hospital and the small pediatric service at the MGH, where transplants of various organs were so few in number that the outcomes were suspect. Despite conversations, no accommodation was ever reached, and I recognized, somewhat painfully, how impotent common sense is in the turf battles that epitomize so much of the health care system in the US.

Nothing substantial emerged from our discussions. The BIDMC continued in a state of turmoil. By 1998 Mitch was replaced by Jim Reinertsen, a physician from Minnesota with a background in managed care. But his efforts to quell the tempests were largely unsuccessful, and he resigned about three years later. This led to a void in leadership at the BIDMC that was filled in sequence by Herb Kressell, chair of the Department of Radiology, and later Michael Rosenblatt, who resigned soon thereafter to become dean of the Tufts University School of Medicine.

Over the next two years I would lead an effort to explore new strategies for inter-institutional collaboration. We examined clinical collaboration along selected service lines, like cancer care. It soon became apparent that such collaboration was too inflamed by vested interests in the individual hospitals, and anti-trust issues were judged to be insurmountable. Efforts for a unified Harvard clinical enterprise were put aside.

One substantial compromise was reached when all the hospitals adopted guidelines regulating cross-institutional recruitments of faculty. These guidelines required documentation of promotion to a new responsibility, in the absence of which the proposed move would require a review by the dean's Faculty Advisory Committee, which was comprised of a senior faculty member from each of the major teaching hospitals. This essentially put an end to inappropriate poaching from one hospital to another and kept the playing field even.

By the beginning of my second year, I had secured an outstanding group of team players in the dean's office. By January of 1998, David Bray had decided to leave to pursue interests in private consulting, as did John Deeley, his internal successor. Good fortune came my way when I was introduced to Paul Levy, who had been for several years the director of the Massachusetts Water Resources Authority (MWRA), highly touted for the successful effort to clean up Boston Harbor. Following his work there, Paul had been consulting internationally for similar projects but was now looking to settle down to a more routine job. Our meetings revealed a remarkable chemistry between us, and in the fall of 1998 Paul agreed to take on a new career in health care. He presciently recognized that health care was emerging as the single most important issue for the US after the failure of the efforts of the Clinton administration to reform health care in 1993 and 1994.

We had an instant trust in each other and for the next three years and four months we worked to create the principal agendas that would define my deanship: securing an improved information technology platform, establishing the new Harvard Medical Collaborative for hospital inter-relationships and, perhaps most important, securing the support of the university to construct a new research building.

Also critical to my new administration was the appointment of Dennis Kasper as dean for academic affairs. Dennis, whom I knew through our joint editorship at HPIM, was a senior member of the Harvard community. He had succeeded Gene Braunwald as interim chair of the Department of Medicine at the BWH and directed the Channing Laboratory of the BWH, with an interest in infectious diseases. Dennis was highly regarded by everyone I spoke to, and for the next five years advised me with remarkable wisdom and support about the workings of the various basic science and clinical activities of the medical school. He was able to recruit Raphael Dolin from his position as chair of the Department of Medicine at the University of Rochester to serve as dean for clinical programs at HMS.[2] Our dean's group was completed that fall when Dan Lowenstein, to my great delight, arrived from UCSF to assume the role of dean for medical education. We were a cordial, close-knit, but entirely uninhibited group. Our weekly meetings as a dean's cabinet were one of the job's highlights for me and I trust also for them.

Recognizing the need for more hands-on leadership in the daily affairs of administrative activities, in 2000, Paul invited Eric Beuhrens, a colleague he had worked with at the MWRA. Eric[3] would prove to be a key leader along with Kevin Hurton, head of facilities management, in riding herd over the planning and eventual execution of construction of the New Research Building, or NRB, as it's often called.[4]

Throughout this early planning stage, I enjoyed invaluable support from Don Gibbons and his staff in the public affairs office. Don had moved to Boston from the San Francisco Bay Area a short time before I arrived. His advice and consent on important issues, both within the academy and especially in relations with the press, was crucial to my reintroduction to the Boston scene. A few weeks after I arrived in Boston, Don had arranged for an interview with Larry Tye of the *Boston Globe*.[5] I'll never forget the complimentary piece, entitled "Harvard Medical Dean in the hot seat" that appeared in the December 29, 1997, issue of the paper. Tye had taken the trouble to visit with my associates in the Bay area to get a take on the new guy. In my interview, I emphasized the importance of peacemaking within the academic scene at Harvard Medical School.

I set out early on to cement longstanding relationships with friends and colleagues whom I recognized would be crucial to many of the collaborative efforts I hoped to shape. A particularly important individual in this regard, given the growing merger realities of Partners HealthCare, was Sam Thier. Sam had returned to Boston first as head of the Massachusetts General Hospital and, following the merger, was appointed the CEO of Partners HealthCare. Sam was a graduate of the medical school at the State University of New York at Syracuse. He had trained in internal medicine at the MGH, gone on to leadership positions at the University of Pennsylvania and Yale before accepting an appointment as president of the Institute of Medicine (IOM). From there, he had moved to Massachusetts as president of Brandeis University, where, after three years, he yielded to the call to return to academic medicine. Together, we forged a number of critical collaborations, including the establishment of departmental reviews and, with the help of his creativity and foresight, the development of the Harvard–Partners Center for Genetics and Genomics, which led to the appointment of Raju Kucherlapati. Our friendship had been cemented through prior professional relationships and while fiercely competitive by nature and in his dealings with other hospitals in the Harvard network, Sam was always sensitive to the academic mission, and I could always count on him for advice and support.

### "Now, With These Doors Wide Open..."

The network of Harvard's affiliated hospitals and the importance of working together as partners would, I knew, pose a major challenge. However, as I prepared for the beginning of my term as dean, another issue I knew would be forefront during my deanship would be the academic community at HMS itself, the various departments and inter-relationships therein. I outlined my plans and priorities at the first meeting of the faculty council. They were arranged around four general principles: strengthen basic science research, broaden relationships with the teaching hospitals, reinvigorate the educational programs, and increase ethnic and gender diversity within all components of the school. I also identified three platforms of execution to support these efforts: improve information technology capabilities for the administrative and educational mission of the school; obtain access to new financial resources; and integrate HMS into the broader community—community service, biotechnology and international health initiatives. These remained my priorities throughout my tenure as dean, and I would report on progresses made—together with disappointments and adjustments—to the faculty, as well as the larger HMS community in my annual state of the school address each fall.

One of my earliest public addresses at HMS was on September 2, 1997, when I set out to welcome the new students in medicine and dentistry on the first day of their orientation week. This was a special ceremony for me. Not only was I meeting my first group of students entering HMS but I also wanted the occasion to be marked symbolically by a gesture to signal the priorities of my deanship. Standing on the top of the staircase leading from the

Quad to the Administration Building addressing the students in their newly acquired white coats, I announced "the opening of the traditionally locked Quad doors of the Administration Building (Building A)," where the dean's office is located. The doors had been locked throughout the school year for several decades, allegedly for reasons of security.

I greeted the two hundred students and society masters gathered on the Quad with the message that they were joining a new community, that the opening of the doors signaled a commitment of the new leadership of the school to an era of openness and transparency and that as we stood amidst the grand buildings of the HMS Quad, our mission was not simply to serve the elite but also the global family, whose issues of health care, poverty and illness were part of our responsibility as health care professionals. The event is still vivid in my memory. By community, I said:

*I mean something much broader than that bounded by this marble quadrangle...That community consists of our neighbors—the community on nearby Mission Hill, the community of greater Boston, the US, and, indeed, the whole world.*

*Although I officially started my tenure as dean of the Harvard Faculty of Medicine on July 1, I join with you today in fully entering this community. As a symbol of my commitment to go with you through your transition into the medical profession, I want to announce today that these front doors of HMS—doors that, for decades, have been locked to you until your graduation day—will be open to you now every day. Well, at least every Monday through Friday from 9 to 5.*

The opening of the doors, I continued, was symbolic:

*It represents my priorities for Harvard Medical School. We, in this building, will be open and accessible to all our communities; at the same time, we will be looking for ways we can be of assistance—to our students seeking knowledge, our affiliates seeking collaboration, or a neighborhood health clinic seeking another pair of hands....*

Later that fall we officially embraced a new mission statement for HMS, which remains in effect today: "To create and nurture a diverse community of the best people committed to alleviating human suffering caused by disease."

## Confronting a Major Illness

The fall term got underway. I was feeling the tempo of a new job and felt ready to begin implementing some of my plans for the school. As October rolled around, I scheduled an annual medical checkup with Dr. Marshall Wolf at the Brigham and Women's Hospital. My medical history was noteworthy for two familial conditions that could potentially impact my future prognosis. One was a family history of cardiac arrhythmias, which had been observed in several of my father's siblings—both men and women—and had affected my father in his later years.

The second familial condition I worried about was prostate cancer, present on both sides of the family, including my father. Given my father's history and the recent diagnosis of a large prostate tumor in a cousin whose condition had led to serious disability and pain at the end of his life, I had been monitoring my prostate-specific antigen (PSA) levels for the last four to five years.

My visit with Dr. Wolf was perfunctory and unremarkable. It was a Thursday afternoon, and I waited through the weekend for the results. On Monday afternoon, I stopped by Dr. Wolf's office to inquire about the results. First to come up on the computer as I gazed over Marshall's shoulder was an elevation in serum calcium to 11.3 meq/l (the normal level is up to 10.5). Next to come up was the startling PSA result—11.5 ng/ml, which had tripled from my former baseline level of 3.5. I was devastated. Since I had not had my PSA level measured in the past twelve or fifteen months and knew that the calcium level had been normal, this combination could only mean cancer—metastatic prostate cancer to bone—which I knew, despite my father's remarkable course, was generally incurable. My world collapsed. I had been dean at HMS for less than four months at this point.

During the radionuclide bone scan, I lay quietly on the bone-hard table in the radiology suite at the BWH as the radioactive chemical mixture was injected into my bloodstream, and we waited for it to equilibrate in the tissues. The scan began as the radiation detector, mounted on an arm above my body, swung to and fro from head to toe recording any focal deposits of activity.

My second moment of transparent panic during my diagnosis came with the technician's communication, some twenty to thirty minutes after completing the scan, that there were suspicious deposits of radioactivity about which she would need to consult with the radiologist. She returned to say that she would need to repeat part of the scanning procedure. After another wait, which seemed interminable, I received the good news that the questionable areas were "periarticular," consistent with wear and tear possibly from an old joint injury or some developing arthritis—but not likely a tumor. (After some further investigation, it turned out that the elevated calcium levels were the result of mild vitamin D deficiency, from lack of sun exposure.)

I was scheduled to visit San Francisco in a few weeks and because of the great confidence I had in the physicians there, I scheduled a visit and arranged for an ultrasound-guided series of biopsies—eight to ten in total—in the UCSF outpatient radiology suite. A single suspicious area revealed itself on the ultrasound, and biopsy confirmed the presence of a small tumor with a Gleason scale—a microscopic grading system of the malignant appearance of a tumor—reading of 2 and 3 for a total of 5 on a scale of 10 (the latter number associated with a poorer prognosis). That was good news.

I returned to Boston, and on December 1 underwent total radical prostatectomy under the skillful hands of Dr. Jerome Ritchie at the BWH. The immediate postoperative period was complicated by excessive blood loss requiring two units of whole blood, and by some hypotension, presenting without any cardiac symptoms of chest pain due to coronary artery ischemia, making it likely that my heart and vasculature were in good shape.

The catheter was removed twenty days later, and Rachel and I attended a pre-Christmas musical event at the home of David and Louise Bray. I was extraordinarily uncomfortable, but we survived the evening, and I returned to work after the holidays.

A few weeks later, near the end of January, I received a call early one Saturday morning from Jack Connors, board chairman of Partners HealthCare. Jack and I had met on several occasions during the early months of my deanship, and now he was asking if I felt like taking a walk in Harvard's Arnold Arboretum, a mile or so away. I did, and as we trudged through the park, covered in four or five inches of snow, Jack described, in vivid strokes, his years growing up in the community and learning the names of the trees and bushes. I doubt he knew how I was feeling on my first major walk after surgery, but the time spent was worth every minute of discomfort. After that walk with Jack, I knew he would be a good friend and colleague, as he indeed proved himself to be, in many projects over the next decade.

## Rethinking an Enduring Legacy

In 1997 the outward appearance of the five marble buildings on the HMS campus remained essentially the same as it had been at their dedication in 1906. The Longwood campus, the result of a grand vision for a center of medical education and scientific research by a few HMS faculty members, was the seventh home HMS had occupied since its foundation in 1782. The first classes had been held in the basement of Harvard Hall in Cambridge, with a handful of students and a faculty of three, and in Holden Hall, the former college chapel in Harvard Yard. It had moved to Boston in 1810 and, after further relocations around the city, had found anchor in the Longwood area at the beginning of the twentieth century. Harvard Medical School had for a relatively brief period found a home adjacent to the MGH. By 1870, however, it moved to Boylston Street near the Boston Public Library. Its relocation to the Longwood Medical Area was a saga in its own right.

The Longwood area was largely open farms and marshland at the time, but it was free of space constraints and offered the potential for future expansion. That potential was realized as several hospitals were soon drawn into the area now known as the Longwood Medical Area. One of the earliest was the "University Hospital," the Peter Bent Brigham Hospital, which opened its doors in 1913.[6]

Finding, purchasing and raising the necessary funds to relocate HMS to the Longwood campus took much effort and commitment from the faculty and a number of businessmen in the Boston area. A leading figure in the effort was Major Henry

Higginson, a Boston businessman and fellow of the Harvard Corporation, about whom I wrote an essay for the winter 2005 issue of the *Harvard Medical Alumni Bulletin*. Henry Higginson, who is well known as the founder of Boston Symphony Hall, was a leading figure in the campaign to raise the necessary funds to purchase the land for the new medical school. In a matter of a few months, Higginson's personal contribution of $50,000 had grown to $500,000, the sum deemed sufficient to purchase the twenty-two acres of land. The buildings of the new medical school were dedicated September 26, 1906.

The five original marble-faced buildings that make up the Quadrangle are still used for classrooms and research laboratories, although all have undergone significant internal rearrangement and transformation. In the original design, the Administration Building, home to the offices of the dean, occupies center stage and is raised seventeen feet above the others. In the one hundred years of its existence, this building has witnessed its share of internal "rehabilitation," although the exterior remains intact and reminiscent of a Greek temple. During the first half of the twentieth century, for example, it housed student spaces, classrooms, an amphitheater, a library, the dean's offices and the well-known Warren Anatomical Museum where students gathered for anatomy lessons. Despite further internal rearrangements in the second half of the twentieth century, when I arrived on the scene in 1997, the six-story structure still maintained its elegant interior design. One striking element of that design is the arrangement of the interior space from the third floor upward beneath an enormous vault that runs across the width of the building, rising like a canopy over the top half of the building, sustained by elegant cast iron columns decorated in classical motifs.[7]

Originally, I was told, the vault had been translucent and together with openings on the flat part of the roof, allowed light to penetrate. This had changed when the United States entered World War II on December 7, 1941, and all higher buildings in the Boston area potentially visible from the harbor were ordered to shutter or black out their windows. HMS obliged, and for the next forty years the atrium remained darkened and illuminated only by artificial light.

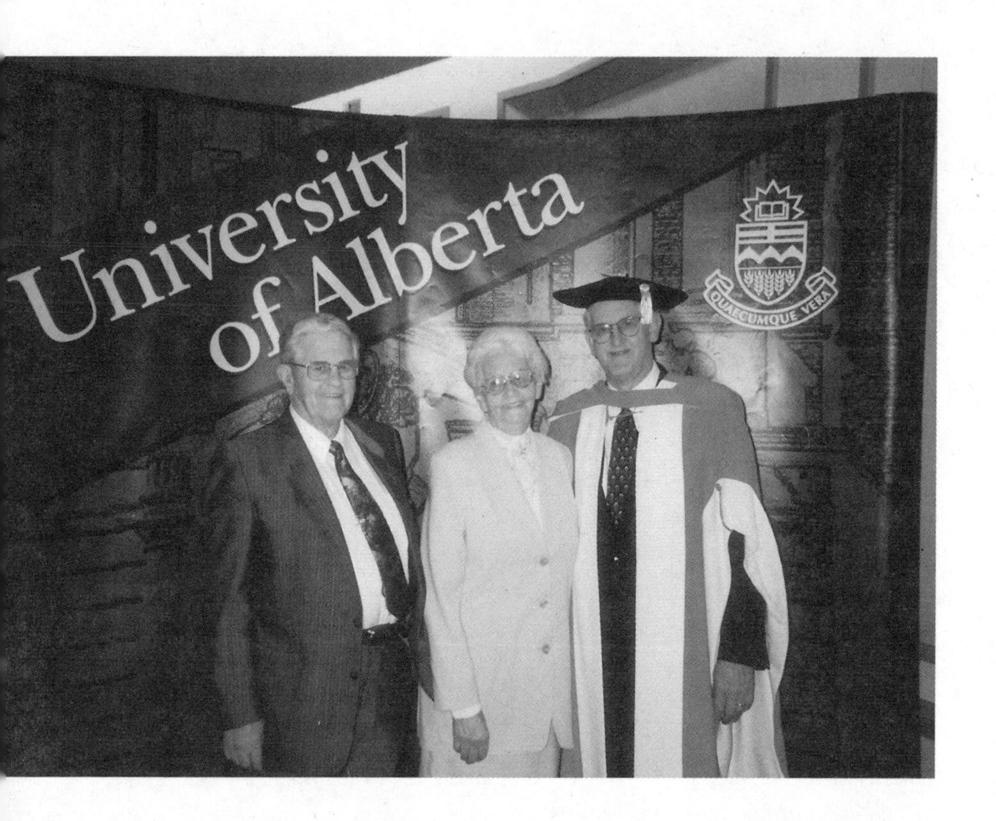


The author and his parents on the occasion of receiving an honorary degree from the University of Alberta, 1998.

Following the decision to open the front door to encourage greater activity in the building, I asked my administrative deans to explore the possibility and cost of reconstructing the atrium. The cost was high, exceeding $1.5 million, for which we had no resources assigned. I pled the case with Ellen and Melvin Gordon, who had already generously funded educational programs in the school and whose daughter, Wendy, was an alumna of the school, to consider an additional contribution for the good of the atrium. In August 2000, we signed a gift agreement, which resulted in a generous contribution with a book value of over $20 million that provided the resources to accomplish this major improvement. We subsequently acknowledged their gift by naming the building the Gordon Hall of Medicine, a tribute that was consummated by then dean for development, Cushing Robinson. Another major need emerged during the ensuing months.

## Francis A. Countway Library: "Equipped to move into the twenty-first century"

The Francis A. Countway Library at the end of Shattuck Street was a fitting memorial to the distinguished tenure of Dean George Packer Berry, who served HMS from 1949 to 1965. Dr. Berry had been educated at Princeton and at the Johns Hopkins School of Medicine. He had trained as a bacteriologist and served as head of the Department of Bacteriology at the University of Rochester before being appointed dean at HMS.

The library, where his profile carved in bas-relief graces the right wall near the first-floor entrance, was opened in 1965. It is an elegant five-story building that houses the remarkable collections of both Harvard Medical School and the Boston Medical Library (BML), the latter founded in 1805 by HMS professors John C. Warren and James Jackson. Oliver Wendell Holmes, dean of HMS from 1847 to 1853, had overseen its rejuvenation and, in 1875, served as its president. It was housed in various locations in the city until 1960, when an agreement was reached to combine the collections of the BML and HMS and share the cost of construction and management of the new Francis A. Countway Library.

By 1997, however, this relatively new library was in need of renovation and updating to keep up with the growing demands of the digital revolution. When I arrived at HMS in 1997, a campaign was already underway led by Amalie Kass, a lecturer in medical history at the library and the wife of a distinguished HMS specialist in infectious diseases, Edward Kass, and Paul Russell, professor and former chief of surgery at the MGH and head of the transplantation unit he founded in 1969. In July 2009 Paul Russell told me:

*After I was asked to assume the chairmanship of the Harvard Medical Library Committee by Jim Adelstein, I consulted with Harold Amos and Alfred Pope, who had preceded me on the committee, about their views of the needs of the library and of its mode of governance...*

*It was, of course, very apparent that the function of libraries was changing with the advent of computerized access to so much information of all kinds. Partly as a consequence of this, as well as budgetary constraints, plans for leasing out as much as two floors of the building were being considered. This raised concern amongst a number of us, especially Oglesby Paul and Amalie Kass, members of the new Joint Library Committee....Thus, we set up a subcommittee of the joint committee to focus on fundraising....*

*Architects and consultants were mobilized and the necessary work was accomplished in a remarkable way with great forbearance on the part of the staff and without ceasing the everyday work of the library.*

The subcommittee raised over $15 million toward an objective of $28 million. I chipped in additional resources, and we borrowed the rest. As part of the renovation, rare books and special collections were housed together in a temperature and humidity-controlled environment. Medical papers, journals and other research materials were cataloged and organized in a way that would make them easier to find, and a new section of the library housed computer terminals to provide quick on-site access to electronic resources.

The library was rededicated on September 28, 2000, at a ceremony that capped its two-year and $26-million renovation, led by then librarian Judy Messerle, who ended her comments on the renovations with the reflection that: "In the end, we will be equipped to move into the twenty-first century." Judy subsequently retired, and the medical school established a formal search committee chaired by Jules Dienstag, director of admissions for the medical school, to search for a new head. The search resulted in the appointments of Zack Kohane, a professor of bioinformatics at Children's Hospital, and Alexa McCray, who gave up her position as deputy director of the National Library of Medicine in Bethesda, Maryland, to come back to Boston.

The combined library resources of the Countway rank it as one of the largest and finest in the world, including an extensive collection of rare books. The library is open and available to students and other health care workers not only at Harvard but also at the three other medical schools of Massachusetts—Boston University, Tufts University and the University of Massachusetts. The renovation served as an example of the commitment of the school's leadership to the educational mission, although the curriculum itself had not been altered greatly since the introduction of the New Pathway in Medical Education in 1985.

## Medical Education Reform: Accepting the Challenges of a New Curriculum

The educational reforms that had been implemented over the previous decade had become well ensconced in the traditions of Harvard Medical School when I arrived on the scene in the summer of 1997. I had great admiration for the perseverance and accomplishments Dan Tosteson brought to the revolution in medical education that became known as the "New Pathway in Medical Education." Students trained in the problem-based, case-oriented, tutorial method of learning performed well on the standardized testing of the National Board of Examinations at the end of the second and fourth years. He deserves credit for introducing new pedagogical approaches, establishing a growing national recognition of the need to engage students actively in the learning experience, and reducing the insufferable hours of didactic lecturing that had stifled so many generations of students.[8]

The impact of this reform on medical education cannot be overstated. The role of Dan Federman, dean of students, and Gordon Moore, professor of medicine, was to be crucial. Federman attributes the reform's success to the hard-nosed persistent engagement of Tosteson, who faithfully attended every planning retreat and seated himself in the front row, combining attentive listening with decisive actions. Over the course of eighteen months a new curriculum was born. Department courses were given new names. Faculty who favored the new direction were given new responsibility for teaching. As Federman states, "It is unlikely that anyone with less determination than Dan [Tosteson] could have pulled it off."

I realized, soon after my arrival, that students fully embraced the new learning format, and some of them expressed concern that I might set about changing the curriculum. It was not entirely unknown that my early experience with the New Pathway reform Tosteson implemented from 1980 to 1985, while I was neurology chief at the MGH, had not been positive. I fell into the category of clinical leaders who were heavily involved in teaching and, like many other clinical chiefs, doubted that the rigors of a classical medical education could be matched by an approach that was more user-friendly to students. At that time,

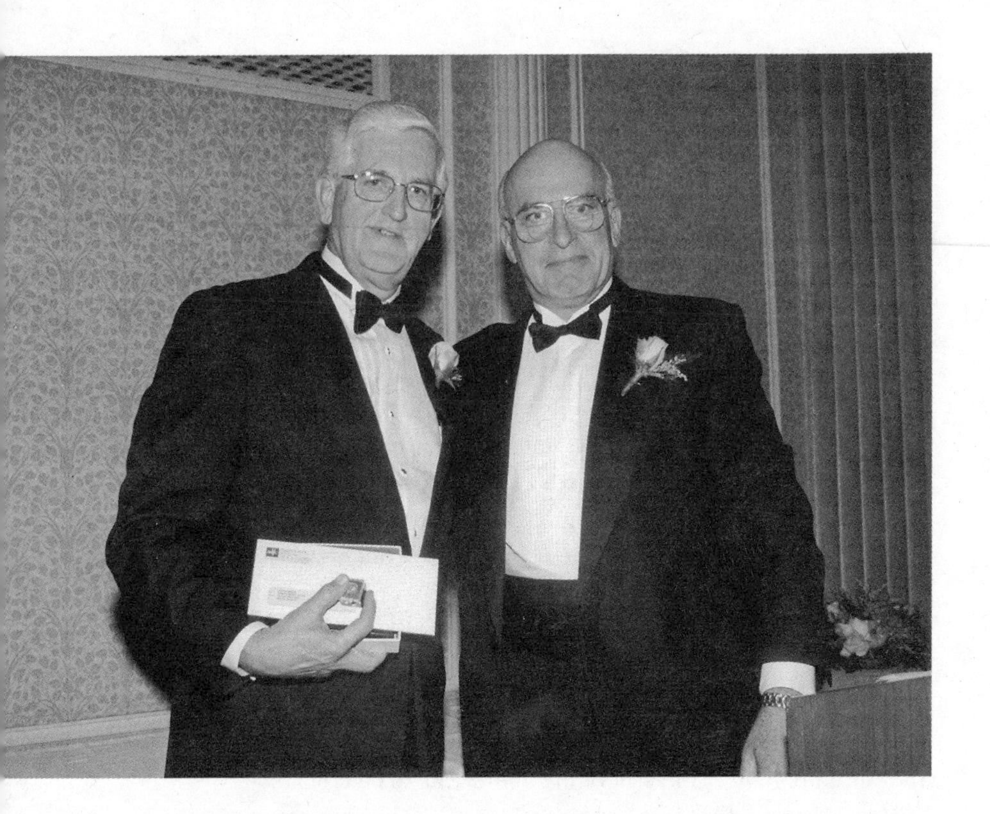

The author and William Peck, Chairman of the Board, Association of American Medical Colleges.

I felt that the education provided in a tutorial setting might be haphazard and that gaps in information would likely occur, not because I felt we taught that much better, but because my tendencies toward organizational detail demanded knowing that the students had been exposed to the basic salient knowledge in an orderly encyclopedic way. That was how I'd been taught and felt that my preparation at the University of Alberta had served me well as I entered the "big time" of American medical school activities.

But despite these lingering reservations, I had no intention of challenging the system. I thought, instead, about ways to attempt to improve it. I had a longstanding interest in medical education fostered by my experiences at UCSF. I was astonished, however, in 1999, to receive a call from Jordan Cohen, president of the Association of American Medical Colleges (AAMC), notifying me that I had been awarded the Abraham Flexner Award, given annually to leaders perceived to have made significant contributions to medical education.

That occasion encouraged me to take a look at how the medical education program was doing at HMS. The opportunity arose soon thereafter when planning began for the mandatory Liaison Committee on Medical Education (LCME) accreditation review that each school in the US and Canada undergoes every seven to eight years. Harvard Medical School was due to submit its self-study review by 2002, which meant that the eighteen-month period of formal internal review would need to begin in 2000.

As we entered this process, I was fortunate to recruit Lorraine Caristo from the Tufts University School of Medicine, where she had worked in the dean's office for nine years. Before that she had been in the administrative ranks at HMS in several positions for more than twelve years, undertaking responsibilities that prepared her ideally for the highly political assignment of leading the LCME preparedness agenda, assisting me in forming the committees required in the process and helping identify key faculty members who could be counted on to deliver the products of review in a timely and thoughtful way.

The process was fully endorsed by my fellow deans and me. Initially, I depended heavily on Dan Federman, who agreed to stay on for another year as dean for medical education until I recruited Dan Lowenstein from the University of California, San Francisco. With Dan Lowenstein's recruitment, I asked Dan Federman to remain in the school in a new position, as dean for clinical programs and alumni relations, a unique perch that served both Dan's and the school's interests. Dan Federman was the most admired alumni representative ever—he was widely respected by alumni, older and more recent, and knew the names of graduates and kept in touch with them on visits that he led for me around the country, rallying their support for the annual fundraiser and other causes.[9]

The LCME site visit preparations began in the fall of 2001, coincident with a private meeting I had with Dan Lowenstein, when he announced the great unhappiness his family had experienced in their transition from UCSF to Boston. Dan Lowenstein's decision to return eventually with his family to California was a serious blow to my plans. I had known him at UCSF where I'd had frequent opportunities during my visits to the neurology service at the SFGH to interact with him as a faculty member who was focusing his efforts in the field of epilepsy. Dan was legendary at UCSF as the quintessential teacher and role model, and I had been thrilled when he told me of his interest to come to HMS as dean for medical education.

Dan promised to stay on at least two more years through the LCME process, but I sensed the pull to return to the West Coast was powerful and unlikely to change. Indeed, by January 2002, his commitment had been reduced to six months, leading me to become intensely engaged in the LCME process. In the end, the process moved forward smoothly, and the January 15, 2003, entry of my journal reads: "The LCME report is nearly ready for submission. The visit is scheduled for April 8–10."

The outcome of the visit was a mixed report on our current programs. The review endorsed the problem-based learning backbone of the curriculum but noted two deficiencies that would require follow-up. The first was the unevenness of our assessment of students in their rotations across the clinical clerkships in our hospitals. The second was a failure to incorporate the tutorial, student-centered learning of the first two years into the clinical experience. The students were increasingly marginalized in the to-and-fro frenetic culture of the modern academic medical center, where patient care was fragmented, admission times reduced and the treatments recommended left the students on the periphery.

The major strengths of the current program included the unrivaled access to the best young people in the world; a successful selection process that admitted an exceptionally talented and diverse student body; a faculty unparalleled in its breadth and depth of abilities and accomplishments; an outstanding dedicated staff that ascribed to extremely high standards of excellence; enormous resources in terms of endowment, buildings, technology infrastructure, etc.; affiliations with some of the best teaching hospitals in the world; excellent curricula in the first two years of New Pathway and the Health Sciences and Technology (HST) programs, the latter being a collaborative effort with MIT established by Dean Robert Ebert in 1970; and, a willing leadership.



As we pondered the LMCE report's conclusions, we identified other weaknesses in our curriculum: the inability of faculty

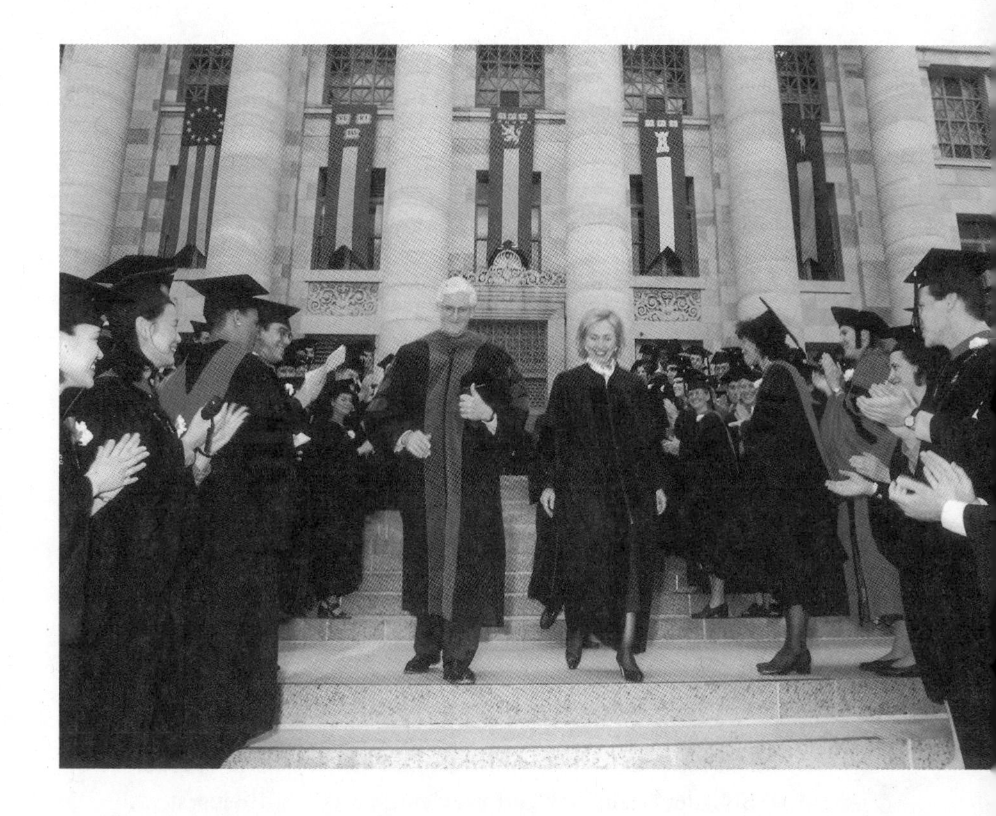

Harvard University Commencement, 1998. Leaving Gordon Hall with commencement speaker Hillary Clinton, the author proudly wears the green and gold of his alma mater, the University of Alberta.

to find supported time to teach, advise and mentor; student indebtedness; lack of coherence in clinical education; too little emphasis on the tempo of disease and treatment over time; marginalization of the students in the clinical setting; failure of the problem-based, or tutorial, system to evolve in the curriculum; and limited training in important aspects of medicine, such as decision-making, errors in care, critical thinking, prevention, culturally competent care, leadership skills, etc.

I took the opportunity to share the LCME report with the faculty in the spring of 2003 and to ask them to invest in a commitment to undertake a thorough review of the entire medical school curriculum, including the pre-medical requirements we used in selecting each class of students. An article in the *Boston Globe* on June 1, 2003, commented on our efforts, describing it as the "first major rethinking of the school's curriculum in 20 years" and commented that while "generally soft-spoken" I had "let faculty know I was upset about the teaching situation."[10] The recognition of these issues led to a sustained effort in education reform that would engage the efforts of three sets of faculty deliberations involving more than three hundred faculty and students and leading to the implementation of a major revision in the curriculum that was introduced in the summer of 2006.

The first step was to engage the faculty in a learning exercise to draw upon their extraordinary talents to formulate directions we might take. We formed two "blue sky" committees. Their report was considered in early 2004 and coincided with the arrival of Malcolm Cox, from University of Pennsylvania, who had succeeded Dan Lowenstein, who in turn had moved back to San Francisco in the summer of 2002.

As we began this lengthy process, I summarized in my state of the school address in September 2004 what I described as the "Five Challenges to Education Reform" or, as they became known, the 5 Cs: Content of the curriculum—what should we teach?; Cost of Education (student debt); Compassionate and culturally competent care; Compensation of clinical teachers; and Chaos of academic health centers.

A second level of review consisted of a task force to recommend the process of revitalization. I asked George Thibault and Phil Leder to chair the effort. George was a cardiologist whose academic career began at the MGH where he led the house staff training program in medicine for many years, followed by a stint as chief of the West Roxbury VA Hospital, and, after my arrival was serving with Partners HealthCare in developing their outreach programs to community practitioners as they moved toward development of a community-based practice. Phil was chair of the medical school Department of Genetics and was recognized for his deep commitment to teaching. He had developed and delivered an extraordinary course in human genetics, in which he himself delivered many of the most important lectures.

The task force concluded that we needed a new model of clinical education and would need to address the developmental needs of the students in order to offer continuity for patient experience, faculty mentoring and student evaluation; that it was necessary to engage the faculty, including the most senior faculty, as teachers, mentors and guides for Harvard medical students; that we should increase the rigor of the teaching of science (basic biologic, social and population sciences) at HMS, and truly integrate the teaching of science and clinical medicine throughout the entire student experience at HMS; and that we should provide the opportunity for all Harvard medical students to acquire in-depth knowledge in one area of inquiry and to produce a scholarly product in their area under the guidance of an expert faculty member.

The implementation of our new plans required new leadership, however. The brief period with Malcolm Cox had turned out to be unworkable, his leadership style provoking concern by many of the key individuals we needed to help us implement further changes. I asked Ray Dolin, an HMS graduate from the class of 1967 and my senior dean for clinical programs, to chair a search committee. From the shortlist of candidates—all of them internal, to avoid the need to bring someone from the outside, given the turnover in recent years—I was thrilled to ask Jules Dienstag to assume the mantle of dean for medical education following up on his very successful tenure as dean of admissions.

Jules was a graduate of the Columbia College of Physicians and Surgeons. Following residency at the University of Chicago, he joined the NIH for a research fellowship in the Laboratory of Infectious Diseases. From there he was recruited for additional fellowship training at the MGH, where he focused on hepatology and infectious causes of hepatitis. He was promoted to full professor in 2002, while serving as dean of admissions and maintaining an active clinical research program at the MGH. Together with Jules we forged a new emphasis on the pillars of medical education reform. These were: faculty compensation, faculty recognition and promotion and faculty development, as well as assessment of educational achievements.

The outcome of this in-depth review was a new curriculum, with plans in place to roll it out in successive stages with incoming classes. The first-year class in August 2006 started off with a new course entitled Introduction to the Profession, a two-week entry into the nuances of the life ahead, with exposure to all aspects of the anticipated learning experience. The course covered clinical and basic aspects of the medical education experience and prepared the students for "what they had gotten themselves into." It was judged to be highly successful and has been continued in subsequent years. In 2010 Jules, a gastroenterologist, and Kate Treadway, a primary care physician in the Department of Medicine at the MGH, worked together to prepare materials to greet the class; this would be the fifth rendition of their efforts.

The curriculum changes included rejuvenation of the basic science courses, enlivened by improved horizontal and vertical integration of subject material around the theme of Fundamentals in Medicine. New required courses in biomedical ethics, health policy and social medicine were introduced into the first-year round of classes. The second-year formal lectures concluded at the end of April, followed by the Principal Clinical Experience (PCE), which begins in May. This initiation of the PCE is perhaps the most dramatic part of the curriculum reform, as it has each student located in one hospital setting for his or her entire third year, thereby eliminating the enervating rotations from one service to another in a range of hospital experiences, which often left students trying too hard to "settle in" to each new experience, particularly in rotations that were as brief as a few weeks. The opportunity to become fully embedded in the culture of a hospital for a full year and to become thoroughly familiar with electronic medical records, and laboratory and radiological procedures, has been powerfully successful. It simultaneously allows students to identify with the hospital and the hospital to take ownership of the student's experience. Students record their choice of hospitals and are then selected for their locations by lottery. The rotations conclude in the spring of the third year to allow time for advanced clinical clerkships in areas of the student's interests, which are required to be taken in part in other hospital settings outside the experience of the PCE.

The most difficult portion of the new curriculum to implement has been the in-depth scholarly experience. Initial efforts in this regard, led by David Golan, professor of biological chemistry and molecular pharmacology, produced an ambitious plan with requests for funding that were unrealistic. At this writing, Jules informs me that the effort has new life, now that David has an expanded role in the dean's office and it is anticipated that it will come into being in 2011.



Being a part of such an intense curriculum revision was a highlight in my tenure as dean. I hope it was my openness—which began with the opening of that Quad door in 1997—to change that made students feel that I was approachable when, in the winter of 2005, a group of students came to see me to complain about the poor quality of the amenities in Vanderbilt Hall and the decrepit state of the lounge. I found money to renovate it, and the students gave me the great honor of naming it the Joseph B. Martin Student Lounge. I was deeply moved by this student initiative.

## Facing the Teacher–Clinical Faculty Challenge: Compensation and Recognition

At my first meeting with Neil Rudenstine in San Francisco in April 1996, I had mentioned that I strongly believed that the next dean of Harvard Medical School ought to "wear a white coat." I still believe that the symbolism of the profession of medicine embodied as it is in the white coat ceremonies at the orientation for new students, where they are given their first white "doctor" coats, should carry over so that students can see their dean not simply as an administrator but also as a doctor who is comfortable with patients and who joins students and house staff in the care of patients on the wards and in the clinics. In my clinical rotations as a teacher and while attending on clinical wards in San Francisco I wore my white coat, and I began my time back at Harvard in a similar fashion, spending a month on the neurology service at each of our major hospitals during the first three years of deanship and then settling into a comfortable time each winter on the neurology service at the MGH. I also took part in the formal educational curriculum each fall by participating in the neuroscience course, where I delivered the lecture on neurodegenerative disorders of the brain focusing on dementias, principally Alzheimer's disease.

My obvious concern for the clinical faculty and the challenges they faced led to the recognition that a new scheme of faculty financial support would be critical to the teaching mission. In the spring of 1999, I approached Neil Rudenstine with an idea that emerged in the middle of the night. I was aware that the hospital-based professorships that made up nearly one-third of the medical school's total endowment had grown substantially with the great success of the university's investment policies. I reasoned that a department-based teaching support fund might be developed by increasing the payout of each professorship by a certain amount. I discussed the plan with Paul Levy, then dean for administration, and Cynthia Walker, dean for finance, and approached the university with the plan. I was very skeptical of the outcome as I met privately with Neil Rudenstine later that month. I knew that the endowment payout was scrupulously attended to by members of the Harvard Corporation and that they were known to be adverse to any exceptions to general policy. But Neil was responsive and asked for more details and concurrence from hospital leaders and chairs.

I approached Neil's request for details first with meetings at the MGH, with the indomitable Jerry Austen, former chief of surgery at the MGH, now head of the MGH Practice Plan. We settled on a plan that would request an additional annual payout of 1 per cent, with seventy-five basis points to be invested in the teaching fund for allocation via a teaching budget for each department. Twenty-five basis points would be allocated to the chair holder for additional academic support but not for salary supplement. Other hospital leaders concurred, a review of the legal impact of such use was viewed to be consistent with donor's general interests, and the corporation took favorable action. A new annual source of about $5 million was now in place to support clinical teachers.

But there was one serious drawback that needed attention. The distribution of endowed professorships varied widely across departments. Some, like surgery at the MGH, had a large number, while others, like medicine and psychiatry at most hospitals, had very few. An expansion of the plan would be critical to the success of the new curriculum to be implemented by 2006.

To generate a new set of options, I asked Cynthia Walker, who had been appointed dean for administration after Paul Levy left, to head the BIDMC, and Peter Slavin, CEO of the MGH, to chair a committee that included financial representatives from each of the major teaching hospitals. The membership of the committee was comprised of Gary Gottlieb, CEO of the BWH; Michael Epstein, chief medical officer at the BIDMC; Dorothy Puhy, chief financial officer at the Dana-Farber; and Sandy Fenwick, chief operating officer at Children's Hospital. I engaged Jay Light, who had just succeeded Kim Clark as dean of the business school, to serve as an outside consultant. Jay had served on the finance committee at Partners, his daughter was a graduate of the medical school and he appreciated the complexities of financing the teaching effort. Jules Dienstag was an ex-officio member of the group, attending carefully to the importance and critical nature of the academic mission and to the importance of the deliberations on the morale of the clinical faculty.

The discussions assumed a somewhat tense but persistent focus on a new range of financial options. The result was a plan that proved to be unbelievably creative, with each hospital agreeing to shore up the teaching fund with additional discretionary money that evened out the asymmetries of support that arose from the endowed chair payout.

## Faculty Recognition and Promotion

An equally pressing issue with the faculty was awareness that teaching carried little academic weight. A large percentage of student teaching was shouldered by instructors, many sequestered in that academic category for decades. In 1998 our faculty affairs office led by Dean Eleanor Shore created a new committee to evaluate service of long duration, chaired by Fred Lovejoy, a dedicated professor at Children's Hospital, whose loyalties to the school placed him in a favorable position to undertake this formidable task. They undertook the effort with serious attention to the inequities of the past and encouraged faculty to consider promotions as rewards for teaching efforts. In 2005, when Ellice Lieberman succeeded Eleanor as dean for faculty affairs, we undertook an additional step. A committee chaired by Ellice established a new set of criteria for consideration by the appointments and promotions committee. In this elaboration of the evaluation process, we considered each of the four parameters of academic effort: research, clinical work, teaching and community service. The outcome was a carefully crafted set of guidelines introduced during the final year of my deanship, which we hoped would transform the culture of medical school scholarship and accomplishments. Specifically introduced was the academic value of medical student teaching. Excellence in teaching became one of the criteria for promotion, along with other activities that included community service.

## Breaking Ground with Neil Rudenstine

During his presidency, Neil had held monthly meetings of the deans and established, as effectively as any recent Harvard president could, a forum to discuss the "every tub on its own bottom" mindset, a longstanding label for Harvard's internal academic competitiveness. The meetings gave me the chance to get to know Jeremy Knowles, a chemist and the dean of the Faculty of Arts and Sciences. During Dan Tosteson's deanship, Jeremy had remained intransigent about the funding of graduate education in the biological sciences, and the two of them had enormous antipathy toward each other.

The friendship that developed between Jeremy and me was important to both of us, before and through the unfortunate suffering he experienced as he progressively failed with prostate cancer. I will always remember Jeremy's sudden appearance at my bedside on the day after my own surgery for prostate cancer when I was feeling the worst effects of the postoperative period. It was a moment I shall never forget. I told Jeremy as much the last time I went to visit with him at his home in Cambridge, just two weeks before he died. By then, he was in a wheelchair, largely immobilized from metastatic prostate cancer to the spine. We enjoyed a tasty lunch his wife, Jane, had prepared and a glass of sauvignon blanc. We had some hearty laughs, mostly about the foibles created by unruly faculty who, more than any other constituency in the university, manage to hasten early retirement plans for endangered deans.

Neil Rudenstine concluded a ten-year term as president of Harvard University in 2001. One of the last public appearances Neil and I held, on February 1, along with Boston Mayor Thomas Menino and Mark Maloney of the Boston Redevelopment Authority, was at the groundbreaking ceremony for the medical school's New Research Building, designed to promote collaboration among researchers at HMS and the hospitals. Neil's support in gaining the endorsement of university leaders for the new

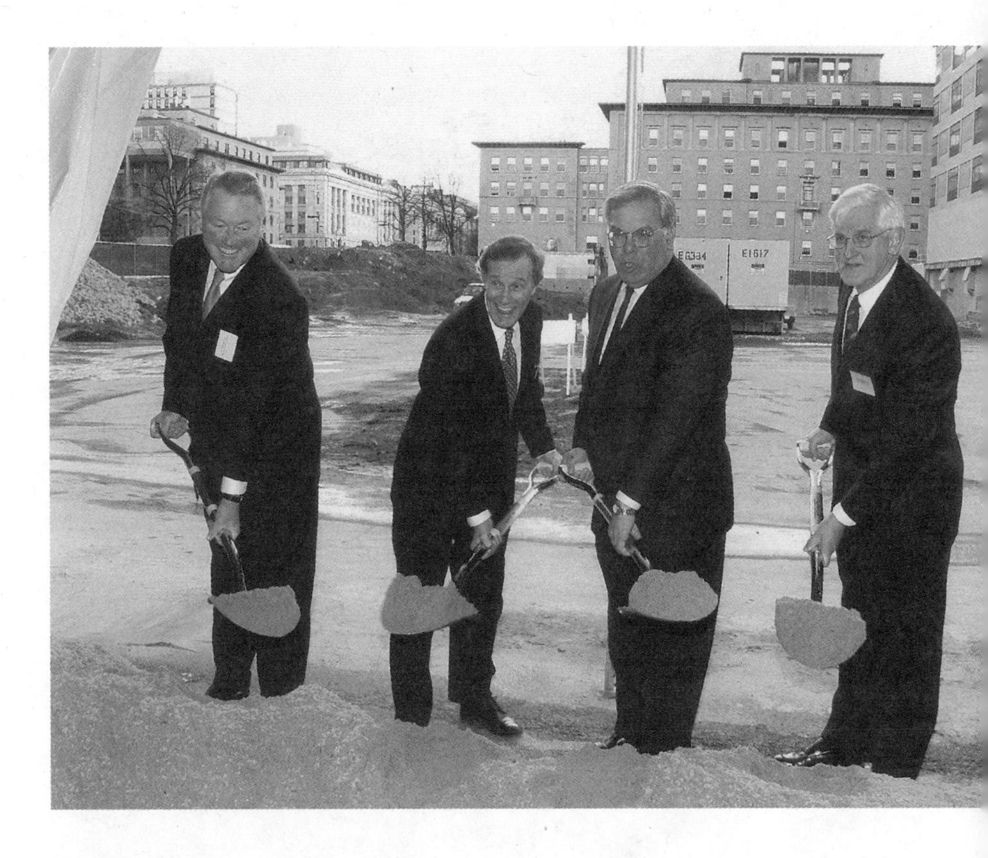

Official groundbreaking for the New Research Building, 2000. From left: Mark Maloney, director Boston Redevelopment Authority (BRA), Harvard President Neil Rudenstine, Boston Mayor Tom Menino and the author.

building had been crucial. He had embraced the importance of interdisciplinary and interfaculty work to face challenges and opportunities in science and medicine, and he imagined a future where science, research, teaching and healing would constitute an integral whole. His vision helped HMS move into an era of unprecedented collaboration with other parts of Harvard and the community at large.

I felt a close friendship with Neil during the four years we worked together. He acknowledged the complex relationships among our hospitals and would often express gratitude for my management of the overt hostilities he had witnessed among the Harvard hospitals during the first six years of his presidency. Dan Tosteson had tried hard to bring together the factions under the umbrella of the Harvard Medical Center but to no avail; he was undermined by successive hospital mergers.

When we broke ground on February 1, we knew that if the mission of Harvard Medical School—to create and nurture a

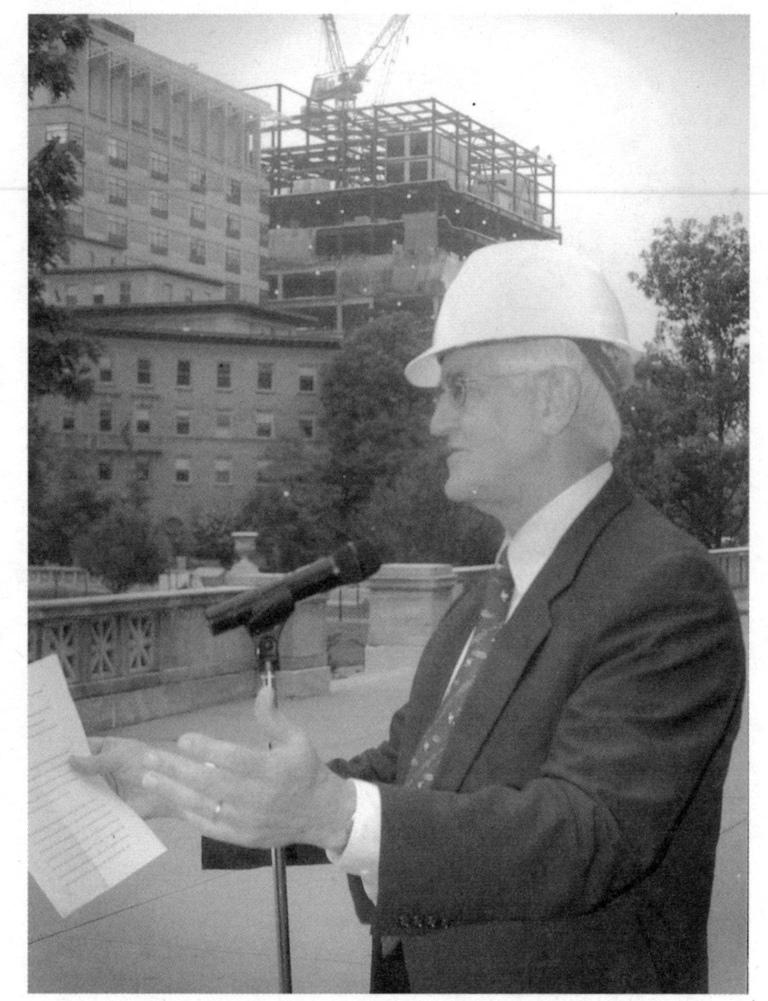

The author during construction of the New Research Building, on the occasion of the 220th anniversary of the founding of Harvard Medical School, 2002.

diverse community of the best people committed to alleviating human suffering caused by disease—was to succeed, old walls that separated disciplines and institutions would have to be torn down. We hoped that the New Research Building would be a step in that direction.

## The World Will Never be the Same Again

Construction on the New Research Building was underway when in early fall the world stood in disbelief as the carnage of 9/11 unfolded before us. I was in my office when I got the news.

Shock and incredulity were soon followed by an urgency to be with our students at the Daniel C. Tosteson Medical Education Center (TMEC). Throughout the day, the students and I watched the magnitude of the loss the country suffered in images that replayed on the television screens set up in the TMEC. We were all trying to grasp the unthinkable, to find words that could adequately describe how we felt. I remember addressing the students, but I can't remember much of what I said that day except that the world would never be the same again. And it has not.

The shock and the aftermath of 9/11 would remain a part of our lives for a long time to come as we witnessed the national and international mobilization of forces to respond to the tragedy. In the November 2, 2001, entry in my journal, (which happened to coincide with my father's birthday), I wrote:

*Tonight we celebrate my father's 88th birthday in the midst of a world gone mad. The events of September 11 and the follow-up reign of terror over anthrax and continued, almost weekly "national" calls for vigilance regarding further terror here, have left the country paralyzed, confused and reactive. The crime is huge, the terror demoralizing, and the fear enervating. But the response is wrong-headed and will result only in years of confrontation, misguided military assaults, and failure to seek understanding of the real causes or to assert "power" in the proper places....*

*We have begun a war in the mountains of Afghanistan that cannot be won...We have no idea how to work on the ground in a war...Our bombing is now "admitted" to be "notoriously" ineffective (remember Cambodia and Vietnam) by our leaders. The extent of civilian damage...has only hardened the hearts of our enemies and cast doubt among our "transient" friends...and the results will be painful to follow and observe...with casualties in the hundreds of thousands...*

I recalled my childhood sense of the futility of war, as images of the tanks and military entourage that passed by our house in 1945 came to mind again. Why is humanity so intent on mutually assured destruction? I found myself thinking about the US's relationship to the principal political entities of the Middle East. I wondered where my original plans to be a missionary doctor might have taken me and what perspectives living abroad might have provided. I was surprised when I felt no regret, thinking about how I had, in my career thus far, been able to help and serve so many students, patients and faculty from one side of the United States to the other. I resolved to continue on my course in the face of what seemed to be a world gone mad.

# NINE

# *Working with Larry Summers*

IN THE SPRING OF 2001, LARRY SUMMERS was introduced to the Harvard deans at a luncheon in Loeb House, the former on-campus residence of the Harvard University president, until it was unceremoniously vacated in 1969 during the student uprisings of the Vietnam War period. He was to begin serving as Harvard's twenty-seventh president in July of that year.

I had arrived four years earlier as the dean of Harvard Medical School. I looked forward to meeting and working with the new president.

## Getting to Know the New President

As a dean, I was invited to make nominations and to discuss candidates on the shortlist with members of the corporation, but I had no opportunity to meet Larry during the search process that led to his appointment as president, although rumors of his candidacy had surfaced in the winter of 2000–2001.

I was aware that Robert Rubin, a New York banker who had been Secretary of the Treasury under President Bill Clinton (and who would later join as a member of the Harvard Corporation) was a strong supporter of Larry's candidacy. As Rubin recounts in his book, *In an Uncertain World*, he and Larry had worked closely during the second Clinton term when Larry, as Deputy Secretary, had been acknowledged for his economic wisdom during the Mexican peso crisis, the Japanese period of stagflation and the Southeast Asia economic turmoil at the end of Clinton's presidency.[1]

My opinion would have served no purpose because I was not acquainted with Larry. I was, however, acquainted with Rick Klausner, director of the National Cancer Institute and the candidate second in line after Larry when Harold Varmus, president of Memorial Sloan–Kettering Cancer Center, withdrew. Rick had called me several times and had come to visit Rachel and me at our home in Brookline to seek my support. At the World Economic Forum in Davos, which Rachel and I attended in January 2001, two months before Larry's appointment was announced, Rick had wanted to meet for a chat. He asked for my support in anticipation of an upcoming meeting he was to have with Hanna Gray, former president of the University of Chicago and now a member of the corporation. I called her on my return to Boston to voice support for Rick, but I could sense that the corporation had already decided to negotiate with Larry.

My first one-on-one meeting with Larry was in July, not long after his arrival on campus. We met in a small office adjacent to the president's in Massachusetts Hall. I was offered a Diet Coke, Larry's standard fare. The conversation was affable and left me feeling that I could work with him. He had prepared for the meeting and knew a considerable amount about the inner workings of Harvard Medical School. He congratulated me, which I perceived to be an endorsement, and said specifically that he looked forward to learning more about the hospital system. We ended our chat about an hour later and walked across Harvard Yard to the Faculty Club for a reception welcoming him to the Harvard community.

"Joe," Larry said abruptly, midway across Harvard Yard, "I was in the Harvard Coop Bookstore the other day and picked up a book by one of your faculty, Walter Willett. Who is he anyway? And by what authority does he propose to modify the

Department of Agriculture food pyramid? What right does he have to make policy recommendations? Does the Medical School endorse his views? Did you review his work before he published it? The cover of the book mentions Harvard Medical School as if you gave an imprimatur to the work."

This was my first encounter with the unnerving quality of Larry's confrontational style, and I immediately realized that every minute with him would revolve around problem-solving. I tried to counter as best I could: yes, I knew who Professor Willett was; yes, he was a very accomplished epidemiologist; no, I had not read the book although I was aware that it had been published; and, actually he was on the faculty of the Harvard School of Public Health, not HMS. The response was: "Get back to me on that. I want to know why a Harvard professor is involved in recommending policy changes. What is the evidence that his proposal is better than the one accepted by food experts over the past several decades?"

We arrived at the Faculty Club and the conversation ended as abruptly as it had begun. I was taken aback by the tenor of Larry's comments and uncertain about how to proceed. I remember thinking that at almost twenty years younger than I, at my age of sixty-four, Larry could have been my son! Walter Willett had written an important book, a bestseller entitled *Eat, Drink and be Healthy*, with a subtitle on the front cover that did indeed state *The Harvard Medical School Guide to Healthy Eating.*[2] The book was endorsed by Tim Johnson, medical editor at ABC News who testified that *Eat, Drink and Be Healthy* was the best book on nutrition for the general public he had read to date. "Dr. Willett," continued Tim Johnson, "is not afraid...to criticize some sacred cows—including the USDA's food pyramid. I urge you to buy this book and read it for yourself; it will be well worth your time."

I relayed Larry's concern to Dean Barry Bloom of the school of public health, who in turn spoke to Walter Willett. Willett sent me an e-mail of explanation, which I transmitted to Larry. I never heard another word about it from Larry, nor did I raise the issue with him again. I had to conclude that he simply wanted to know the background facts about the issue. I also sensed the impact a decade in federal government had on his reactions to policy and amendments to it. But the event lingered on in my memory as an example of Larry's style, which I came to appreciate was driven more by curiosity than animosity.

From that first encounter onward, we developed a very open and interactive conversational style from which I benefited. During our meetings over the next few years, he taught me economics, and I tried to teach him aspects of health care delivery and the intricate relationships HMS had with its hospitals—which it did not own. At an early stage in our discussions, I tried to impress on him how tragic it was to have uninsured patients seek out care in our hospital systems, where reimbursement came from state financial pools for the uninsured, and how catastrophic medical events often resulted in personal bankruptcy. I soon learned that Larry had had a stark experience with his own health before he had turned thirty, when he was diagnosed with late-stage Hodgkin's disease at the Brigham and Women's Hospital and had then undergone prolonged chemotherapy. He would often talk publicly about his personal experiences to audiences at our hospitals, including a very emotional recall of how important the doctor's communication style had been while informing him of the prognosis of his condition. He would describe how he had hung on every word as the doctor placed his life in the balance.

It was in December 2001 when the news broke about a contentious meeting he had held with Cornell West, an African-American professor whom Larry had challenged to account for his teaching commitments and aspects of his recent sabbatical that included time spent producing rap music CDs. Reports of the meeting made the headline news, and soon Professor West noisily decamped to Princeton. This was the first of many ill-fated events that would culminate in Larry's resignation at the end of his fifth year as president, an outcome I personally regretted.

I recall another event that fall that reminded me of how powerless I felt in the health care maze of Harvard Medical School. After completing a couple of sets of tennis with a chap on Cape Cod, Summers learned that his opponent was a professor in one of our hospitals that belonged to the Partners HealthCare network, which included the MGH and Brigham and Women's. The two of them agreed to stay in contact, and when the doctor e-mailed Larry with an Internet address of Dr.xxxx@partners.org, Larry was annoyed and confronted me at our next meeting: "Joe, why don't 'your' hospital faculty use their Harvard address on e-mails? Aren't they Harvard faculty?" All I could think was, "Larry, welcome to the complexities of my life as dean of Harvard Medical School."

Early on in the second year of his tenure as president, Larry would summon the deans of the four largest schools—Arts and Sciences, Business, Law and Medicine—to his house once a month on a Friday morning. Also present at these meetings was Provost Steve Hyman. We met several dozen times over the next four years, and, over orange juice, bagels, muffins and coffee—and Larry with his Diet Coke—we discussed the issues that Larry raised in order to gain our perspectives and insights, which I believe he valued. The issues we discussed were always substantive, like the turnover at the Harvard Management Company, a wholly owned subsidiary that is responsible for investing Harvard's endowment, when the legendary Jack Meyer decided to form a private investment firm. Larry was furious. He did not want Meyer to take money along to manage when he was abandoning the Harvard ship. We could not tell exactly what led Jack to leave, but the corporation did end up providing a substantial investment portfolio for him to manage "on the outside." Jack's exodus was followed by several aborted efforts to find a competent successor over the next five years.

I realized at the Friday-morning sessions that Larry had a genuine need to speak candidly to a group he could trust. He introduced the topics and asked each of us for our comments. He was a good listener, and I felt very close to the pulse of his presidency. I learned more about the inner workings of Harvard from these exchanges at our informal times together on those Friday mornings than from the monthly meetings Larry continued to hold with all the deans. One Friday morning, the topic was the challenges at the Harvard School of Public Health and the enormous grant, exceeding $100 million, the faculty had been awarded as part of President Bush's Emergency Aid Package for an African HIV-AIDS relief program (PEPFAR). The PEPFAR grant to Harvard, an important legacy of the Bush administration in the fight against HIV-AIDS, was announced in the *Boston Globe*. Larry was incensed that, given the enormous size of the award, he had not been included in the application process and was even more concerned that the reputational risk involved with working in East Africa was excessive, if not insurmountable. The project envisioned delivery of better treatments to indigenous populations of the region without a clear academic plan of education and research. Larry was concerned about the appropriateness of this project being led by a faculty member of the Harvard School of Public Health who was trained as a veterinarian. The issue would linger on in Larry's mind for months, and he threatened to put the project on hold. The grant was eventually implemented, but as dean of the school of public health, Barry Bloom felt the pressure of a potential Harvard presidential interdiction not only on the grant but of his leadership of the school as well.

## Envisioning the Unconventional: At What Cost?

As I now reflect on the important issues Larry Summers and I faced together, I place our joint effort to address the financial straits of the BIDMC near the top. The financial mismanagement of the hospital over many years, with capital and operating losses running into the hundreds of millions of dollars, had depleted nearly half of the hospital's endowment. Bonds financing the hospital's capital expenditures were up for renegotiation in the summer of 2002, and agreements to prevent default had to be in place by the end of September. Because the hospital is a nonprofit entity, drawing up these agreements fell under the jurisdiction of Massachusetts's attorney general, who was actively engaged in assessing the impact of financial failure of an entity serving the public good.

The crisis had led to the appointment of a succession of administrative leaders. Dr. Jim Reinertsen, a well-meaning and compassionate man, had failed to rally the troops into more efficient interactions. Dr. Herbert Kressel moved into the position from the chair of the radiology department, but he lasted only a short while. As tensions mounted over the summer of 2002, there were several meetings in my office with Tom Reilly, the Massachusetts attorney general, and one meeting with Reilly and me in Larry's office. The outlook was bleak for the hospital: the immediate cash requirement was about $100 million, which was about equal to the value of a lease the hospital had with Harvard for research space in one of the medical school's buildings. I recommended that the university consider purchasing that agreement. The attorney general looked favorably on it, and Larry carried the request to the corporation, which gave its approval in time to prevent default on the hospital's bonds.

I came to appreciate the impact that the failure of a major hospital would have on patient care, research and the teaching of our students. HMS would almost certainly have had to reduce its class size of 165 students—then and now—each year, and the status of tenured faculty, whose positions were guaranteed by Harvard University–hospital agreements, would lead to unprecedented legal challenges. An additional concern arose over the potential purchase of the hospital by a for-profit entity, which would have severed the longstanding relationships between HMS and its hospitals.

I saw Larry at his very best during this difficult period. He instantly understood the economic and political issues and appreciated their impact on the programs of HMS. Larry brought his experience at the International Monetary Fund to apply economic principles for a bailout, namely to provide support but with conditions. The rescue package provided time for the hospital to re-establish its operations and seek new leadership, with the medical school close to the action. I worked closely with Bob Meltzer, chairman of the board of the Beth Israel Deaconess Medical Center, who asked me to co-chair the search committee with incoming hospital board chairwoman, Lois Silverman, to find a new hospital CEO. I was somewhat reluctant to agree to part with Paul Levy, my senior administrative dean for the past three years, but I knew Paul would succeed in leading the hospital out of the doldrums into a "going concern," as he did.

Larry's commitment to engage the university more deeply in the biological sciences was front and center in his mind as strategic plans unfolded. His approach had both academic and economic arguments. In his public speeches, he often lamented that Harvard College graduates were unlikely to have trouble describing the plots of several of Shakespeare's plays, but they might not be able to explain the difference between a gene and a chromosome. He pointed, possibly to the detriment of relations with the college faculty, to the strengths in biomedical research at HMS and the hospitals, and he admired the reputation of HMS's graduate programs, which recruited students in competition with Stanford, UC Berkeley, UCSF and MIT, while Harvard College programs remained relatively out of the running. College programs, he believed, tended to act in silos; graduate programs were fragmented, and students often applied directly to faculty members in fields like chemistry. For its part, some in the Faculty of Arts and Sciences accused him of "medicalizing" the university.

Then there was the issue surrounding the growing influence of Harvard Medical International (HMI). When Larry took charge in July 2001, a major change in emphasis was put into play on the international opportunities that the university was to undertake. Larry was very sensitive to the disaster that had emerged earlier with the Harvard International Institute of Development (HIID) in Russia, which had led to federal charges of mismanagement of funds and to a lawsuit charging Harvard faculty with misappropriating money.[3] Neil had been aware of the charges and despite all efforts had not been able to solve the crisis before Larry came on board.

Larry was personally acquainted with and had been a mentor to some of the principals involved in the HIID scandal. Early in his term, he had placed the large HSPH PEPFAR grant on hold while he and the provost examined the implications of all the risks involved. They both began to look anew at the risks of international collaborations and commitments. While we, at HMS, had no clear idea of what the objections were, Larry asked members of the corporation to resign from the HMI Board, pointing out that they were not appropriately placed in such administrative positions. But since Ron Daniel was retiring from the corporation, Judith Hope had already done so and Conrad Harper, an attorney, was frequently a dissenter in much of HMI's activities, we seemed in some ways the better off. The first five years of my deanship (1997–2002) saw HMI become a force admired by many within and beyond the HMS orbit. Larry Summers personally took great interest in our work and

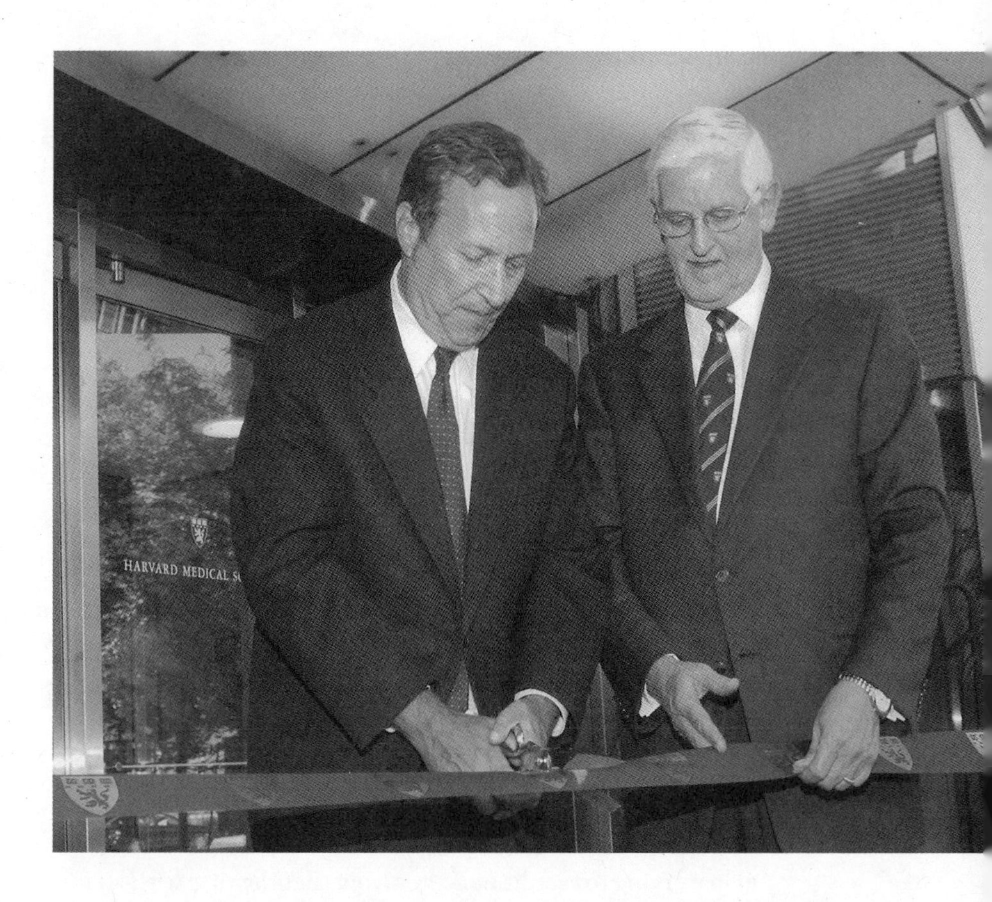


Larry Summers and the author at the ribbon cutting ceremony for the NRB, 2003.

accepted an invitation to visit Dubai, where HMI had operations, to meet with His Highness, Sheikh Mohammed bin Rashid Al Maktoum. While there, he participated in a symposium and continued to encourage our activities during his remaining days as president. Things were to be quite different when Derek Bok took over after Larry's exodus, as you will see in the next chapter.

In the meantime, though, in September 2003 I joined Larry at the ribbon-cutting ceremony to officially open the medical school's New Research Building, the largest single construction in Harvard's history, and a project that Neil Rudenstine had supported. President Rudenstine had gone to considerable lengths to ensure the support of the Harvard Corporation. The rationale for the new building was the need for the integration of Quad-based scientists in the Departments of Genetics and Pathology with hospital-based scientists, primarily from the Brigham and Women's Hospital and the Dana-Farber Cancer Institute (DFCI).

The basic science chairs at the medical school engaged with the dean's office planning group to make a recommendation that two departments relocate to the new space, freeing up space for the expansion of the remaining departments at their old sites on the main campus. We established a campaign to note that HMS occupied a South Quad, which had opened in 1906, and now, nearly one hundred years later, a North Quad, where the New Research Building was located near Vanderbilt Hall, the medical students' residence.

## The Establishment of the Broad Institute and Emphasis on Translational Work

Larry took great risks in supporting unconventional arrangements. The most remarkable, I believe, was the agreement with MIT to establish the Broad Institute. At first, when the promise of a major investment from Eli and Edythe Broad in the work of MIT's Eric Lander seemed likely, Larry raised the issue of recruiting Eric to Harvard and asked Steve Hyman to explore the matter. The Broads were interested in forging effective research collaborations with Harvard's teaching hospitals, and an agreement with Harvard would facilitate that. I strongly advised against trying to recruit Lander, saying that the rifts with MIT would disadvantage both institutions and the region. After all, there were many effective inter-institutional programs, like the Harvard–MIT Health Sciences and Technology (HST) program, so why not add another one? I also strongly urged the formation of an independent entity that would serve the broader constituencies of the region to provide research programs to facilitate the biological impact of the post-genomic era.

I recall vividly when the issue of university-matching funds arose. To complete the arrangement with the Broads, the two universities were to agree to raise $100 million over five years. Larry worried about the impression this gave to the university's main campus. I told him he could not afford not to do the deal because Harvard needed to be part of the initiative. The formation of the Broad Institute of Harvard and MIT was announced within a few weeks.

Larry spoke passionately at every opportunity about the need for the Boston area to adopt strategies for economic development in the marketing of biological advances, which he compared with Silicon Valley and the development of computers two decades earlier. Boston lost a great deal in that competition as computer development moved from the large models of IBM and Digital Equipment to Sun Microsystems, Apple Computers, Oracle, Hewlett-Packard and so on. He feared that the same fate might befall the therapeutic development of biological and engineering devices if universities and business communities did not act in concert. His approach was highly acclaimed by the business community and the Boston Chamber of Commerce, venues where he brought forward specific proposals. His approach also won friends with the medical faculty, who generally worked to advance translational opportunities. But such was not the case at Harvard College, where it met with dissatisfaction among many scientists who had disdain for any focus on "practical" work.

Larry's concepts had a great deal to do with the establishment of the stem cell program, the efforts to develop a new site for advanced interdisciplinary work, and the setting in motion of the development of a new school of science and engineering at Harvard. Each of these new programs was to be integrated into a new science campus located in the Allston section of Boston, across the river from the university near the Harvard Business School (see Map 6 in chapter ten). The university had quietly acquired an extensive portfolio of land over the previous decade—more than two hundred acres—that promised to be the focus of new academic programs for the twenty-first century. Larry made his plans for greater integration of science graduate programs explicit by supporting the development of a new Department of Systems Biology at HMS, with a substantial commitment of new funds and plans for it also to be located at the Allston site. He urged the coordination of the university-wide application program for graduate students with a single website and a new title—the Harvard Integrated Life Sciences Program (HILS)—and asked Christopher T. Walsh of HMS to chair it. These exciting plans were unfolding at a remarkable pace when other events overtook the attention of many in the university.

## Propitiation

Larry gave his infamous speech about women in science and engineering in January 2005. By then, he seemed to be offending many of the traditional-minded professors in the Faculty of Arts and Sciences. Indeed, his challenges of faculty scholars presented for tenure at the ad hoc sessions he chaired in the college were unusual for a president. Neil Rudenstine had taken a more placid approach. Derek Bok, on the other hand, was known for the close personal attention he had paid to candidates for tenure during his term as president from 1971 to 1991. But not only did Larry take it to another level, he often belittled faculty and department chairs with his scathing assessments of the contributions made by the candidates in question. In some cases he was relentless, despite his lack of expertise in the work of the candidate under consideration.

The level of animosity toward Larry grew and, I think, contributed in large measure to the instantaneous reaction—like powder ignited—when the issue of disparities of the innate ability between men and women broke open that January. Nancy Hopkins, a distinguished professor from MIT who had worked effectively to improve women's status within that institution, walked out of the meeting in disgust. The meeting was at a small luncheon of about forty people, to which Larry was invited to deliver a welcoming address. He was acquainted with the organizer of the symposium, who encouraged forthright and open discussion of challenges facing women in academic circles. Before long, the issue was front-page news in the *Boston Globe* and, shortly thereafter, in the *New York Times*. Initially, Larry turned down requests for the full transcript of the speech, only to later relent and publish the full text on the university website.

I believe it only fair to recognize the setting of this unfortunate event and to understand the intellectual exercise that I think Larry perceived himself to be engaged in. It is also important to carefully read the full text of his comments. Larry clearly put aside his role of university president and took on the role of an economist, looking at the issues from the perspective of statistics and epidemiology. In the context of his overall comments, the issues he suggested as relevant to the underrepresentation of women in science and engineering were clearly intended to be provocative, as was his style in general. He summarized his talk in three points. First, success is determined by how hard people are willing to work at their professional pursuits, which represents special challenges for women raising families. He next considered the faculty selection process, noting that at the extremes of intellectual ability (in mathematics and the sciences), boys and men have a wider distribution of capability, ranging from common developmental abnormalities, including autism and mental retardation at one end of the spectrum, to measures of the "innate" mathematical and theoretical abilities at the other extreme. For Larry, this simply meant that compared to women, men were overrepresented at the extreme ends of the spectrum. In his third point, he recognized that women face "cultural" challenges by way of discrimination, but he considered these to be of lesser importance, although requiring attention to assure that no discrimination occurred. Provocative he was; the reaction was instant, and his position as university president was openly challenged from that occasion forward.

One participant in the conference, Cathy Trower, head of the Collaborative on Academic Careers in Higher Education, based at the Harvard Graduate School of Education, commented recently, "I thought Larry was setting us up for a discussion of the issues women faculty face. But instead he appeared disengaged and left the room without inviting real dialogue."

Reflecting on Larry's apparent insensitivities, I find it peculiar that little recognition has been given to appointments Larry made of women to senior academic posts at Harvard. Notable among these was the appointment of Elena Kagan as dean of the law school. Kagan, herself a graduate of the law school, was appointed at age forty-one, charged with pacifying a contentious faculty divided along ideological lines that had fractured the school. She skillfully changed the culture without taking sides and among her own appointments were several faculty members who bridged the political divide between left and right. Kagan was appointed Solicitor General of the US by President Obama in 2009 and is, with the announced retirement of Justice Stevens, now the fourth woman appointed to the Supreme Court.

I recall vividly from the experiences at Larry's Friday-morning gatherings of senior deans, Kagan's fearlessness in disagreeing with Larry on certain points and defending her view, which he clearly respected greatly.

Another distinguished appointment was Kathleen McCartney, dean of the Faculty of Education. These were examples, I felt, of Larry's open-mindedness about appointments, and his always making the effort to find the best person.

Larry never recovered from the onslaught of hostility that followed his comments at that meeting in January 2005. I watched him enter into a shell, lose much of his animation and, despite apologies, regrets and the formation of a committee to correct issues adverse to women's careers in science at Harvard (including dedicating funds to right the wrongs), he could not do enough to pacify the Faculty of Arts and Sciences. His leadership continued to be challenged, and a majority of the school's faculty attending a jammed meeting in the Faculty Room of the college called for a vote of no confidence and asked for his resignation. The students by and large defended him, and members of the Harvard Corporation, especially Robert Rubin, who, perhaps better than anyone else knew Larry's great strengths and weaknesses, were very reluctant to take action. I remained an ally to the very end, together with Jay Light, who had recently been appointed dean of the Harvard Business School, and Venky Narayanamurti, who was setting up the newly formed school of engineering and applied science.

At HMS, except for a contingent of women faculty who expressed deep resentment over Larry's comments, there was great support for the entire course of his presidency—among both women and men. About a month after the crisis over his comments on the "innate differences between the sexes," Larry called me to ask if he should accept a lunch invitation at the medical school to address the HMS Joint Committee on the Status of Women. I encouraged him to do so and joined him at the luncheon along with about forty faculty members. He listened carefully to the presentations on the progress being made at the medical school to further academic opportunities for women. When asked to respond, Larry took the podium and spoke humbly and apologetically for any misunderstanding that his previous comments might have created. He was so different from the man I'd known a few months earlier. I also couldn't help but notice that his comments were deeply healing and his efforts very much appreciated by the group present.

### "Let me say something slightly outrageous...."

Despite widespread perception that Larry showed insensitivity in interpersonal relationships and an impersonal attitude to ordinary events, he was a brilliant communicator. Arriving minutes before the scheduled time, often quite disheveled, he could immediately capture his audience. Without any formal notes and without PowerPoint to illustrate his presentation, he would typically introduce three or four ideas and weave them into a seamless story. The Seidman Lecture he gave at HMS in 2004 was one of those instances. After Barbara McNeil, chair of the Department of Health Care Policy, had introduced him, Larry set out to outline and define the main elements of the health care crisis facing the US, beginning, as he often did, by recounting his own experience with a life-threatening illness. He then drew on C.P. Snow's famous lecture, *The Two Cultures*,[4] a lament on the breakdown between the sciences and the humanities, and Michael Lewis's *Moneyball* on the techniques Billy Beane and the Oakland As used in selecting high-performance players at lower cost,[5] and then went on to describe what he called, "...the art of diagnosis and treatment for patients presenting with given symptoms," detailing his thoughts on the matter:

*Let me say something slightly outrageous. Whenever it is proudly asserted by practitioners of an activity that that activity is an art rather than a science, they are describing an activity that is still in relatively primitive form, and where great progress will follow the application of more scientific techniques.*

*I was struck, and I have to confess somewhat worried, by a conversation I had with an advanced medical student and a junior resident a year and a half or so ago as I accompanied them on rounds in the Brigham. They went in and saw a patient, and they had a variety of tests and they discussed what to do. And then they said, "We're going to do X." And I said, "Gee, this must be one of the thousands of patients the world has seen who had this combination of symptoms. Isn't there any database where you could plug these symptoms in and learn what the possibilities were, and just in case you've possibly forgotten what the right thing to do was, test your intuition against the systematic experience of thousands of cases like this?" The young resident explained, "No, no, no, no, no. Medicine is an art not a science, and to reduce it to something mechanistic would just be wrong. That's done, but not at really good institutions like Harvard. And at other institutions sometimes they use computerized diagnosis, but that is not where it's at." And I said, "Well, is there a possibility you could perhaps check what you were doing, just in case you might have made a mistake or that there was a resident who wasn't as good as you or it was in an area you weren't familiar with?" "Well, no, no. We really need to understand the science of this particular patient with this particular disease."*[6]

My colleague Dan Federman said it was the best lecture on the topic of health care he'd ever heard. I could not help but reflect on how a conversation like that would have been interpreted if Larry was addressing a time-worn senior FAS faculty member whose sacred ground was being unceremoniously tramped upon.

Praise for Larry's speeches was not limited to Harvard audiences. I remember a comment made by Warren Hellman, a venture capital investor in San Francisco and a graduate of the Harvard Business School. Warren had heard Larry speak at an alumni gathering at the University of California, Berkeley, and told me later that it was the best speech by an academic leader that he had ever heard.

In June 2003 Larry gave the Blackfan Lecture at Children's Hospital. He told the story I often heard him relate about how, when first being introduced to the deans at Harvard by the Fellows of the Harvard Corporation, he was placed between Dean Jeremy Knowles of FAS and me:

*I asked Jeremy, "How many members of the faculty are there in the Arts and Sciences?" He said, "630." I turned to Joe, "How many full-time cancer researchers are there at the Harvard Medical School?" Joe said, "Do you mean in the Quadrangle or in the hospitals?" And I looked blank. And Joe said, "Do you mean basic science or clinical science?" I said, "Joe, it's my first day. I mean people who wear white coats, use pipettes, and try to fight cancer." Joe thought for a second and said, "800." I have to confess that was seven times the estimate I would have given if Joe had asked me to guess. It says something very powerful about what a modern university is, and it says something very important about the role of things medical at Harvard. It is something I have not forgotten and have retold frequently because there is nothing that I think is more important to what is happening at the University than at the medical school and in its affiliated hospitals.*[7]

Such a statement would not have appeared on the lips of most other Harvard presidents; small wonder that I liked the man and what he stood for. In that same speech, his concluding comments were:

*If you think about the three points that I have made—the central importance of health care, the need to balance the drive toward market efficiency with the assurances of the availability of the very valuable (assets) that the market does not actually support, and the central role of scientific progress in the health care system—they really point to a common conclusion that there are few, if any, institutions that do work that is as profoundly important as the teaching hospital, the modern medical school, and the academic medical center. And that is why I am so pleased to have a chance to be here today and to affirm their very central importance to Harvard University.*

Larry's thoughts mirrored a seminal statement by the great William Osler in an article in the 1911 issue of *The Lancet*:

*The truth is, we need an active invasion of the hospital by the universities. But—and here comes the rub—the universities must be willing to undertake their share of the expenses, and...pay enough for its hospital privileges.*[8]

Larry understood the significance of Osler's thought, as had Neil Rudenstine—who had helped implement the payment system that allowed for medical education reform lying before us—and supported the rethinking of the curriculum at HMS and the hospitals.

## Harvard after Summers...Summers after Harvard

Larry resigned in the spring of his fifth year. The medical school and hospital-based faculty turned out in large numbers for a celebratory "Thank You" in May at the Harvard Club in Boston. We gave Larry a standing ovation to signal our appreciation for his interests in the activities of the medical complex, and I presented him with a photomontage of the significant events he'd participated in at the medical school during his leadership. A few months before the celebration at the Harvard Club, I had sent an op-ed piece to the *Boston Globe* entitled "Summers's Bold Vision for the Life Sciences," which appeared a few weeks after his publicly announced resignation. The editorial stated:

*During the 4½ years of his presidency, Larry Summers championed a bold vision for life sciences at Harvard—and that process has the potential to have major impacts on Boston, the region and society as a whole. We must assure that this robust new way of looking at scientific opportunities will continue and accelerate during the last four months of Summer's tenure, and it is critical to Harvard and the region that the process continue long after he has begun his next big challenge.*

*Spurred on by Summers, Harvard is re-examining its entire scientific enterprise. It is now focused on the integration and collaboration critical to interdisciplinary discovery, the aspect of research that most observers would say is the ripest for results that can transform health and promote well-being...*

*Biologists and physicians working with those trained in chemistry, physics, and mathematics are opening new approaches to identifying disease mechanisms and novel drugs in cancer, Alzheimer's disease, and heart disease....*[9]

To replace Larry Summers, Harvard set about finding a new president, while Derek Bok took the reins as interim president, returning to the helm after fifteen years, at the age of seventy-five, to manage the complexities of a world that had changed profoundly and in so many ways. On the eve of his interim term, I sent Derek a somewhat arrogant and, in retrospect, probably unnecessary missive making the case that the medical school was in a strong position at the end of Larry's term and that as it moved forward, the university might benefit from looking at some of our accomplishments. I shared the text of my comments, constructed over a couple of days, with my fellow deans—Ray Dolin, Cynthia Walker and Nancy Andrews, each of whom concurred with the thrust of the message. It drew a measured, nearly angry response from President Bok and led to a difficult year as I watched a new administration take on the legacy of Larry's efforts with a different focus.

In the letter to Bok, which I also shared with Jamie Houghton, the senior fellow of the Harvard Corporation, I lamented the fact that the corporation knew very little about the inner workings and complexity of HMS and that most of the members of the corporation had never set foot on our campus and had held very few meetings with me and my fellow deans. I was especially concerned that the planning strategies for the development of cross-university science that Larry had initiated in January 2006 were about to be implemented by taking away commitments made to HMS, such as the support for the new Department of Systems Biology. I was also concerned that the Allston planning process as proposed by the University Planning Committee on Science and Engineering (UPSCE), an interfaculty committee that Larry had charged just six weeks before his announced resignation and that made its report public in June 2006, sought to take away many HMS initiatives and relocate them to Allston without concern about their impact on our planning.

In 2007, in the epilogue to his book entitled *Avoid Boring People,* James Watson lambasted Harvard University's failure to keep up in the world of science when compared to MIT and blamed Larry Summers for his misguided focus on the Allston development at the expense of science support to the Faculty of Arts and Sciences. He blamed the late Jeremy Knowles for skimpy research funding for FAS and decried the mediocre performance of the medical school science establishment. Then, he added "Summers's...proposals for the future of science...figured more critically in his vexed relations with the faculty than any clumsy words that marked his ultimate undoing."[10]

I personally doubt that most Harvard faculty members understand it was the strained relations with the elite science faculty at FAS that contributed as much to Larry's eventual downfall as his dealings with the FAS faculty in general. Support for Larry's approach to interdisciplinary biology was appreciated by some esteemed scientists like Doug Melton, whose work had turned to practical problems in biology after two of his daughters developed type 1 diabetes mellitus. Doug led the world in the promise of stem cell research and worked with new FAS Dean Bill Kirby and me in proposing that the Allston science initiative include a new stem cell institute and a new integrated Harvard-wide Department of Regenerative Biology. But other faculty members, such as Physics Professor Daniel Fisher, were outspokenly critical of Larry's approach to making science more translational.

The last time I saw Larry on the Harvard campus was in May 2006, less than a month before his leaving the presidency. The occasion was the unveiling of President Neil Rudenstine's portrait by E. Raymond Kinstler. I watched the ceremonies from the back of the room, in the very faculty room where Larry had received so much harsh criticism from the FAS faculty and where he had humbly apologized. He stood alone by the buffet table chomping on nuts as Neil thanked the artist and those in attendance for their friendship and support during his decade as president. Larry looked forlorn and anguished. I left the ceremony feeling deeply saddened. We will never know what might have become of Larry's dream for a twenty-first-century Harvard, focused on life sciences and the contribution that new interfaces between the academy and industry, might have produced.

The economic disasters that have ensued came to trump any such ambition under Harvard's new administration. And so, in the spring of 2011, the Allston initiative was put on ice and the building of the first science Quad was on hold, unlikely to be resurrected in the next five years. The stem cell institute headed for relocation to the northwest corner of the Harvard Campus, as far from the medical school and its hospitals as it could possibly be. The initiative in bioengineering is located in a space at the medical school on the Longwood campus, a good location for those of us here in the medical world, but, once again, keeping separate the activities that Larry hoped would integrate our communities across the university.

When Larry assumed his responsibilities with President Barack Obama in 2009, Sharon Begley in her column in the February 23, 2009, issue of *Newsweek*, described him as a fox, not a hedgehog:



*Larry Summers is seldom accused of having a modest personality, but he displays the fox's cognitive style: in briefing the president, he assigns numerical probabilities to possible outcomes of economic policies, rather than saying "This will (or will not) happen."*[11]

The analogy captures, I believe, the aspect of Larry's style that began the downfall of his presidency: he was too analytical, which was his proclivity, without an appreciation of the potential emotional reactions his approach might draw. He did not deserve the treatment he was given. He was and remains a great man and a grand thinker. I often think of his vision for Harvard University and Harvard Medical School as I watch him negotiate, now from afar, the thickets of federal politics centered on health care reform and the economy from his current vantage point in the White House. And, I will always treasure the letter he wrote me shortly before I completed my term as dean in 2007, about a year after he had stepped down as president. The letter read, in part:

*Working with you was one of the joys of my years as Harvard president. Beyond appreciating your loyalty and support in good times and bad, I developed enormous admiration for your commitment to Harvard Medical School and beyond HMS to what scientific progress can mean for the reduction of human suffering. You, more than anyone else I worked with always led with a sense of purpose that recognized that budgets, plans, administrative structures and other rituals of university life are not ends in themselves but means to the ultimate of education and knowledge creation. That I believe is why you were able to do so much to renew Harvard medicine in the New Research Building, in its curriculum, in its scientific approaches and leadership, and in its relationship to the teaching hospitals.*

*From our first meetings together where we discussed getting the BI (Beth Israel) back on track, through your steadfast recognition that the right if not always the comfortable thing to do was to help create the Broad Institute, through our many conversations about Allston you have always been wise, strong and visionary.*

Today as I reflect on the problems Larry Summers faced during his tenure of five years as president of Harvard, I appreciate the fact that Larry was not a politician. The remorse he showed over the fallout of his speech on "innate differences" between men and women was genuine, but mainly because of the impact on Harvard's reputation as he came to appreciate that there are limits to freedom of speech for a president. As an intellectual, Larry could synthesize brilliantly complex situations into a concise package that would be understandable to a knowledgeable audience. He was intellectually honest but inept at displaying an appearance of flexibility.

What Larry lacked was the politician's skill of reading between the lines and connecting with the emotions of the audience. After the disdain expressed over his speech, he succumbed to appearances of repentance with promises of initiatives to examine and adjust for any discrimination that was taking place, but his personal capacity to adjust to the "political" impact of what was taking place led to a progressive teetering on the edge and eventual resignation.

Despite Larry's profound intellect, there were hints that he wanted to be grounded in the context of a given circumstance. I was surprised on many occasions when Larry would ask after he had completed a talk: "Did I do okay? Was that what you wanted?" It was an intellectual query about the success of the message delivered more than curiosity about the impact on the listeners.

I still think Larry was the best boss I ever had. I was pleased in 2011 to welcome him back to Harvard after his two-year leave working with President Obama. He returned to his position as University Professor.

# TEN

# *Harvard Medical School, 1997–2007*

THE DEAN AT HARVARD MEDICAL SCHOOL occupies a complex and challenging position. On the one hand, there is the bully pulpit and the power of the brand name that grants the dean access to many forums: the dean is invited to lunch; people within the academy and without return his telephone calls; he is invited frequently to serve, for example, on community not-for-profit organizations; and regular opportunities arise to serve on national policymaking bodies. The dean seems to be on lists for potential commencement speakers, often with the promise of an honorary degree. Yet, as dean I often felt that the symbolism wasn't so overwhelming to HMS alumni and couldn't help but sense that my presentations to them were often met with skepticism. With so many illustrious HMS graduates, why had Joe Martin been selected for the job? What was his claim to fame? Needless to say, such questions were never made explicit, and, in a way, I blame mostly myself for feeling apologetic.

On the other hand, in sharp contrast to the symbolism of the job is the relative impotency that comes with it. The day-to-day

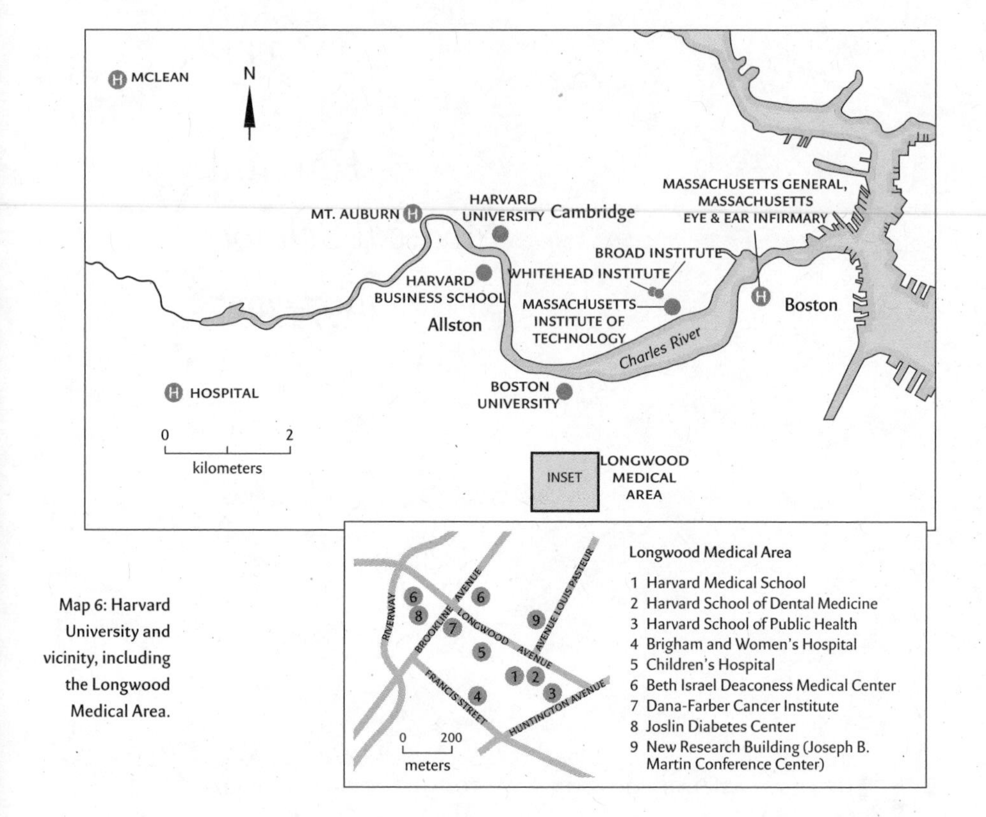


Map 6: Harvard University and vicinity, including the Longwood Medical Area.

encumbrances deriving from the school's position in the governance structure of the university and its position *vis-à-vis* the hospitals leave the dean feeling quite powerless. HMS is the largest school at Harvard in terms of number of faculty, yet only a small number of its faculty receive benefits in salary or perks from the university. Most of the physicians at the seventeen Harvard-affiliated teaching hospitals and research institutes hold academic appointments—from instructor to professor—but their salaries are paid by the hospitals. The enormous budgets and capacity for research support, clinical trials and the ever-expanding specialty services of the hospitals dwarf the HMS budget. Now that I've left the job, I am somewhat surprised at the respect faculty express toward the dean's role. And what's even more ironic is that now I, too, have a certain sense of awe when visiting the present dean in his office. Did I underestimate the influence the symbolism broadcast over the Boston medical establishment?

## The Complexity of Institutional Relationships

There are examples that illustrate the reality of the school's position, placed as it is, in a matrix of institutions with formidable powers. Consider philanthropic efforts. Every year over the past decade, Harvard has announced that is has generated between $500 and $600 million in philanthropic support, with HMS contributing about 15 per cent of that amount, or around $100 million, annually. Similar ratios emerge when comparing the school's efforts to combined hospital philanthropies. In this instance, the five largest hospitals in the Harvard orbit together raise about $500 million annually, and again, the HMS effort is about 15 per cent of their total.

The school also faces challenges in fundraising due to lack of access to grateful patients, who are for the most part interested in supporting the hospitals. HMS graduates, while supportive, are by and large not very capable of large gifts, nor is there much inclination on the part of the Faculty of Arts and Sciences or the schools of business and law to encourage their alumni to consider health-related gifts to HMS. And, with a few negotiated exceptions, these schools do not generally give alumni class credit for their gifts to HMS.

The challenges that result from the structure of governance can be illustrated in another way. The HMS budget is approximately $500 million, nearly half of which comes from grants and research contracts, most from federal sources. The research budget of Partners HealthCare (which includes Massachusetts General and Brigham and Women's Hospitals) alone exceeds $1 billion, and the five largest independent hospitals of the Harvard medical community are all listed in the top rung of independent hospitals and research institutes funded by the National Institutes of Health. The total support of the research enterprise of the Harvard medical complex exceeds $4 billion annually. The medical school's budget comprises about 10 per cent of that total.

## Working with the Hospital CEOs

It should not come as a surprise that an effective hospital CEO spends very little time thinking about the HMS mission

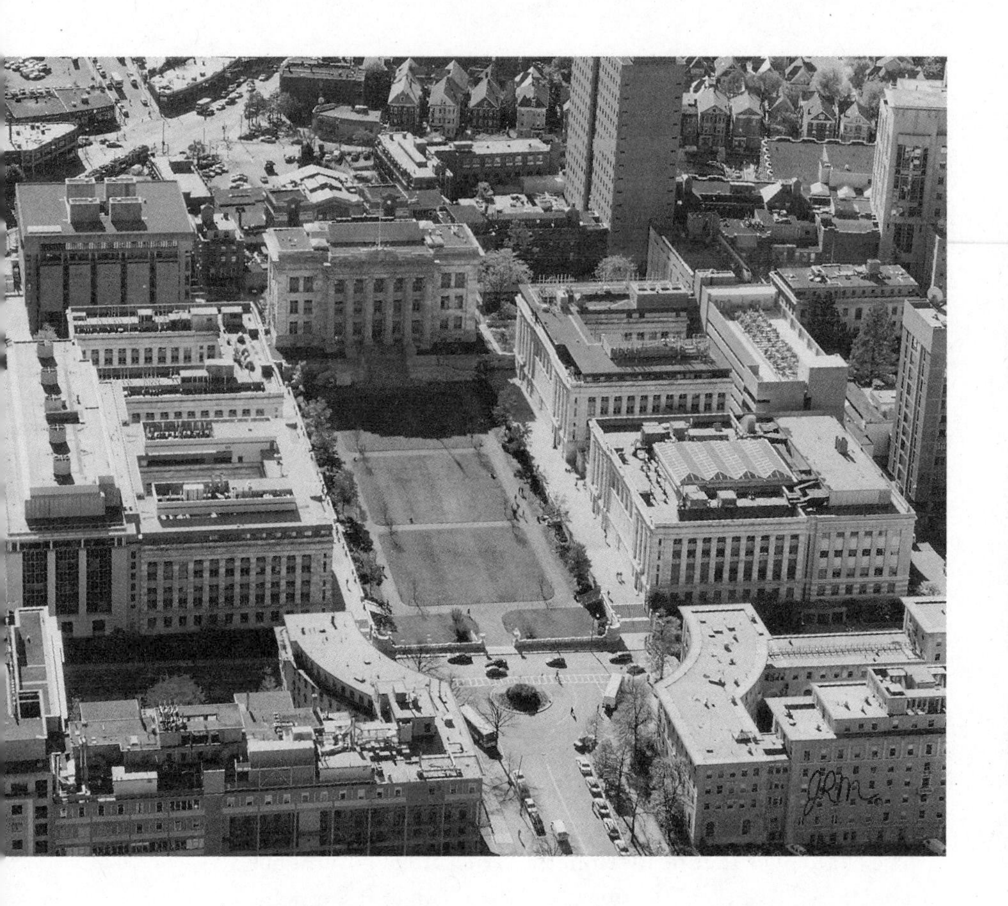

Aerial photograph of Harvard Medical School, 2003. The dean's office is located at the end of the Quad, on the left.

of education and research or about the teaching obligations of hospital-based faculty. The CEO is mostly, and quite appropriately, concerned with the bottom line and the way clinical care activities and efficiencies will result in a positive margin for the whole activity, a margin nearly always in the low single digits in Massachusetts. The CEO is also quite interested in the indirect payments accompanying federal grants that can be applied quite leniently to offset costs involved in research and for capital projects in support of research activities.

Hence, the relationship between the HMS dean and the hospital CEO, while polite, is at risk of being quite perfunctory. During my time, I was fortunate to be deeply involved in the transitions in leadership at each of the five large affiliated institutions: the Brigham and Women's Hospital, the Massachusetts General Hospital, the Dana-Farber Cancer Institute, the Beth Israel Deaconess Medical Center and Boston Children's

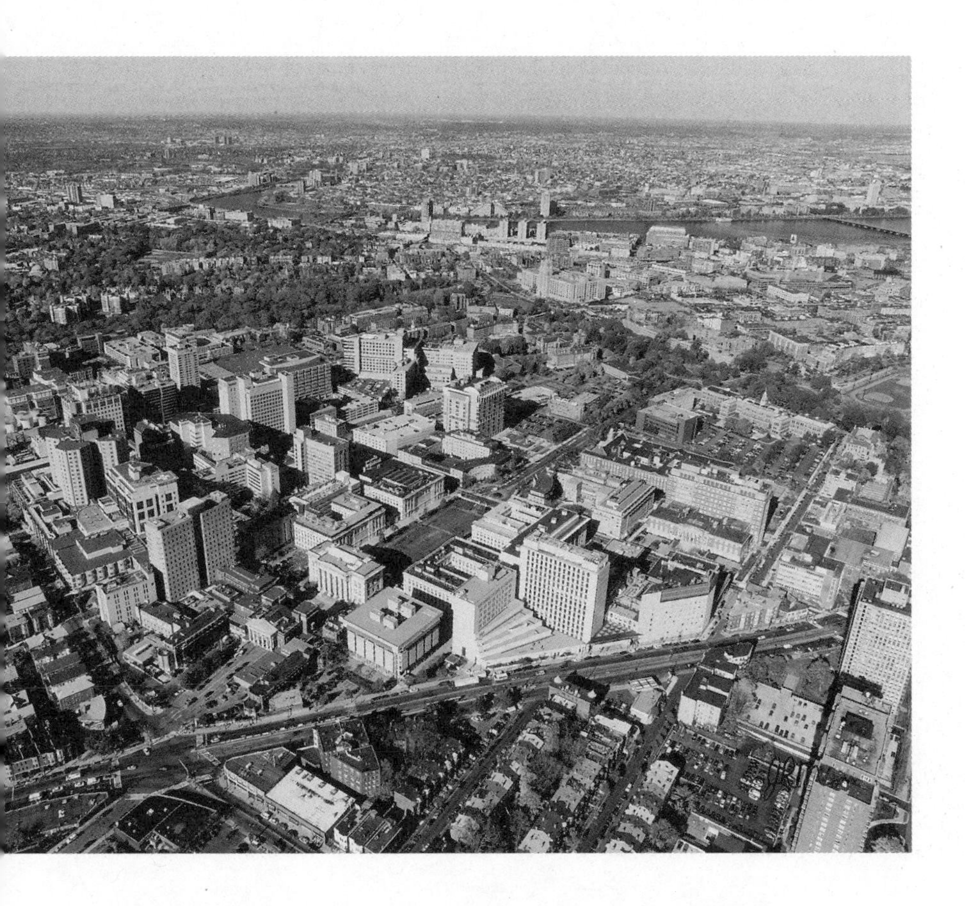

Aerial photograph of the Longwood Medical Area.

Hospital. I made a special effort to meet with the chair of each hospital's board of trustees before or shortly after my arrival in 1997, and much of the collegiality and comfort I enjoyed during the decade I served as dean was due to relationships cultivated early on. As a result, when leadership searches took place, I was invited in most instances to be co-chair of the search committee. The outcome of these searches was a powerful adjunct to my efforts at HMS. These folks were, in many ways, my buddies, eager and willing to take on issues that had not been satisfactorily addressed in previous administrations.

I held monthly one-on-one meetings with each of the CEOs, alternating between my office and theirs. We were frank and honest with each other. Telephone calls between us were frequent, and we alerted each other to impending news—good and bad. We shared victories and setbacks, and together we plotted the best ways to send out messages, including on how, for instance, to encourage faculty to show respect for our students. Most of the hospital leaders had appointments in the professorial ranks of the school, which I believe they valued greatly, and each taught courses or gave lectures to HMS students. We worked together on the unpleasant issues of faculty misconduct or forming responsible faculty committees to make recommendations to us. Discipline of a faculty member over scientific misconduct or sexual harassment was delivered conjointly, giving strength to the force of the findings and gaining assent for the recommendations made.

A particularly important decision I made early on was to spend one day each month at the MGH, where, because of the distance, the faculty historically felt isolated from the main Longwood campus. I set up meeting hours there in the administrative section of the hospital and met regularly with department chairs, senior faculty and administrators. Those visits served to ground me in current matters affecting the institution and brought back nostalgic memories of my earlier time there in the 1980s, when I was chief of the neurology service and for nearly a year served as the hospital CEO, or general director.

Following is a June 1998 entry from my journal that reflects on how I was feeling after a year as dean of HMS:

*What then are some of the conclusions of my first year back at Harvard? Certainly I did not come here because I believed that HMS was manageable. There are many faces to this great and unique institution. The strength of HMS is its complexity. The weakness of HMS is its complexity. Perceptions vary enormously throughout our ranks.*

*For the medical student, HMS is a two-year undergraduate curriculum followed by hospital rotations. For many, the intimacy and self-assurance (even self-adulation) that derives from the tutorial experience is rapidly diluted by the complexity of our affiliated institutions. Almost as soon as students begin their core clinical clerkships, they are pressed to plan their future. What do they like and why? What can be discarded or what preferences emerge—a life in primary care? An academic career? A life as a clinician-teacher? The concerns about growing indebtedness limit the options for many.*

*Viewed from Building A, the medical school appears as an administrative jungle. We have our work cut out with little time and attention given our affiliates. Viewed from the perspective of the Quad departments, emphasis appropriately is placed on balancing research and teaching, recruitments, promotions and retentions. From the perspective of graduate training, there is enormous competition to get the best students—the very best!*

*Viewed from a hospital position, particularly as a junior faculty member, HMS seems remote, formal, uninvolved and often more of an obstacle than a help.*

*Balancing teaching with increasing pressures to deliver more patient care, or balancing a research laboratory with clinical obligations, creates enormous challenges and often anxiety.*

*I view HMS from the "adminosphere" as having primarily a service function—to establish conditions, circumstances, opportunities to allow for the greatest creativity, ingenuity and clever devices that talented people can produce. Get the best people, provide them with adequate but not excessive resources, and give them the time and freedom to accomplish their ambitions and goals.*

*What a wonderful life to be part of! Cheers.*

It would seem that I felt I was off to a good start.

## The Imperative of Collaboration

As nearly as I could tell, my appointment as dean of HMS was in general well received. Chief among the expectations for my deanship was that the currents of competition and of faculty migration among the hospitals would diminish and academic and hospital leaders would welcome a more deliberate approach to the role of HMS in these matters. To this end, and early on in my tenure, I launched a comprehensive initiative to create opportunities whereby all Harvard-associated hospitals and research institutions could increase academic collaboration. My goal was straightforward: to ensure that the mission of HMS and the entire Harvard medical community would not be unduly compromised by a turbulent and highly competitive health care environment and hinder our academic mission.

In September 1997 I gave the first of what would become my annual "State of the School" addresses to the entire HMS community and outlined the priorities I would follow during my tenure as dean. Each fall thereafter, I reported on the progress we had been able to achieve, along with disappointments, realignments and new directions. More than any other factor, the priorities I outlined—strengthening basic science research, broadening relationships with Harvard's teaching hospitals, reinvigorating educational programs and increasing ethnic and gender diversity within all components of HMS—were anchored in and depended on collaboration among institutions affiliated with Harvard. Harvard Medical School, I often pointed out, was not embodied in a piece of real estate but in its faculty. Since the founding of the school, the faculty had not only grown in numbers but had also spread across the vast medical landscape that had grown around the school where research was conducted, patients were treated and medical students were taught. I further argued that at a time of rapid change and ever-increasing complexity in all aspects of health care, a time of managed care and failed reforms, it was imperative that collaborative relationships among the entities that constituted the Harvard medical orbit replace earlier posturing. For this to happen, I pointed out in my first address, we needed to reflect on the meaning of "community":

*Community implies working together, bridging divisions and committing to a common mission. Admittedly, these efforts have been eroded to some degree in recent years and deserve particular attention...*

*In the months since my appointment, I have given considerable thought to the task of sustaining and strengthening this extraordinary community, and, in particular, to creating synergy among our many individual efforts and to building and healing sometimes fractured relationships.*

I reached the conclusion that to advance the shared mission of a vast community dedicated to research, medical education and patient care, it was important to launch overarching, collaborative, programmatic initiatives to gain enhanced effectiveness for our patients, as well as to serve the interests of our faculty and students. So, as the uncertainty of establishing a unified Harvard Medical Center became apparent, I turned attention to areas of research collaboration, working closely to bring together the hospitals and the university. The result included seven new initiatives: the Dana-Farber/Harvard Cancer Center (DF/HCC), the Harvard Center for Neurodegeneration and

Repair (HCNR), the Harvard Clinical Research Institute (HCRI), the Broad Institute (BI), the Harvard Stem Cell Institute (HSCI) and Department of Stem Cell and Regenerative Biology, the Department of Systems Biology, and the Harvard Clinical and Translational Science Center (CTSC).

*The Dana-Farber/Harvard Cancer Center (1999)*

Dana-Farber Cancer Institute, the most widely recognized center for cancer care in New England, had gone through its own purgatory in the years leading up to my tenure as dean. Medication errors in the administration of a chemotherapeutic agent had led to the death of Betsy Lehman, a prominent *Boston Globe* reporter. Christopher T. Walsh, then the CEO of the DFCI, resigned as a result. DFCI's independent board of trustees had been strongly urged to appoint Walsh to succeed Nobel laureate Baruj Benacerraf as CEO. Walsh's extensive academic career, first at MIT and then as chair of biological chemistry and molecular pharmacology at HMS, qualified him to head a research institute, but he had not previously held a managerial role at a clinical institute. Walsh was succeeded by David Nathan, a senior hematologist, who at age sixty-five had retired as chief of the children's service at the Children's Hospital. In that role, and previously as head of the Division of Hematology and Oncology, Nathan had served with great distinction for over three decades. The DFCI had been forced to close its small inpatient service after Betsy Lehman's death and had negotiated collaborative agreements with the Brigham and Women's Hospital for adult patient care. In addition, the DFCI operated the pediatric outpatient oncology program, the famous Jimmy Fund, with the beds all located at the Children's.

Here, I realized, after consultation with David Nathan, was a possibility to expand the existing system within the framework of Dana-Farber's leadership, to strengthen our academic community's ability to attract research support and to provide more efficient care to our patients. A telephone call from Rick Klausner, director of the National Cancer Institute (NCI) in Bethesda, Maryland, came just in time and made the effort easier. The NCI, the largest and best funded of the NIH's twenty-seven separate disease-associated institutes, provides funding to the nation's Comprehensive Cancer Centers. Rick and I had met on several previous occasions. While I was at UCSF, I had approached him about emerging plans to submit a proposal for Comprehensive Cancer Center status there.

Rick was calling me to deliver a direct challenge to the HMS community. The DFCI, one of the oldest of the Comprehensive Cancer Centers in the country, had been funded for thirty-four years without interruption, said Rick, and it was now in the process of renewing its grant. He then went on to say that several other Harvard-affiliated hospitals, most notably the MGH, had decided to apply separately, in competition with the DFCI. Rick's message was clear: the NCI had no interest in evaluating parallel competing grants from the Harvard community and urged us to "get our act together."

He delivered the same message to the leaders at the MGH, in particular to Kurt Isselbacher, who headed the developing MGH Cancer Center at the pristine new research space at the Charlestown Navy Yard, and to David Nathan, at the DFCI. Implicit in Klausner's message to each of us was that a collaborative HMS effort would likely fare better financially and held the possibility of doubled core grant support, and that combined efforts would benefit cancer research progress for the ultimate benefit of our patients.

Rick's call did cause some internal strife at HMS. Peter Howley, chair of pathology, had been recruited by Dan Tosteson with the promise of establishing a cancer center based at HMS. It was deemed that such a center would be of interest to patients with family histories of cancer and could serve as a potential fundraising target. This agreement had to be abrogated in the plan to proceed with a unified effort. Fortunately, Peter joined in with Ed Harlow, chair of the Department of Biological Chemistry and Molecular Pharmacology, to give full HMS support to the effort.

David Nathan was eager to pursue the possibility of a Harvard-wide collaboration that would include the Harvard School of Public Health, where most of the faculty providing epidemiology and biostatistics were located. But he insisted on one condition that was nonnegotiable with the board of the DFCI: the Dana-Farber name would have to precede the Harvard logo.

I tried to anticipate the impact of this condition on the huge research operation at the Charlestown Navy Yard of the MGH and was not surprised at the intensity of the discussions that followed. But in the end, everyone agreed to the demands of the DFCI to call the new entity the Dana-Farber/Harvard Cancer Center (DF/HCC). No one expected collaborations to extend to every aspect of patient care, but improvement in patient access to clinical trials became possible by developing a single institutional review board (IRB) for all patients who entered into trials. A skeptical "mock" site visit team convened to review details of our Harvard proposal for an expanded NCI-designated cancer center. During this practice run, we sought advice from cancer scientists and clinicians from around the country. After incorporating changes based on their advice, the final application was sent to the NCI. David Livingston, a senior investigator at the DFCI, played a key role in organizing the approach to an innovative administrative design for the center. He described in the grant application "nodes" intersecting basic science, clinical and epidemiological research where Harvard was outstanding, as well as areas of weakness that were therefore in need of improvement.

At the "official" site visit a few months later, in early 1999, each hospital CEO made a strong pitch for the new advantage of a joint effort. For me, it was and remains the single best example of the power of collaborative efforts. DF/HCC went from no Specialized Program of Research Excellence (SPORE) grants (intended to promote interdisciplinary cancer research and move findings from the lab into the clinical setting) to eight with expanded program project funding, and a number of new collaborations among investigators located in independent venues.

On April 7, 2009, DFCI President Ed Benz, who was also the principal investigator for DF/HCC, reported on the progress achieved over the previous eight years. The DF/HCC now includes over 1,000 investigators. Harvard Medical School and its affiliated hospitals now received over $500 million for DF/HCC-related research activities from the NCI. These include support for 36 project grants and the 8 SPORE grants mentioned above. There are currently 564 active clinical trials. The total number of patients enrolled in these trials now exceeds 14,000.

Nine programs are under development to build on the already strengthened collaborative efforts. In January 2011, the results of ten years of effort were summarized in the third five-year renewal application submitted to the NCI with high expectations for continued funding.

The center grant is now considered a national model of a consortium grant and has been adopted by several other institutions as a model for interactive science, fashioned along the ideas of nodes of intersection, so brilliantly devised by David Livingston, which was a key to the success of the initial application. Rick Klausner was right when he called us to pull our act together—tough love worked. We were all forced into greater interactions. Hopefully, our patients have benefited as much as our investigators have. Certainly, the dramatic increase in patients entering into clinical trials, a potential benchmark of the center's impact, should, in time, signal improved opportunities for better cancer treatment. I was particularly proud of the role played by three of the basic science department chairs at HMS: Ed Harlow, whom I had recruited from the MGH Cancer Center to chair the Department of Biological Chemistry and Molecular Pharmacology, Peter Howley, chair of pathology, and Joan Brugge, chair of the Department of Cell Biology, each of whom worked diligently over the years to make the collaboration real and productive.

*Harvard NeuroDiscovery Center*

In 2000 we received a generous gift of $37.4 million from an anonymous donor to establish the Harvard Center for Neurodegeneration and Repair. The center's funding stabilized over time with annual support from donations, private and philanthropic, and through funding from the NIH. The HCNR was established as a separate, independent, 501(c)(3) organization at the request of the donor, and, from the beginning, the plan was not to fund it through the endowment but instead to expend the original funds donated over the course of the first five years.

The donor has since made additional contributions that assisted in establishing centralized brain imaging facilities in the Longwood area, including a magnetic resonance imaging center devoted to patients with neurological diseases. In 2003 the center's Laboratory for Drug Discovery in Neurodegeneration (LDDN) received a $9 million federal grant to take its drug discovery model national. Additional funds have been contributed recently toward the establishment of a cyclotron/positron emission tomography unit at the Brigham and Women's Hospital.

The HCNR has provided support for students by way of tuition benefits, has established early-phase clinical trials where other resources have been lacking and it has expanded the LDDN. Despite its success, the future of the center needs to be carefully studied with respect to the model of a separate center to assure that its role is most effective in bringing in collaboration in the field of neurodegenerative diseases across our extraordinary community.

By the spring of 2007, the center had established a board of advisors that worked to position it in a more favorable public role by choosing a new name, less cumbersome and more in alignment with its expanding mission, working not only with neurodegenerative disorders like Alzheimer's disease, Parkinson's disease and amyotrophic lateral sclerosis (ALS) but also through establishment of an international consortium to study the genetics of multiple sclerosis. The new name, the Harvard NeuroDiscovery Center (HNDC) was embraced and the designation was blessed by the university and Jeff Flier, the HMS dean who followed me.

The current structure of the HNDC consists of three pillars. The first focuses on neurodegenerative disorders: Alzheimer's disease, Parkinson's disease, multiple sclerosis, ALS and Huntington's disease. The second pillar consists of interdisciplinary and multi-institutional collaboration, and the third of translational research. To accomplish the collaborative interaction, the center has core facilities in optical imaging and biostatistics, a tissue center, a biomarkers program and a centralized mouse behavioral testing facility.

A genetics program in multiple sclerosis is another key component of the center. A global initiative involving Harvard, the University of Cambridge, England, UCSF and universities in Australia and New Zealand was formed in 2006. The goal is to identify genes associated with disease risks.

By the spring of 2011, the center had 700 investigators listed on its website. It has raised over $80 million in support and has an annual budget of about $8 million. More than 1,000 projects have been supported by core facilities: 150 publications in peer-reviewed journals have been published, and the LDDN is noteworthy for a national program providing support to promising leads for new therapeutics from applicants around the US.

Dean Jeff Flier serves as the designated "sole member" of the not-for-profit entity. Dennis Selkoe, the Vincent and Stella Coates Professor of Neurologic Diseases at BWH, and I serve as co-chairs of the governance committee. For future stability, the HNDC needs to strengthen its relationship with the Department of Neurobiology. At this writing, it appears that issue is being addressed by the appointment of Professor Michael Greenberg as chair of the department. Michael is designated to have a major role in the center's future activities.

*Harvard Clinical Research Institute*

The notion of a Harvard-wide initiative to facilitate the interaction between evolving clinical research ideas and their translation into clinical trials was launched in 1998 in an effort to create a single gateway for industry-sponsored research between HMS, BIDMC and Partners HealthCare. Working together with hospital leaders and my fellow deans, I proposed an aggressive method to facilitating such an approach. Initially, the efforts to create a clinical research organization (CRO) model within the academic setting depended primarily on the efforts of the BIDMC group led by Rick Kuntz. The result was the formation of a non-profit 501(c)(3), the Harvard Clinical Research Institute, with joint governance provided by the HMS deans and hospital spokespersons. It has undergone several changes in leadership and its stated goals, but by 2007 it had become a "going concern" with bottom-line profitability. Critical to its early success were the management tools put in place first by Paul Levy, while he was my senior administrative dean, and subsequently by Eric Buehrens, dean for facilities management, with strong support from Ray Dolin, dean of clinical affairs, and members of the board Eugene Braunwald from BWH; Jay Piper of Partners HealthCare; and Victor Dzau, former chair of the Department of

Medicine at BWH; then later, Joe Loscalzo, when he took over as chair of that department.

Spencer Goldsmith, who has led the effort since 2002, reports that HCRI now employs approximately 180 people, with an annual operating budget in excess of $30 million. Goldsmith sums up the institute this way, "We work in a decentralized medical community. Clinical research infrastructure is increasingly expensive to build and maintain, and HCRI provides medical faculty with access to turnkey resources to efficiently run multicenter clinical trials. Our hope is to facilitate the design of these trials and the analysis of the results by providing resources that are not economically feasible to sustain within each department at every hospital. It is also important for us to provide a bridge to industry sponsors of research in order to create a research paradigm that assures the participation of academic faculty in a scientifically credible way."[1]

The hope for the HCRI is that it will facilitate expanded academic faculty efforts in designing clinical trials and analyzing results.

### *The Broad Institute*

As mentioned in the previous chapter, a remarkable opportunity arose in 2001 when Eli and Edythe Broad of Los Angeles became aware of the power of the genomic assessment of human conditions and the potential of the new technology to define the molecular bases of diseases and seek new therapies. They had initially come to appreciate the potential of this approach after a family member was treated at the MGH for inflammatory bowel disease. The Broads were introduced to MIT's Eric Lander, who now directs the Broad Institute, and discussions rapidly progressed, culminating in the formation of the institute in 2003 and its launch a year later. The Broad Institute was initially funded through a unique relationship with Harvard and MIT, put into effect by the president of MIT at the time, Charles Vest, and agreed to by Harvard's then-president Larry Summers.

The Broad Institute, whose development HMS strongly supported from the outset, has now entered a new phase, with additional contributions to establish an endowment. The institute has allowed faculty members in each of our hospitals to explore clinical innovations in seeking the post-genomic role of genes in disease development and progression. Several of our faculty members on the HMS Quad, including Dr. David Reich, Dr. Christine Seidman, Dr. Jonathan Seidman and others in the field of genetics, have benefited greatly from collaboration with the Broad Institute. Many hospital-based faculty members have joined the Broad Institute as associate members, and four of the institute's primary appointments are HMS faculty—Drs. David Altshuler, Todd Golub, Vamsi Mootha and Deborah Hung.

In 2008 the Broad family donated an additional $400 million, increasing the total amount of their support to $600 million. The recent donation converts the institute into a permanent, not-for-profit, biomedical research organization. The universities will continue to exert a role in the governance and the dean of HMS remains a member of the board of directors. The total commitment exceeds that of any other reported single philanthropic donation to a university-based enterprise.

In its next iteration, I believe it will be important to more clearly delineate the rules of engagement for the services provided by the Broad Institute. Some HMS investigators feel disadvantaged because the selectivity of projects and the funding of activities have not been sufficiently transparent to provide the types of interactions that are most desirable. Nevertheless, support for the institute remains strong at HMS and in the hospitals, and the possibilities for additional recruitments in human genetics afforded by the connection to the Broad will have a positive influence on strategic planning in genetics and genomics both at Harvard and MIT.

*Harvard Stem Cell Institute and a New Department*

President Bush's decision in 2002 to limit work on stem cell lines to those already available placed a serious limitation on the study of the utility of stem cells as therapeutic targets when using NIH funding sources. The outcome was the development of many models for private or public support that would allow work to continue, but only in research spaces separate from NIH support. In California, the establishment of the California Stem Cell Initiative, now called the California Institute for Regenerative Medicine (CIRM), was funded by state bonds. At Harvard, we worked to raise private money to support the efforts of individuals working at the university and in our teaching hospitals. The outcome of these efforts was the establishment of the Harvard Stem Cell Institute, launched in April 2004, which not only engaged faculties at FAS and HMS but also those at the business, law and divinity schools.

The initial plan evolved into an agreement during the tenure of Derek Bok in 2006–2007 to establish a new interfaculty department. Jeremy Knowles and I debated these issues privately and agreed to support the notion, working closely with Provost Steve Hyman to appoint Douglas Melton of FAS and David Scadden (of HMS and the MGH) as co-chairs. Members of the new department were expected to migrate to shared space at the new Allston campus, by 2011 still on hold given the exigencies of Harvard budget issues.

During the 2006–2007 academic year, Jeremy Knowles and I gave approval for junior faculty appointments. The result, as summarized in the July 2009 issue of *Boston Magazine*, was the appointment of three new superstars—Kevin Eggan, Konrad Hochedlinger and Amy Wagers—who are each leading the way in understanding stem cell differentiation. The new department was given an interdisciplinary name, the Department of Stem Cell and Regenerative Biology.

After the initial plans for the institute and department to be located at the Allston site were abandoned, space was found on the Cambridge campus, to be occupied in 2011. According to David Scadden, this has the disadvantage of separating the hospital-based faculty from the proximity to HMS envisioned for the Allston site.

Despite the obstacles from the dislocation of a joint effort at one site, morale remains high and the objectives that led to forming the institute and department remain intact. There are currently over seventy faculty members, called associate members, who collaborate together in stem cell biology, of which about thirty are very active. There are fifteen primary appointments in the department, and currently several active searches are underway to recruit new faculty to space available at Harvard and the affiliated hospitals.

*Department of Systems Biology*

An outcome of the process of evaluating programmatic and departmental activities to occupy the New Research Building and to backfill the space freed by the relocation of the genetics and pathology departments led to a strong recommendation by Bruce Alberts, then president of the National Academy of Sciences (whom I had asked to chair a committee on the future of science at HMS), suggested a new thrust to align cell biology with emerging computational analytic approaches. After consideration of these recommendations and further review and discussion with several chairs, including Ed Harlow and Marc Kirschner, I chose to work through the process of developing a new department. We decided to name it Systems Biology, a designation that was emerging to define this area of science, and launched it in September 2003. It was the first new department at HMS since the 1993 merger of the anatomy and physiology departments that created the Department of Cell Biology, an effort led so ably by Marc Kirschner after his recruitment from UCSF.

Marc appeared to be the logical leader for the new undertaking in systems biology but agreed to take that role only quite reluctantly, with concerns over leaving the Department of Cell Biology. The resources to establish a new department required a university-wide commitment, which we envisioned as an interfaculty effort between the Faculty of Arts and Sciences and HMS. The plan was supported by Larry Summers, who agreed to assist in funding its start-up. Joan Brugge accepted a position of interim leadership of the cell biology department, but after a very successful year and following a very positive external review, I asked her to take charge for a five-year term. Marc moved his operation to the Warren Alpert Building on the Quad campus and enthusiastically set about recruiting new faculty.

I was delighted when President Drew Faust honored Marc Kirschner in 2008 with appointment as a University Professor, the highest honor granted to a Harvard faculty member. He was at the time the only person to hold this distinction among professors at the medical school, and it has enabled him to join an elite university-wide group of about twenty others.[2]

The choice to ask Marc to lead a new effort in systems biology resulted from a spectacular moment at the HMS department chairs' retreat on Cape Cod in March of that year. I had asked Marc to address the group after dinner that Saturday evening on the evolving relationships between cell biology, a "new" physiology of systems regulation and the promise it held for new understandings of disease mechanisms. Marc labored hard to prepare the material and his presentation stunned the audience with new concepts and approaches. Andy Warshaw, chair of surgery at the MGH told me the talk was informative and provocative.

A review of the new department's activities indicates that the concepts that led to its formation are playing out in a positive way. The leadership of the department is executing a plan to establish more quantitative measures on the molecular level to understand the regulatory networks of gene products (proteins) and their influences on one another. It is critical to understand how cellular events involving multiple protein interactions control the function and fate of cell dynamics; such knowledge will enable the search for new therapies for diseases where, as in cancer or heart disease, these mechanisms go wrong.

To accomplish this, the department has recruited faculty capable of combining actual experiments with highly theoretical approaches, with the belief that this is the best way to ensure that theory can be tested in real experiments.

The department currently has seven senior faculty and ten junior faculty. The majority have received outside research funding, and, to my deep satisfaction, many have joint appointments in hospital departments. The department is presently seeking additional space to expand to a total of twenty to twenty-five faculty members.

I believe that the department has a commanding position as one of the most visible and exciting systems biology departments anywhere in the world. But the proof of the experiment requires that its activities deliver by providing clarification on the biological pathways being studied, so that treatments of a new variety can be realized.

### *Harvard Clinical and Translational Science Center*

The Harvard Clinical and Translational Science Center is perhaps the most complicated and ambitious collaborative project ever undertaken primarily by HMS, with the help of other faculties of the university and the affiliated hospitals. To stimulate a "transformation" of the conduct of clinical and translational research, the NIH has formulated a new Clinical and Translational Science Award. This mandates that the currently established General Clinical Research Centers (GCRCS), of which there are four at the Harvard-affiliated hospitals, be replaced by a single, broadly directed center. For Harvard, this means that an annual level of support of $17 million would need to be transitioned to a new organizational structure along with the additional support provided by a CTSC award.

A broad-based effort to respond to this request for proposals was initiated, first with a planning grant, led by Dr. Daniel Singer, professor of medicine at the MGH, and Dean Ray Dolin from HMS. Over one hundred faculty members soon were involved, including representatives from FAS, the school of engineering, the school of public health, the school of dental medicine, and the Harvard-affiliated hospitals (BWH, BIDMC, MGH, DFCI and Children's). The planning grant proposal described establishment of a virtual center intended to: offer education and training in clinical and translational research; accommodate "think tanks" for connection between basic and clinical investigations to support collaborative pilot projects; offer bioinformatics capabilities to access Harvard-wide databases to link investigators; reconfigure current GCRC activities to emphasize transformative technologies; and expand community engagement with patients and physicians in clinical research.

After the planning grant was funded in 2006, we began working toward submitting a full proposal with an annual budget of $55 million, of which $23 million would be requested from the NIH and the remainder drawn from a combination of university, HMS and hospital sources.

The CTSC proposal we worked on had the potential to not only transform the conduct of clinical research in our community but also have a positive impact on the relationship between the hospitals and Harvard University. Leadership from HMS, along with sustained commitment from the participating institutions in the CTSC, would be essential for the ultimate success of this extraordinary project.

By the fall of 2007, Dean Jeffrey Flier had replaced Danny Singer as the principal investigator with Lee Nadler, professor of medicine at DFCI. Lee organized an ambitious program, and in May 2008 the center was funded with a strong recommendation from NIH. Nadler energized a new inter-institutional effort called the Harvard Catalyst, which provides numerous community-wide academic activities, lectures and study groups to facilitate research collaboration. I was very pleased when he and Jeff Flier appointed Ann Klibansky, professor of medicine (neuroendocrinology) at the MGH, to organize the collaborative arrangements among the four GCRCs. I can think of no one more capable of integrating these efforts.

I have been gratified to observe that our planning for new leadership of the Countway Library (Issac [Zak] Kohane and Alexa McCray) has led to the library playing a key role in the activities of the Harvard Catalyst. The bioinformatics group, led by Kohane, has proven critical to the emerging coordination of data sharing across the entire Harvard medical community. This includes providing capability for uniform patient entry across four HMS-affiliated hospitals with a full listing of individual faculty, their interests, publications and research plans.

## Departmental Reviews

The interdisciplinary initiatives outlined above were only part of my plan to increase efficiency and communication between departments and institutions in the Harvard medical community and the university. By 2000 I was also searching for meaningful ways to interact with the large assembly of clinical department chairs. As organized, the HMS community was divided into executive committees in each of the clinical specialties of medicine, surgery, pediatrics, radiology, psychiatry, neurology and so on. Representatives—typically the clinical department head—from each of the major hospitals met monthly to consider the issues of medical student teaching and faculty recruitment and promotion. The committees functioned quite independently but, I thought, very effectively with the chairmanship rotating annually, from one leader to another. While I was welcome to attend the meetings, doing so with forty-six departments was somewhat impractical.

I had brought up the idea with Sam Thier, head of Partners HealthCare, of establishing departmental reviews to benefit each department and allow the hospital leaders and the dean to work more effectively together. Both Sam and I had experience with the format of external reviews—Sam from Yale, and I from UCSF. I assigned the responsibility to Executive Dean Dennis Kasper, who suggested that Ray Dolin, then dean for clinical programs, develop an orderly process for the external reviews. Three nationally recognized leaders in the field of the department were invited to visit for two days. The department responsibility in preparation for the visit was to do an in-depth internal evaluation assessing financial, clinical, educational and research programs. The document was shared with the outside reviewers.

Critical to the process, which was initially deeply resented by many of the clinical chairs, was the unequivocal support by myself and the hospital CEOs. The hospital leaders and I met jointly with the external review committee at the beginning and received at the end of each visit an oral communication about the outcome of the visit. This report was followed by a written set of conclusions, usually within four to six weeks, and the results were shared with the department head at a meeting convened in my office. A formal redacted report was prepared for the department head, who was then free to pass on any or all of the findings to members of the department.

As time went on, the benefit of the reviews began to pay off, improving the culture of relationships between hospital department leaders, hospital CEOs and myself. The growing awareness and the self-evident sharing of the power base made an impact on the dynamics of the complex relationships of each component of the clinical interface. The reviews had real teeth: accomplishments were formally recognized, empowering the clinical chair to seek additional support; problems were acknowledged, leading, in some instances, to a recommendation for new leadership.

By 2007 a total of thirty-nine reviews had taken place. Most of the hospital leaders pitched in to support the process, and the clinical chairs, some of them new in their roles, sometimes urged reviews to help them in forging an effective leadership style and setting priorities for departmental initiatives. There was one troubling exception: Children's Hospital. Resentment persisted on the part of some of the chairs there about the "intrusion of the dean into our clinical affairs." The result was that fewer reviews were undertaken at Children's, although in orthopedics and pathology reviews were conducted at the request of the individual chairs.

From my own perspective, the reviews allowed me to develop a personal relationship with the department chairs. That relationship could not have emerged at individual meetings, and certainly not at the quarterly meetings of all the HMS chairs, which were in general poorly attended.

In my second year, I initiated an annual off-site department chair retreat held over a weekend during the winter or early spring on Cape Cod. These retreats were meant to address another serious problem in the relationship between department heads, namely the distance felt between the nine basic science chairs on the Quad, who received their budget and administrative reviews from Harvard on an annual schedule, and the clinical departments who had little to gain in the formal quarterly meetings scheduled for all departments. The annual retreats were remarkably successful with full attendance and active participation. We broke into small groups for discussions on specific issues and concluded the meetings on Sunday morning with committee reports and my summation of the critical issues facing the school, with a focus on the collaborative efforts being made with the clinical entities. Hospital CEOs were also invited, and many attended. Curiously, given the complexity of relationships with Children's Hospital, I was delighted at the support I received from James Mandel, the CEO, and by other attendees, notably Fred Lovejoy, professor of pediatrics, from that part of the Harvard community.

By 2003, my fellow deans and I succeeded in extending the departmental review process to the basic science departments at HMS, and established a sequence of five-year reviews that became part of the culture of the Quad-based faculty and chairs. The reviews changed the dynamics of expectations from the leadership of Quad departments with the establishment of formal five-year renewable appointments depending on the accomplishments of leadership. As Ray Dolin summarized the effort and the outcome in May 2007:

*The Department Heads Retreat was initiated in 2000 and was so successful that it became an annual event. Over the past seven years, the medical school has also undertaken a systematic review of clinical and basic science departments. The extension of the clinical department reviews, which now total approximately 39, to reviews of the basic science departments, has yielded important information with respect to strategic planning and leadership assessment. With the recent review of microbiology, five basic science departments have been completed with the full cycle anticipated to be finished in five to six years. Despite their general success, it is important that the mechanisms of such reviews be institutionalized by the next leadership of the medical school.*

*In addition to these five-year reviews, we have, for the past decade, carried out annual reviews with each Quad department chair and the administrative staff to outline strategic planning with a five-year rolling commitment of resources allocated for space and recruitments and promotion of faculty. These sessions have been effective in offering guidelines for recruitment of new faculty (timing and slots available), assessing mentoring and junior faculty promotion, and guiding us with respect to space requirements and educational opportunities.*[3]

## The New Research Building: Collaboration through Research Program Development

During the fall of 1997, just after I arrived, HMS's faculty were pessimistic about meeting scientific initiatives and opportunities. The emerging Institute of Chemistry and Cell Biology (ICCB) showed promise for combining Stuart Schreiber's brilliant work on combinatorial chemistry with Marc Kirschner's strong Department of Cell Biology. The downside of having committed 10,000 square feet to the institute was the virtual elimination of other research expansion. The recruitment of Carla Shatz in 2000 to chair the Department of Neurobiology required major reconfiguration in space to meet her needs and those of others in her department in the Goldenson Building. Phil Leder's Department of Genetics had filled available space in the Warren Alpert Building, the most recent research building added to the campus

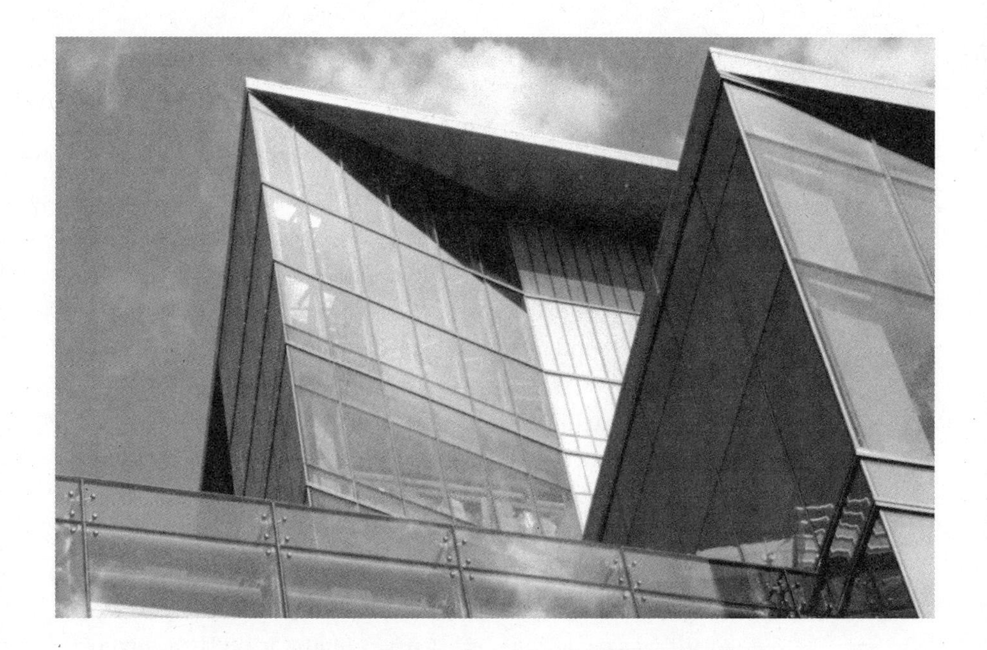

The New Research Building.

five years before, and the Departments of Microbiology and Molecular Genetics and of Pathology were crowded in Building D, the fourth of the original buildings on the Longwood campus.

I initiated planning efforts to explore the feasibility of constructing a new research facility adjacent to the Harvard Institutes of Medicine, where newly renovated laboratories were created within the walls of the old English High School. Dean Tosteson's administration had carefully planned for a possible expansion onto the four-acre parking lot at the time the building was acquired, with rights for possible future research development negotiated with the City of Boston. The agreement stipulated a requirement for the provision of equivalent parking space within the boundary of the plot of land, which necessitated two levels of underground parking in a region below the water table, creating great additional expense to the project.

I asked Paul Levy, my experienced dean of administration, to lead the effort, which he undertook with the assistance of Associate Dean Eric Beuhrens. We examined the potential for a ten-story building that would be equal in height and possibly be connected at each level with the HIM facility. We organized a small coterie of department chairs led by Ed Harlow and Phil Leder to assist in the evaluation of candidate designs, which came from an open competition with local and national architectural firms. The charette led to a number of preliminary designs that were carefully evaluated; Architectural Associates of Cambridge won the draw with a magnificent structure of exterior-glass-paneled design drawn together floor to ceiling by a newly crafted set of cables that crisscrossed the interior of the individual glass panels: it would be held together by tension.

I was eager to move the space assignments in the new building beyond the condominium-leased space arrangement that had made the HIM project possible. More than half of that building was rented to hospital-based scientists whose research areas and interests were disparate and not centered on a particular theme. I intended a different structure for the new building and engaged in extensive collaborative arrangements with BWH, and later DFCI, to develop programs in both genetics and pathology that would complement the two departments we had relocated. The result was a vigorous interactive cohabitation that encouraged the development of new initiatives. With an expanse of 525,000 square feet, the New Research Building remains the largest construction ever undertaken by Harvard and awaits a generous donor to place a name over the front door.

## International Outreach: The Armenise-Harvard Foundation, Harvard Medical International, and The Harvard-Dubai Foundation For Medical Research

Among the less publicly visible responsibilities of the deanship in our academic medical centers is stewardship of bequests, given to provide assistance to our academic efforts. Among those that I inherited was a remarkable agreement forged by Dean Tosteson that came from Count Giovanni Auletta Armenise. Count Armenise—affectionately called Nino by all who knew him—came to the Harvard community to seek treatment for his wife, Nora, at the MGH, under the auspices of neurologists Verne Caviness and Fred Hochberg. She succumbed inevitably to glioblastoma multiforme, a rapidly growing brain tumor. The relationship that developed between Count and Countess Armenise and her doctors was unusually personal. Her doctors would even travel multiple times to Rome, to the home of the Armenises, to assist and advise in her management.

Before Nora's death, Count Armenise recognized that hers was a disease for which there was no present cure. As owner of the largest private bank in Italy, the Banco Nazionale del Agricultura, as well as other commercial interests, he responded by endowing a program of study of fundamental neurobiology. It was through the remarkable administrative skills and vision of Tosteson that the Armenise-Harvard Foundation was created. The bequest was large, exceeding $50 million over the course of the decade of my deanship. It had two general components; one was to support work on brain tumor research at the MGH, which included funding a professorship to which Caviness was named as the first incumbent.

The second and major portion of the endowment went to establish four centers of excellence in basic research at Harvard Medical School. From these funds, fellowships were created to support young US and Italian investigators. These included postdoctoral studies for young Italians and support for joint projects in research with Italian collaborators.

After my succession to the deanship, Dan Tosteson remained with the foundation as its director, while I served as a close advisor, taking part in joint programs and seminars where the progress of the foundation was monitored. In 2002 we renamed Building D (of the original HMS Quad) the Giovanni Auletta Armenise Medical Research Building. In 2006 I attended a symposium in Catania, Sicily, to celebrate the foundation's decade of achievement.

Harvard Medical International was also the brainchild of Deans Tosteson and David Bray (executive dean under Tosteson), who had conceived of it as an instrument for exploring international health issues. Its earliest shape, in 1994, was framed around a consulting initiative that would generate revenues to support other academic activities of the medical school. The recruitment of Robert Crone, a Harvard-trained anesthesiologist, was seen as a successful step in the implementation of HMI's strategic plan.

By the time I arrived in 1997, HMI was struggling to pay back loans to the university, and while engaged in projects throughout the world, it was not apparent that there was any faculty ownership. Many felt that HMI's activities were questionable within the framework of the academic mission of HMS. Several steps were taken to remedy the situation. First, the board of the non-profit corporation was expanded to provide internal cohesion as well as external expertise and included: George Thibault, a representative of Partners HealthCare, which had also established an international effort; Robert Truog, an ethicist at Children's Hospital; Benjamin Sachs, chief of obstetrics and gynecology at the BIDMC, who had international public health interests; and Steve Sallan from the Dana-Farber Cancer Institute. I chaired the board and attended every quarterly meeting faithfully. Initially, there were also two members of the Harvard Corporation on the board—Harvard University Treasurer Ron Daniel and Judith Hope—and I invited a third, Conrad Harper, who had recently been appointed to the corporation. They took an interest in the expanding portfolio and provided a link to the university to assure continuity of purpose and to inform the university leadership of our activities. I also benefited from the wisdom provided by former Harvard FAS Dean Henry Rosovsky, who offered academic and strategic input.

The HMI portfolio grew and came to include traditional medical consulting around hospital developments in several countries, advice regarding the implementation of new educational programs in medical schools, invoking the New Pathway problem-based program at HMS, and providing venues for regional continuing medical education (CME). The activities expanded to include many hospital-based faculty members, who appreciated the opportunity to travel and to serve the school's mission.

A major opportunity for further development arose in February 2001, when Bob Crone received a call from Dubai as we traveled in India together, requesting a consultation in the United Arab Emirates about the development of a new initiative in health care to match some of the other business opportunities under development. We stopped in Dubai for a short visit on the way home from India, and subsequent visits and negotiations led to the possibility of a major collaborative effort around the development of the Dubai Healthcare City.

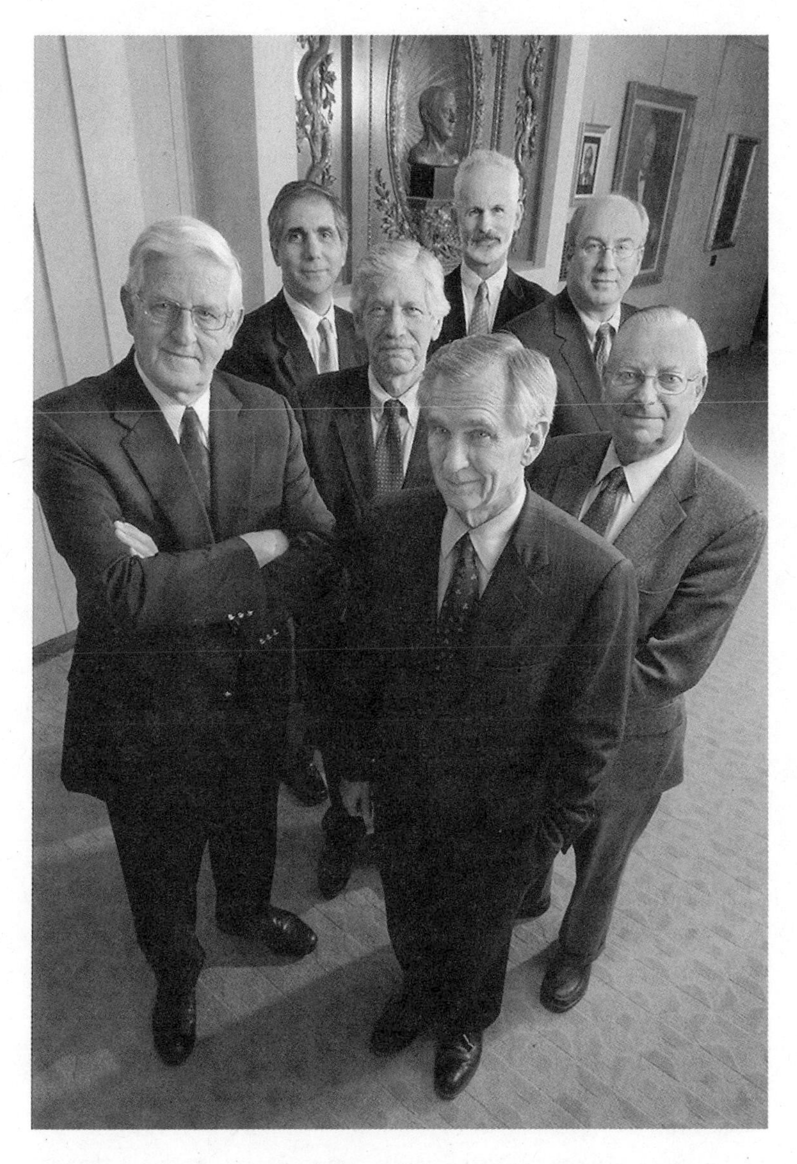

Founders of the Dana-Farber/Harvard Cancer Center, 2007. From left, clockwise: the author; Gary Gottlieb, CEO of Brigham and Women's Hospital; Paul Levy, CEO of BIDMC; Peter Slavin, CEO of the MGH; Barry Bloom, Dean of HSPH; Ed Benz, CEO of DF/HCC; and James Mandell (center), CEO of Children's Hospital.

HMI leadership became aware, when Larry Summers took charge in July 2001, that a major change in emphasis was introduced at Harvard, with respect to undertaking international collaborations, and that possible reputation and financial risk factors in international collaborations and commitments were under closer scrutiny. In line with the new level of caution he introduced, Larry asked members of the Harvard Corporation to resign from the HMI board because, he believed, they were not appropriately placed in such administrative positions.

The next five years saw HMI become a force admired by many within and beyond the HMS environment. Summers personally took great interest in our work and accepted an invitation to visit the Dubai scene and meet with Sheik Mohammed bin Rashid al-Maktoum. While there, he participated in a symposium and continued to encourage our activities during his remaining days as president. At my suggestion, Steve Hyman and I had commissioned an external review that suggested new mechanisms to separate the consulting functions of HMI from its more academic parts. But Derek Bok, advised by a new provost for international programs, Jorge Dominguez, decided that HMI had to go, and by the end of the 2006–2007 academic year, negotiations were proceeding to move the controversial parts of HMI into the Partners HealthCare network, where it fortunately finds a comfortable home today. However incoming Dean Jeffrey Flier became painfully aware of the loss of discretionary income to the medical school resulting from this migration to another business arrangement.

At the same time we set about expanding our academic activities in the Gulf Region and engaged in negotiations with the leadership of the United Arab Emirates in Dubai. This led to the successful modeling of the Harvard Dubai Foundation for Education and Research after the effective not-for-profit model Dan Tosteson had put in place for the Armenise-Harvard Foundation. By 2007 we had raised close to $50 million for the support of the academic activities of the Harvard Dubai Foundation for Medical Education and Research. Sheik Mohammed bin Rashid al-Maktoum contributed $13 million and a successful gambit to Riyadh, Saudi Arabia, to meet Prince Al-Waleed bin Talal bin Abdulaziz al-Saud resulted in a $5 million gift.

## Continuing Challenges



The changes in relationships between the individual entities of the Harvard complex since 2000 have been at once constructive and problematic. New adventures in collaborative work are

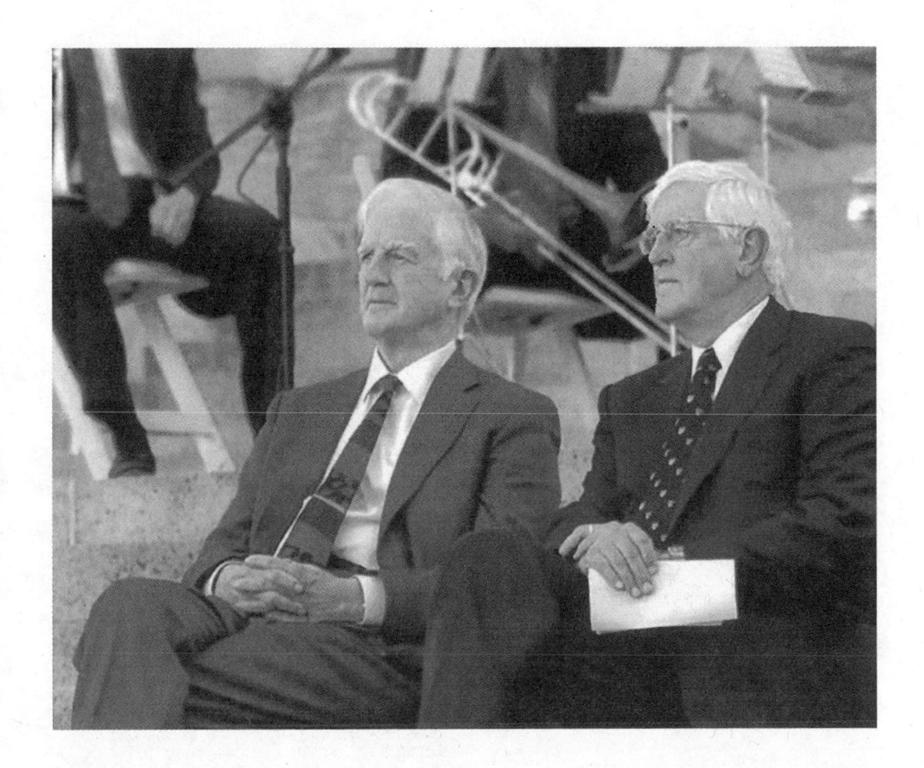

Harvard University President Derek Bok (left) and the author at the celebration of the 225th anniversary of the founding of HMS, 2007. This was the author's tenth year as dean; he had worked with three Harvard presidents.

promising: the Broad Institute, the DF/HCC, a new trans-Harvard Department of Stem Cell and Regenerative Biology, and formation of a new university committee to coordinate program review and expenditures for new science initiatives have each added potential value to the whole enterprise.

At the same time, these relationships place the medical school in a new balance between Harvard University, the provost's office and the hospital networks. The overall impact has been to reduce the leverage of the medical school in some of these efforts. For example, negotiations to establish the first four faculty positions at the Broad Institute included detailed discussion between the provost and the hospital CEOs because two of the four faculty members had clinical department appointments. The dean's role in allocating resources to sustain this part of the program was essentially nil, whereas the hospital CEO had to deal with intellectual property issues and the use of grant revenues (indirect costs).

I served on the coordinating committee of the Broad Institute chaired by Provost Steve Hyman and strongly favored the model

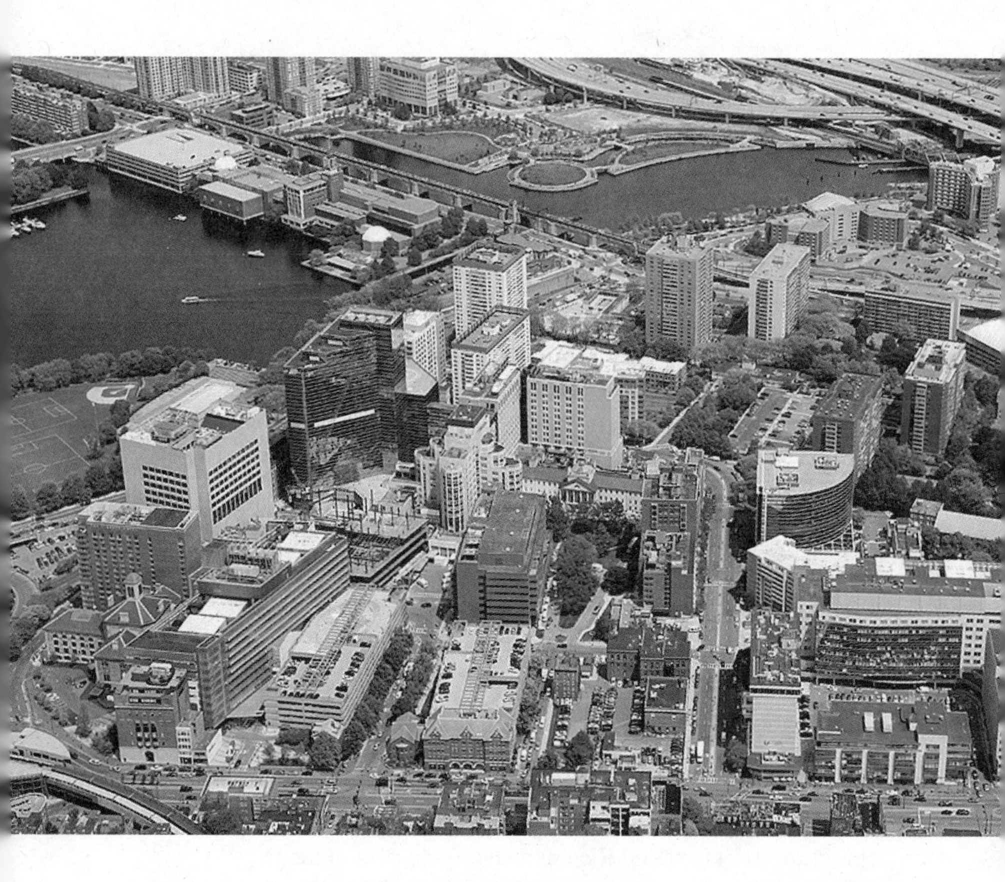

Aerial view of the Massachusetts General Hospital complex, 2009.

we developed for governance, recognizing that the impact on HMS is real in isolating the school from the day-to-day practical elements of management and oversight. I have no regrets and believe firmly that the direction taken in forming the Broad Institute was the correct one; I only wish to point out that it added another venue whereby administrative assignments left the school relatively stranded.

In May 2007, as I was ending my final year as dean, I submitted a detailed account of my activities to Derek Bok—at his request. It was a broad-ranging document with commentary on every aspect of the school's mission and accomplishments, drawing his attention to the growing complexity of new projects and some of their implications for HMS. In my conclusion I urged:

*It is very difficult to project or predict the best outcome for these efforts and to assign definitively the medical school's current stance and planning in this regard. Indeed, I believe that a renewal of strategic planning efforts will be critical....Everyone has agreed that bold plans that integrate trans-disciplinary research are critical to success. The continuation of this planning initiative over the next year will be crucial in defining these objectives.*

## Reflections on Leadership, or Leading by Listening

During the last year of my decade-long tenure at Harvard Medical School, I began to receive more than the usual number of invitations to share with audiences—medical and otherwise—my thoughts on leadership and the lessons I had learned in the course of four decades of academic leadership. Those familiar with the topic of leadership are aware that many volumes have been filled—from antiquity to the present era—and continue to be filled, by attempts to define the essence of leadership and the attributes an ideal leader should possess. In fact, in the early 1990s, Joseph C. Rost in his book, *Leadership for the Twenty-First Century*, cited more than two hundred definitions of leadership coined just between 1920 and 1990.[4] There are, of course, attributes of leadership that remain constant over time and without which no leader can have a lasting impact. One of the oldest attributes, and one that I find relevant today, is in Plato's *Statesman*, where an analogy is drawn between leaders and weavers.[5] A good leader brings together, weaves people of divergent and sometimes conflicting interests around a common mission, including those who do not necessarily care for each other or for the leader.

Rather than offer my audiences yet another catalog of attributes with which a good leader should be endowed, I decided instead to focus on the lessons I had learned throughout the course of my career. Invariably, this involved reliving and recapturing moments and people who have been part of my journey and have shared with me the challenges and rewards, the follies and accomplishments of my leadership. From that retrospective emerged many lessons, but one lesson in particular eclipsed the others: the ability and will to listen to others, to try to understand what others are saying, even when it lacks clarity. The need to be heard is a basic human need, one that is remarkably crystallized in the words of the shipwrecked sailor in Gabriel

García Márquez's *The Story of a Shipwrecked Sailor*.[6] As anyone who is familiar with the story knows, the shipwrecked sailor is the only one of nine Colombian sailors on a destroyer to survive the voyage home. The lone sailor drifts in a small half-inflated raft without food or water for ten days until he is finally washed ashore. Half-conscious, still lying in the sand, he is approached by a man who asks what has happened. The sailor recounts later, "When I heard him speak, I realized that more than thirst, more than hunger, more than despair, what tormented me most was the need to tell someone what had happened to me." The powerful message here is that everyone has a story to tell, and a lot of times, leadership begins with, and is about, listening to people's stories—stories told by faculty, students, staff, administrators, the community within and outside of one's immediate world. Decisions and judgments, to be lasting, should always follow careful listening.

In June 2007 I recounted the story of the shipwrecked sailor to the graduating class at Harvard Medical School as they prepared to enter their careers in medicine. Then I added:

> *All of your patients will have a story and that story will be inextricably linked to the healing process. As professionals we are expected to be good listeners—we are expected to listen to the stories that our patients tell us and to reach conclusions that will lead to the best recommendations for their care. Your ability to communicate—listening and telling, will determine in large measure your gift for healing.*

The singular importance of listening was the lesson I shared with my audiences, especially with the HMS class of 2007 and with the returning alumni—as I delivered my last addresses to each as dean of Harvard Medical School.

# ELEVEN

# *Issues Facing Academic Medical Health Centers Today*

WHEN I ASSUMED THE POSITION as dean at HMS, I never envisioned extending my term beyond ten years. Harvard has no firm rules on the length of service of deans and there are no regular reviews of performance. So decisions are made with consultation between the dean and the president. When I indicated an interest in retiring during the last year of Larry's presidency, he urged me to remain in place for the transition, which I did. Since I left Gordon Hall and the dean's office in 2007, my days are spent teaching medical students, supporting the efforts of the Harvard NeuroDiscovery Center, with particular focus on clinical research in Alzheimer's disease and Parkinson's disease, and serving as a faculty member in the Department of Neurobiology at Harvard Medical School and the Department of Neurology at the Brigham and Women's Hospital. This perch provides a remarkable opportunity to view and reflect on the issues that continue to challenge the mission of our academic institutions. Of the many issues large and small, three remain important to me: diversity and affirmative action; challenges of academic-commercial relationships, particularly with respect to conflicts of interest; and the question of the citizen's right to health care, most recently coming to the fore with US health care reform. In this chapter, I offer some of my personal experiences with these issues, together with some perspectives gained over time.

## Diversity: A Lifetime of Listening and Learning

For more than six decades I have observed, and not always with pride, the evolution of my own outlook on diversity, especially as it refers to gender, ethnicity and sexual orientation. That evolution was slow and grew as I listened to the many voices around me and the messages sent my way. Some of these voices were gentle, others less so, and a few of the messages had to be sent more than once. But, thankfully, during my tenure at the University of California, San Francisco, and as dean at HMS, I did manage to evoke appreciation from staff, students and faculty for the essential "rightness" of pressing for diversity, for which I am grateful. At UCSF, I was pleased in 1996 to receive from staff and faculty the Dr. Martin Luther King Jr. Award for support of underrepresented minority students and faculty.

### *The Lingering Issue of Gender*

While in elementary and high school in Alberta, I found that the best students were often girls. Among my extended family, it was the girls who showed the most interest in reading and in preparing their schoolwork, and many went on to a university education. I was soon to discover, however, that the professions favored men over women and that few of my colleagues seemed troubled by that or by the gender imbalance. In my medical school class of fifty-three students, only three were women, each of them high achievers.

One of the earliest messages sent my way as a physician was during my years as a junior professor at McGill. It came from a young graduate student, a mother of four children, who had returned to university for a master's degree in psychology. She was interested in the emerging field of physiological psychology, and she approached me about the possibility of doing a PHD.

I struggled with the issue: Would she be able to keep up with the pace required? Would she be able to compete with the "full-time" students and postdocs in the lab?

As I mentioned in chapter four, in the end, I accepted her application and she did, indeed, prove equal to the task in every aspect. As far as I was concerned, the issue was closed, but apparently not for her. One day, just as I had entered the lab, I was totally taken aback when she confronted me and accused me, in the presence of others, of giving more time and attention to the men in the laboratory than to her. To this day, I'm not sure if I was guilty as accused, but I do know that the encounter sensitized me, in an abiding way, about perceptions that are, wittingly or unwittingly, part of gender relationships.

Over the years, my daughter, Melanie, played a central role in moving me to a new appreciation of the issues. While she was a medical student at Stanford in the late 1980s, she was active in changing the school's sensitivity to gender issues. I felt I had "made the grade" when, as a senior resident in the primary care internal medicine program at Stanford, she invited me to present grand rounds and began her introduction by saying, "I have known the speaker for a long time. And I am very proud of him. He is my father." By the time I had finished my lecture, I was emotionally drained–and very proud of her.

I realize only now in retrospect how dominant the male culture was at McGill University and at the Massachusetts General Hospital. It seemed that everyone in a position of power was a man. I note with sadness that this continues largely to this day at the MGH, with only two women chairing a department: (my successor, Anne Young, and Jeanine Wiener-Kronish, who was appointed chief of the Department of Anesthesiology at the MGH from UCSF in 2008). My failed attempt to recruit Susan Leeman after my arrival there in 1978 confirmed the existing biases. I was able later as chair, however, to recruit several junior women faculty to the neurology department and watched with great pride as they successfully advanced to full professorial status.

It wasn't until San Francisco, however, with the influence of the dean's office, that I was able to take actions to provide new leadership opportunities for women. I recall vividly a decision

I had to make to appoint a successor to Leon Leventhal, who had very ably chaired the Department of Microbiology and Immunology. My choice for Leon's successor was Elizabeth Blackburn, an internationally renowned scientist who had discovered seminal aspects of chromosomal telomere structure and function with the identification of the enzyme telomerase. She was reluctant when I first approached her with the idea, expressing self-doubt, concerned that a woman might not be accepted in a department with so many distinguished male faculty members, including Nobel Prize–winner Mike Bishop. In the end, and with encouragement, she did take on the task and proved to be a tremendous leader. We kept in close contact over the years as I observed her leadership emerge internationally. I was delighted in October 2009 to learn that she had been awarded the Nobel Prize in Physiology or Medicine; hers was the third Nobel Prize awarded to faculty at UCSF since 1989.

When I returned to Boston, there were numerous opportunities to improve women's stature as leaders at Harvard Medical School and to make a direct statement of appreciation toward women faculty members. I thought of one such statement early on in my tenure as dean, as I sat in the Benjamin Waterhouse Faculty Room in the Administration Building (now Gordon Hall), a few feet from my office. The walls of the room were lined with portraits large and small of white males who had served the school. I wondered: Had any women occupied chairs of HMS departments, past or present? If so, who were they? I asked around and was startled to find that there had only been nine *in toto*, or at least that was all I could discover. One, the Viennese-trained psychoanalyst Grete Bibring, who had served as chair of the Department of Psychiatry at the Beth Israel Hospital, was deceased. Another four—Shirley Driscoll, Mary Ellen Avery, Betty Hay and Lynn Reid—were living in retirement from their chair positions. The current chairs included one from the Harvard Medical School basic science departments (Barbara McNeil) and three from the hospital departments: Anne Young, chair of neurology at the MGH; Mary Ann Badaracco, chair of psychiatry at the BIDMC; and Carol Warfield, chair of anesthesiology at the BIDMC.

I devised a plan to acknowledge the services of Bibring and those living in retirement, sought advice from my colleagues and arranged for a distinguished portrait photographer to prepare photographs of all five past women chairs to hang on the walls of the faculty room. We arranged an induction ceremony, attended by Shirley Driscoll, Mary Ellen Avery, Betty Hay and Lynn Reid, among others, where I was able to express appreciation for their many contributions. The responses they gave were emotional and left everyone in the room teary-eyed.

The five portraits, together with two others we installed of the first two African-American professors at HMS—William A. Hinton, who had developed the test for syphilis, and Harold Amos, who was twice chair of the Department of Microbiology and Molecular Genetics—continue to grace the room where all important administrative decisions and discussions for the school and its hospitals are held. I think of them as a new signal of the commitment to diversity that HMS rightly ought to be proud of.

Another opportunity to make a statement regarding the importance of woman at Harvard came with the establishment of the Archives for Women in Medicine at the Countway Library of Medicine. A committee was established in 2000 with fundraising efforts led by Dean Eleanor Shore (MD, class of 1955) and Professor Nancy Tarbel; I was pleased to provide some initial support from school coffers. The first public event occurred in November 2007, and it focused on the career of Grete Bibring, the first woman to be appointed a full professor at HMS. The activities of the archivist, Jessica Sedgwick, and support from the hospitals allow the center to continue an active in-depth documentation of the contributions women have made as Harvard faculty. I was pleased in the spring of 2010 to be present at a Countway Archives for Women event honoring Patricia Donohoe, who had ably led the division of pediatric surgery at the MGH for two decades. Back in 1993, Pat had accepted my invitation to address the audience as the keynote speaker at my inauguration as chancellor of UCSF.

For my support for the Joint Committee on the Status of Women (JCSW), I received a personal letter from the committee on the occasion of my retirement, acknowledging, very touchingly, the progress we had made together, one component of which was a survey of salary equities between men and women faculty, led by Eleanor Shore of our faculty affairs office. The results of the survey, while underwhelming, show favorable trends that merit continued scrutiny. To my immense surprise and gratitude, the JCSW honored me by naming an annual faculty award to an individual active in support of women at HMS after me.

Before I left the dean's office, I made an effort to assess the role women were currently playing in leadership positions throughout the school and its hospitals. The results were mixed. The total number of chairs occupied by women at the hospitals was five: there was Anne Young at the MGH; none at the BWH; Mary Ann Badaracco and Carol Warfield at the BIDMC; Orah Platt at Children's Hospital; Joan Miller at the Massachusetts Eye and Ear Infirmary; and none at the Dana-Farber Cancer Institute. Of the nine departments in the basic science areas of HMS, three women—Carla Shatz in neurobiology, Barbara McNeil in health policy and Joan Brugge in cell biology—were serving very effective leadership roles. In my own area of responsibility in the dean's office, three of the six senior deans were women: Cynthia Walker, dean for administration; Nancy Andrews, dean for basic science and graduate programs; and Joan Reede, dean for diversity and community partnership.

What does one make of this? In my experience, women leaders have in every way been comparable to men and, in some areas, were superior to them. I have found women to be more generous with their time in mentoring and in listening to the strategic whole rather than their own vested interests.[1] I have concluded that we too often fail to take the "risk" of appointing women because our targeted recruitments and the recommendations we get about candidates are driven primarily by the old boys' network.

### *Ethnic and Racial Diversity*

My views on racial issues while growing up in Alberta were narrowly confined, to say the least. I grew up with suspicion about Native Canadians, who were often labeled as alcoholics too lazy to take on responsible jobs. I was keenly aware that the Trans-Canada Highway from Brooks to Calgary traversed the reaches of the First Nations settlements, now reserves. I thought of the "Indians" as we passed by Gleichen, where a sharp drop-off in the prairie landscape afforded by a narrow cluster of hills provided their past hunters with a place to conclude their buffalo drives. It was said that there were vast graveyards of bones at the bottom of the hill where the animals were herded from above to their deaths.

Later, during my first years at university, I encountered very little ethnic diversity—a homogeneity broken only by the large Ukrainian community of Edmonton, which had expanded following the Bolshevik Revolution that drove large numbers of immigrants to western Canada. In medical school, my classmates came from a mixture of religious and immigrant roots, typical of western Canadian populations.

The political events in Cleveland and Montreal that Rachel and I experienced within only a few years of leaving Edmonton would go a long way toward dispelling the racial and ethnic myths I had grown up with. In both cities, we witnessed the most dramatic expressions of racial and social inequity, as well as violent reactions to the status quo. The Hough riots, as well as the civil rights movement, were afoot during my residency in Cleveland, while the FLQ Crisis in Montreal coincided with my tenure there. Each experience, in its own way, was to leave a permanent mark on my thinking and would shape my perspectives.

Dramatic racial and apartheid encounters were especially painful during my visit to South Africa with Rachel in 1977. Bernard Pimstone, a scientist colleague I'd met first in Milan, Italy, had invited me to visit several medical schools as a visiting professor of the South African Medical Research Council. Bernard's laboratory, like mine, was focusing on development of radioimmunoassays to measure small peptides, notably somatostatin, and we had shared reagents and research developments. During the visit, which lasted two weeks, I visited medical schools in the English and Afrikaans universities in Johannesburg, Pretoria, Bloemfontein and Cape Town. It was during this trip that I met the late Helen Sussman, a phenomenal political foe of apartheid and a leader of the liberal party. The full impact of apartheid impressed us on a visit to the town of Soweto outside Johannesburg.

On the last evening of our visit before our return home, Rachel and I attended a wonderful banquet in Johannesburg, where I was asked to make some remarks about my visit to the country and about its medical schools. I complimented the quality of the science I'd seen and acknowledged the esteem with which South African medical schools were held. But then I remember deciding during the last few minutes of my talk—and quite impulsively—to tell a story that I felt summarized my feelings about the place. It was the man-suit-tailor joke, which I told with some trepidation, but that I thought then, was appropriate for the occasion. The story goes like this:

A man enters a shop to buy a suit and, trying one on, finds that it needs some alterations. "The right sleeve is too long," he says, to which the tailor responds by hitching it up and suggesting that the man hold it there with the chin against the shoulder. The man next notes that the left pant leg drags on the floor: "Pull it up and put your elbow against the hip to keep it there," advises the tailor. "But the left sleeve of the suit is too short," the man continues to complain. "Grab hold of it and tug it down with the right hand," instructs the tailor, and then adds, "There, you see it looks great." Upon leaving the shop, the man is met by two nuns. One of the nuns remarks that the man must be suffering from a strange malady, to which the other nun says, "Yes, it's too bad, but he is wearing a lovely suit."

That, I said, reminded me of South Africa.

### *Affirmative Action: Great Progress or Misplaced Focus?*

Although my cousin Freddie Martin left Canada for a couple of summers during the African-American Civil Rights Movement in the American South to join demonstrations, march in protests and help register voters, I did not give much thought to racial inequities when I was at university. One of the earliest instances of racial strife I recall was the famous Boston school busing controversy that arose after Judge W. Arthur Garrity's 1970 ruling that students be transported across the city to make integration real. The result was two decades of turmoil. Living in the bedroom community of Belmont at the time, we were not directly involved with the busing issue, but we did participate in the Metropolitan Council for Educational Opportunity (METCO) program that brought a small number of students from inner-city schools to suburban classrooms. Our sons Doug and Neil in particular, came to appreciate the efforts of the program and the friendships they developed with some of the students.

My arrival at the University of California changed my perspectives on inequality irrevocably as I observed and participated in a decade-long reassessment of the impact of affirmative action on student admissions and faculty hiring. By the fall of 1995, I was witness to a new form of entrenchment at the University of California. Regent Ward Connerly, a successful Republican businessman, set out to abolish affirmative action as a guiding principle in UC admissions, influencing the other regents. Connerly, an African American who had come from an underprivileged background, was proud of his own success. He postulated that affirmative action led to personal recrimination and did not serve the best interests of the university community or the underrepresented minority students.

I was aware, of course, that this debate was triggered by a lawsuit from a pre-medical student who was denied admission to medical school at UC San Diego. Together with his parents, he had requested and obtained the admission data for the class members accepted in the fall of 1995. The graph of the data clearly showed that college grade point averages plotted against MCAT (Medical College Admission Test) scores for white students, when compared to those of underrepresented minority students, yielded two overlapping but statistically significant different clusters. The student applicant compared his grades with the minority students selected for admission when he was rejected and concluded that he had been discriminated against. The facts of the case were presented to the regents shortly thereafter, with the outcome a sophisticated media awareness campaign led by Connerly to challenge current admission procedures and press for the total abolition of consideration of race, per se, as a criterion for admission.

Later that fall, I found myself attending obligatory meetings of the UC regents, where Regent Connerly was systematically unraveling the decades-long support of affirmative action that had been effectively used to increase minority enrollment. His efforts continued until California state law was changed through a public referendum, Proposition 209, which notoriously, in my view, set new barriers for admission, with much of the effects lingering to this day. Enrollment of underrepresented minorities has tumbled.

I reacted strongly and vocally to the pressure being imposed by the regents, most of whom had been appointed by Republican governors Ronald Reagan and Pete Wilson. I joined the academic senate of the UCSF campus in protesting the action, as did the academic senates of the other eight campuses of the UC system.

Connerly's actions led to a majority vote at the January 1997 meeting of the regents, permanently damaging the university's future efforts to provide educational opportunities to the underrepresented minorities of the state. This occurred at a time when actuarial assessments indicated that within a few decades white citizens would be a minority in the state.

### *Should Diversity Be a Goal at Academic Institutions?*

When I returned to Harvard in the summer of 1997, I was very pleased to note the tremendous diversity of the HMS student body, which was the outcome of a dramatic admissions policy change initiated in the 1970s. Three days after the assassination of Martin Luther King Jr., a small group of HMS faculty that included Ed Kravitz and Jon Beckwith, working together with Leon Eisenberg, took action on the local scene and convinced then-Dean Robert Ebert to expand class size in 1970, to extend opportunities to underrepresented minorities.

While transitioning from San Francisco to Boston, I was deeply impressed by an article in the *Harvard Gazette* by President Neil Rudenstine, where he addressed the question of educational values that derive from cultural diversity.[2] Using examples that dated back to the nineteenth century, he convincingly argued that whatever case might be made for or against selective favoring of minorities, no one disagreed with the premise that diversity of experience has educational value. Neil Rudenstine's brief treatise, entitled "Diversity and Learning at Harvard: A Historical View," filled me with a sense of pride in my new employer, Harvard University. The address had been delivered to the Massachusetts Historical Society at the Harvard Club on November 6, 1996. For me, it was very timely. Rudenstine's arguments were compelling. There were advantages to the

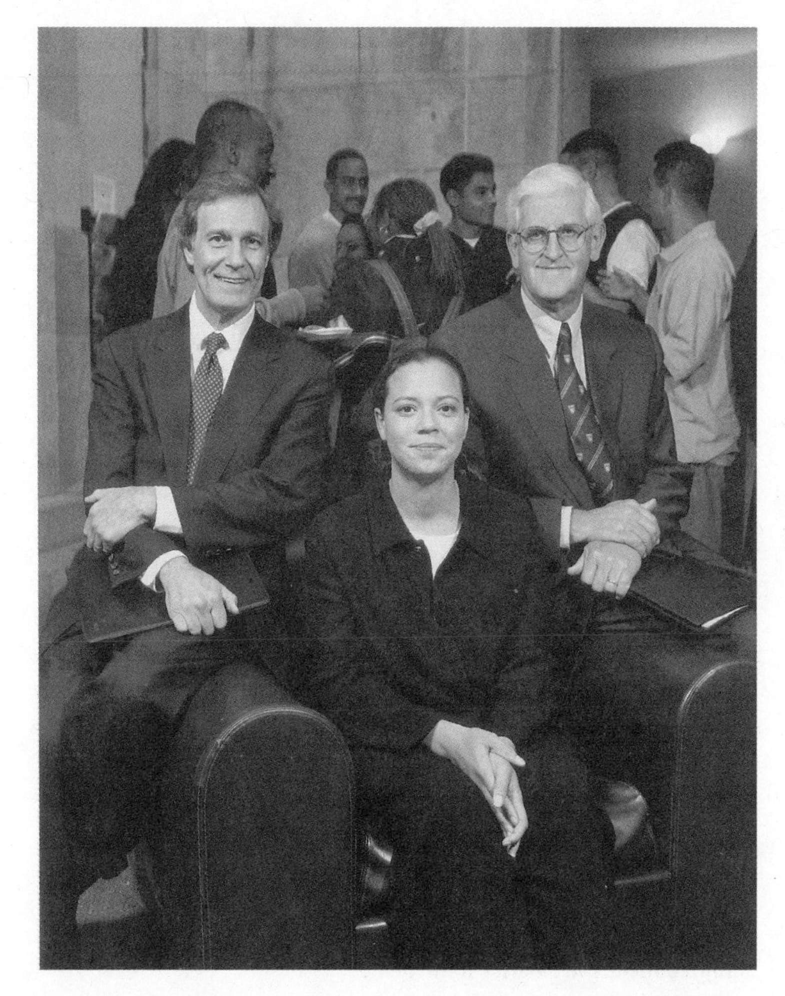

The author (right) with Harvard President Neil Rudenstine and HMS student Donella Green (HMS 1999) on a day celebrating Harvard Medical School's commitment to diversity.

educational experience gained by students coming together from diverse backgrounds. The secret to ensuring diversity lay in how one exercised admission actions that produced a diverse class without breaking the law extant by the Supreme Court's 1978 Bakke decision, a California case, and in view of an emerging case involving the University of Michigan Law School, where a female applicant who had been denied admission was suing Dean Lee Bollinger.[3] In both cases, the essence of the Supreme Court decision was that race could be considered in determining which students would be admitted but that a quota system could not be used.

In medical schools, highly qualified minority candidates continue to be selected through an interview-driven admission policy. But the Supreme Court ruling regarding the University of Michigan Law School admission policies changed our practice of using a separate committee to consider the admission of minority candidates. Fortunately, the effectiveness of the individual interview has permitted HMS to maintain a highly diverse student body. In 2008, 23 per cent of students who matriculated to enter medical school came from underrepresented minorities.

Other methods have also been used at HMS to foster a diverse student body. When I arrived as dean, Joan Reede was working closely with Bill Silen, invited into the dean's office by the previous dean, Dan Tosteson. Silen, a distinguished surgeon and former chair of the Department of Surgery at the BIDMC, had been a mentor to Joan. A graduate of Johns Hopkins and a pediatrician, Joan had many ideas on how to promote diversity within and outside the walls of the medical school. She had established an extraordinary effort to bring high school and college students from the New England region to Boston every other year to attend the Biomedical Scholars Program held over two days in February. Faculty from the medical and nursing schools in Boston contributed to the event with noteworthy results, as students from minority backgrounds were successful in entering college and medical school. It was quite remarkable to watch Joan at work with a breadth of activities that spanned middle-school content to faculty mentoring.

I assured Joan of my firm commitment to the efforts she was undertaking and found resources to support her office. In 2003, when Bill Silen took retirement, she was appointed Dean for Diversity and Community Partnership and since that time has performed many noble tasks, not only in the region but also nationally. In 2009 she was elected a member of the Institute of Medicine, the highest honor within the medical academy, in recognition of her national stature in promoting diversity. I am very proud of what she has accomplished.



### *The Culture of San Francisco*



The move to San Francisco was liberating in many ways. There is a certain temperament there that some call permissive and others might label as a high propensity for risk-taking. But whatever the description, upon arrival the feeling emerges almost instantly, when compared to Boston, that you are in a more tolerant, accepting and forgiving cultural context. The free expression of views is evident in all spheres of the city's culture, and one isn't there long before an emerging sense of "ordinariness" challenges and then banishes one's biases and prejudices. The openness and friendship felt so easily there was a distinctive change for Rachel and me from the conservative-mindedness of the Boston scene. The academic community at UCSF reflected the San Francisco culture of thought, as well.

San Francisco's openness is predicated in part by the city's rich ethnic complexion, which invariably affects everyday practice and experience. There is a remarkable contiguity and overlap between the old guard, whose origins often date back to the late nineteenth century, and the "new arrivals," typified by the flower children of the 1960s and the expanding gay and lesbian community of the 1970s continuing to the present time. The annual June gala of the gay pride march and festivities has to be amongst the most outrageous and provocative anywhere, and Halloween in the Castro district is an event requiring participation at least once. I remember going there with Rachel one Halloween evening during our eight-year "sabbatical" in San Francisco. I wore a Lone Ranger outfit with a cowboy hat and a mask; Rachel was less dramatically decked out. Standing by the parade I was shocked to be greeted by a participant who called out, "Hello, Dean Martin." It was one of my medical students. I joked with him later about what he was doing there.

I don't remember facing the issue of sexual orientation with respect to academic matters before my time in San Francisco. My first personal challenge came shortly after my term as chancellor began. I was asked by the gay, lesbian, bisexual and transgender (LGBT) community to speak at one of their meetings and to give my opinion regarding their important role in the UCSF community, something the chancellor before me had been reluctant to do. I accepted their invitation after some hesitation. When I took the podium, I simply expressed my willingness to learn of their experiences and to exercise my authority to assure that their rights for equality were an official part of my administration's commitment. My frankness and openness with the community was to serve me well in the years ahead. I came to admire and appreciate the honesty that the group demonstrated.

Our experiences in this regard were not limited to the workplace. In San Francisco the First Mennonite Church had a unique position in the transitions that the Mennonite Church and its colleges were undergoing. Its franchise rights within the broader Mennonite constituency were tested early on when the issue of whether or not the LGBT community was welcome to attend, or to become members, became defining issues for the local church. The relationship with the larger Mennonite Church was retained during this evolution of radical liberation from the older tenets of the tradition. There was constant testing of the limits that would allow more freedom of expression and yet enable this particular church to remain "credentialed" by the mainstream church. There were a number of openly gay relationships within the community, and the pastors selected to lead the group were familiar with and sympathetic to their concerns. For Rachel and me, it was a new adventure that opened our vistas of recognition and appreciation for the struggle that many of our friends faced within and without the church.

Within our Mennonite community, there were two openly gay brothers who came from a family of five children. One of their sisters was gay, as well. The family had grown up in South America, where the parents had served as missionaries. Each of the three gay members of the family became part of our inner circle while in San Francisco, and we treasured their friendship.

The LGBT community challenged me again, when I returned to Harvard. I agreed to meet with them and to address their group in public. I think I knew more about their issues than they might have realized; the experience in San Francisco had been invaluable.

LGBT issues were also frequently discussed at the Mennonite Congregation of Boston (MCOB), which Rachel and I attend. The concerns were thoughtfully captured in a note I found recently, penned by Jacob Yost, a Mennonite graduate student at Harvard University. It is addressed to a pastoral candidate who was being considered to lead our congregation:

*MCOB has several openly gay members, as well as at least one family with a gay child. Indeed, one of our gay members is pursuing graduate study in religion and sexuality at Harvard Divinity School, and thus, I am confident, has a sophisticated understanding of the theological issues that I probably couldn't do justice to.*

*As a congregation, we start from the assumption that all people are invited to participate fully in the life of the church, regardless of sexual orientation, and we live accordingly....Members of the church are active in church-wide organizations and campaigns that advocate for sexual inclusiveness....So, for instance, the perspective that homosexuality is a sin, or a deviation and aberration from God's redeemed/shalom natural order, is one that if articulated bluntly could be very hurtful to people....As council thinks about introducing you, or any other candidate who is closer to the mainstream of Mennonite theology than to our own minority position,...we think about how both sides can use language that will allow them to build a relationship based on their enormous commonalities and shared beliefs and convictions, rather than fracturing or stunting that relationship over this single issue.*[4]

The candidate, who graduated from one of the Mennonite seminaries with an employment history of several years of teaching in a Bible College in West Africa, was hired by the congregation after assurances that she would be comfortable serving the congregation by "welcoming" everyone who wished to attend. After nearly two years of service our hopes for her leadership have been fully realized.

## Academic–Commercial Relationships, Including Issues of Conflicts of Interest

Academic–commercial interactions are critical for development of effective new therapies, whether drugs or medical devices. These relationships have undergone intense scrutiny in recent years, in some instances threatening the productivity that is essential for improving the health of the citizenry.

In 2011 Hamilton Moses and I summarized these issues in a paper in the *New England Journal of Medicine*:

*The biomedical-research enterprise in the United States soon became the envy of other nations, as well as the primary source of the world's new drugs and medical devices. Since 1945, biomedical research has been viewed as the essential contributor to improving the health of individuals and populations, in both the developed and developing world.*

*Today, the primacy of biomedical research and technology development is being challenged. Patients, physicians, insurers, and policymakers are all questioning the slow pace of advance, escalation cost, dubious clinical value, inappropriate commercial exploitation, and lure of false hope for patients with serious disease. The backdrop is growing skepticism of the value of science itself as a solution to global problems.*[5]

My first introduction to the pernicious aspects of academic–industrial collaborations occurred at UCSF in 1994 when I was chancellor of the campus. A faculty member, Betty Dong, had signed a contract with a company called Boots Pharmaceuticals to study thyroid hormone replacement using the company's widely prescribed form of thyroxine: Synthroid. The study protocol compared efficacy of their drug with less expensive generic forms of the hormone. As the trials reached conclusion, it became apparent to Dong that the generic forms were equally potent and effective, a result that had potential devastating financial implications for the company. (Synthroid was the company's main product, and it was widely prescribed and marketed as highly effective.) The company forbade Dong from publishing her findings even though a manuscript had been accepted by the *Journal of the American Medical Association* (JAMA).[6] Post hoc review of the contract that Dong had signed confirmed the company's contention that publication was to be permitted only after the company granted permission.

The matter became public news in the medical community and JAMA made a big issue about the squandering of academic freedom. Strong allegations were made concerning the university's reluctance to stand up for the faculty member and to challenge the company. The UC lawyers were accused of complicity. University counsel argued that the costs of litigation, since the contract would be held in breach, were potentially very large. The likelihood of losing the case was too hazardous to permit publication. In their review of the documents it was apparent that the investigator, Dong, eager to gain support for the clinical trials, had signed the agreement with the company without obtaining university legal review. Dong was not to be blamed; there were no clear guidelines for faculty disclosure of academic–industrial contractual arrangements.

The matter dragged on for several years. Eventually the data were published, but there were no winners—the company lost market share, the university stood blamed for acquiescence to industry demands and the investigator experienced a delay in academic productivity. Painful to me was the strong criticism leveled at UCSF's administration over impacts of the loss of academic freedom.

A Canadian example, still in legal challenge since the late 1990s, is the case of Nancy Olivieri of the Hospital for Sick Children at the University of Toronto. In this case, the investigator was denied publication of results she interpreted to show that the agent, deferiprone, a treatment for the blood disorder thalassemia, being developed by a company called Apotex, was more toxic and less beneficial than the company was willing to accept. This legal interchange precipitated a *New England Journal of Medicine* commentary in 2002 by David Nathan of Harvard Medical School and David Weatherall of Oxford University about the failure of the university to provide appropriate protection to an honorable and well-meaning faculty member.[7] The university stood in a duplicitous position, having received substantial gifts from the company. The case was settled eventually for close to $1 million, with agreement by the university and Olivieri to discontinue "disparagement" of the company. In November 2008 the company reopened the legal proceedings, alleging breach of the agreement, claiming that Olivieri had not fully complied with the conditions. Her immediate defense, supported by faculty colleagues, was that she had attended meetings where the matter had been discussed, but this did not vacate the terms of the agreement.

The dean of the Faculty of Medicine and now president of the University of Toronto, David Naylor, as recently as 2008, called-for "moving on"—beyond the issues. (Olivieri was awarded the Scientific Freedom and Responsibility Award by the American Association for the Advancement of Science in 2010.)[8]

*Relations with Foundations Can also be Problematic*

I recall another traumatic example from my days at UCSF where entanglements with funding of research by not-for-profit foundations also led to misunderstandings and the potential for lawsuits. Mike Merzenich, a neuroscientist, was renowned for experimental findings in monkeys that showed brain plasticity—the capacity for brain rewiring after injury or change in sensory inputs. His group documented changes in the neuronal wiring within the cerebral cortex. Together with Paula Tallal, a psychologist from Rutgers University, he championed the notion that the underlying defect in some cases of reading difficulty (dyslexia) and other learning disorders might be treated with protocols that would "rewire" the brain. They speculated that acoustic stimuli coming too closely together were encoded incorrectly by the brain, leading to perceptual errors in sound interpretation. They went on to devise a system of retraining auditory inputs by changing the timing of auditory signals. The computer-based games they devised rewarded children for correctly identifying speech intervals.

Based on this work, Merzenich and Tallal decided to start a company called Scientific Learning. I became aware of their efforts both because I understood the science behind the idea and because they went to the intellectual property office of the UC system to patent their ideas for licensing to the company. Venture capital funds were raised, and employees were hired to work at an off-campus site. Every aspect of the arrangement followed university guidelines for technology transfer.

I thought little more about the matter until one October morning in 1995 while Rachel and I were attending a neurology meeting at the Broadmoor complex outside Denver. I received a call from James Watson, co-discoverer of DNA, about the new company and its developing products. The Dana Foundation, a not-for-profit based in New York City, on whose advisory board Watson served as a consultant to David Mahoney, the president of the foundation, had not been informed of the commercialization plans, and Watson asserted foundation rights to the discovery because it had provided funding for aspects of the experimental work. The foundation threatened to sue Merzenich and UCSF for breach of contract. It turned out that a modest proportion of the funding that Mike had used in his work came from the Dana Foundation, but the agreement had not included any legal rights to discovery as was now being claimed.

Watson accused me and the university of probable illegal activity and said, "If this goes to court, the issues of academic–industrial relationships will be set back for a generation." He went on to say that William Safire, a columnist for the *New York Times*, who was a board member of the foundation, was aware of the way the university had "taken advantage of the foundation" and that he was prepared "to write about it as an example of bad-faith relationships between scientists and those supporting the research that gave rise to commercial potential, in which the scientists personally profited financially." Watson indicated that my job would be on the line, and that, if uncorrected, the matter would embarrass the scientists and the university.

I did not know Jim Watson well, although we had had friendly interactions at meetings I had attended at Cold Spring Harbor Laboratories, where he was president. I called Bruce Alberts, president of the National Academy of Sciences and a former colleague from UCSF for advice. He remarked that Jim was known for his outbursts and that he would call him for more details.

As it turned out, the matter was not resolved despite many hours of discussions with the foundation and with Ed Rover, their attorney. UC lawyers entered the deliberations. Their review of the research award from the Dana Foundation concluded that it did not contain any definitive binding agreement with the foundation for disclosure of intellectual property or any mechanism for sharing licensing fees or royalties with them. The matter continued for more than a year and was resolved finally when the university returned the money to the foundation that Merzenich had used to support his work.

Later, when I came to Harvard as dean, I would have an opportunity to engage in a number of activities with David Mahoney, his wife, Hillie, and the Dana Alliance for Brain Initiatives. Ed Rove became a close friend during these years. I came to appreciate that misunderstandings of the sort I had at UCSF can be transitory, and I have treasured the friendships that followed.

These examples emphasize the need for clarification and transparency of all arrangements regarding commercialization of science and the assurance by faculty that they will not enter into contracts without explicit university review and approval.

### *Facing a New Challenge at Harvard Medical School: Conflict of Interest Policies and For-profit Entities*

Shortly after my term as dean began in 1997, I was approached by hospital faculty who requested revisions to Harvard's conflict of interest (COI) policies regarding relationships with for-profit entities. The policies at issue had been put in place in the early 1990s by a faculty committee assembled by Dean Tosteson and chaired by Professor Barbara McNeil, head of the Department of Health Policy and a radiologist at the Brigham and Women's Hospital, who had been charged with the responsibility of developing a comprehensive policy. A vociferous debate had ensued, with objections voiced principally from clinical faculty at the MGH who thought the proposed new guidelines were unnecessary and that faculty could be trusted to "do the right thing." These faculty members objected to what they perceived as excessively protective academic rules that constrained innovation and the development of academic–industrial relationships. Despite the objections, the faculty council, with one dissenting vote, eventually approved policy guidelines.

The guidelines had remained in place for nearly a decade, but the debate had lingered on. The issues were still unresolved in the minds of several hospital faculty members when I arrived, and I was given the dubious honor of handling the situation.

Before taking any action, I took a careful look at the evolution of the issues involved, particularly as they impacted policy at Harvard. The notion that universities should contribute to the development of technology and, in the case of the biomedical sciences, to new treatments for disease has gone through decades of revisions. The postwar period had seen the development of an entire computer-based industry framed around relationships with universities, notably with MIT, Carnegie Mellon and Stanford. These institutions had long histories of engineering applications critical for technology development of new products, devices and collaborations regarded as advantageous by most parties in the academic and for-profit sectors.

By around 1970, universities and the private sector were deploying intellectual property (IP) agreements in the biological sciences, whereby academic faculty were allowed to file patents owned by the university, to license them and share income, albeit with a number of restrictions. There were also IP agreements between the universities and their faculty. In general, while patents could be filed in the inventor's name, inventors did not actually retain ownership of the patents. Rather, they were assigned to the university in exchange for a share of the income. These arrangements allowed successful technology development and served as useful vehicles for payback to support the academic mission.

At Harvard University, these developments had gone through a long incubation period and gradual implementation. The first granting of a patent at Harvard occurred in the 1970s, when President Derek Bok and General Counsel Daniel Steiner were pressed by the Children's Hospital about pending agreements between Monsanto and two faculty members, Judah Folkman and Bert Vallee. Joyce Brinton, now a retired director of the Office of Technology Licensing (OTL) at Harvard, recounts the development of these arrangements with faculty and outside interests:

*A new patent policy was adopted by the university in 1975 (approximately at the same time that the funding agreement with Monsanto was signed). That policy provided that the university would own patents in the health and medical therapeutics fields and that it would share income with inventors on the following basis: First $50K, inventors received 35%; next $50K, inventors received 25%, and above $100K, inventors received 15%—shares also went to the inventor's lab and departments as well as his or her school and the university. (The same sharing was also in place at the MGH at the time or soon before or after.) This sharing arrangement was modified (I think in the mid-1980s) so that the inventors received 35% for the first $100K, and 25% for all income above that amount.)*[9]

One of the hallmarks of the Monsanto agreement was the establishment of an outside (international) advisory board that could march in if Monsanto was not working to develop inventions for which they held a license.

Meanwhile, with the emerging promise of molecular biology and recombinant DNA technology, tremendous advances were being made in biomedical research in the 1970s. These discoveries led to the establishment of Genentech in San Francisco in 1976, followed by Biogen in Cambridge in 1978. Amgen in Los Angeles and Chiron in the San Francisco Bay Area were founded in 1980. The technologies for promising new protein-based therapies, such as insulin and growth hormone, arose from recombinant DNA technologies developed at academic institutions: UCSF/Stanford (the Cohen/Boyer patent on recombinant DNA technology), Harvard, the City of Hope Cancer Center in Los Angeles, and MIT.

These new potential therapies and their implications differed from prior experiences with engineering and computer technologies in three very important ways. First, they had to do with life and death matters, involving patients with serious illnesses whose lives depended on the successful outcome of these new therapies. This demanded development of safety and efficacy standards for testing potential drugs in human subjects, necessitating the formulation of new ethical contracts between doctor and patient, requiring the informed consent of patients facing real or potential dangers.[10]

Second, the promise of new drugs derived from basic science discoveries encouraged academic–industrial partnerships, which required new policies about the conduct of research in academic laboratories. Companies, recognizing that they could not match scientific efforts at a level found in academic institutions, sought partnerships that involved many leading institutions. These arrangements were perceived as beneficial to the scholarly enterprise of hospitals and medical schools.

At HMS, we witnessed the evolution of several large academic–industrial alliances. The experience with Hoechst (described in chapter five), which resulted in the founding of a new Department of Molecular Biology at the MGH, proved to be a great success in the opinion of hospital leaders. But by 1997 Hoechst support was winding down. From a corporate perspective, there was little commercial value to show for their basic science investment. Other agreements were implemented, most notably one between the MGH Department of Dermatology and

Shiseido, which was signed in 1995 and lasted nearly fifteen years, once again without significant development of new commercial products.

Third, over time, there emerged the recognition that development of new therapies and devices required consideration of a new cost-base structure of what the public—patients and insurers—were willing to pay. The cost-benefit ratio of each new treatment ought to be compared with therapies already available. The debate continues about the level of patient benefit that needs to be demonstrated regarding a new biologic in cancer treatment, for example, in order to receive approval, as well as what price could be demanded for the drug. In many instances, benefits have been very marginal, extending life by only a few months, even though the costs may run into tens or hundreds of thousands of dollars for each patient treated. The ideas behind such vigilance and cost awareness have been popularized as comparative effectiveness research, and the issues remain highly relevant today.

### *The Role of NIH and Government Emerges*

The evolution of the critical role of the National Institutes of Health in the developments related to academic–industrial partnerships raised a number of issues. The expanding research enterprise in our medical schools and universities came to surpass educational budgets; the *Bayh–Dole Act* of 1980 gave license to universities, research institutes, medical schools and hospitals to accept federal support and transition it to patents, licenses and royalties. The intention of the law was to encourage companies to take advantage of scientific discovery and develop federally funded inventions; small companies were to be given preference if they were equally (or perhaps almost equally) able to carry out that development.

Other regulatory factors followed: the establishment of the gold standard for translational medical research in the form of the "double-blind" clinical trial, where neither patient nor physician know the treatment given, whether agent or placebo; the development of institutional review boards (IRBS) that allow inside members of these institutions to work with non-conflicted outside community members to establish rules and give permission for clinical trials; the interesting double standard imposed on the development of surgical devices and techniques that often allow their experimental use through extenuating patient-care needs without imposing the burden of a "controlled" clinical trial; and, finally, the emergence of the successful academic entrepreneur who can make a fortune from medical discoveries through the formation of privately held companies supported by venture capital entities.

These evolving concerns and the development of standards increasingly came under the jurisdiction of the US Food and Drug Administration (FDA), which became subject to growing criticism on both sides of the equation: for failing to move with dispatch in the regulatory approval process, on the one hand, and for the delayed withdrawal of approved drugs when subsequent deleterious side effects were revealed, on the other. A genuine no-win dilemma.

In 1995 the NIH and the National Science Foundation (NSF) promulgated rules that for the first time regulated the relationships of NIH- and NSF-funded investigators working in academic institutions. Investigators were required to disclose "significant financial interests" of more than $10,000 to their institutions at the time of grant submission. Institutions were then required to take steps to review the disclosure and, if a determination of a conflict was made, to manage or eliminate the conflict before the grant funding was released. For a number of institutions, this requirement represented their first serious look at potential conflict of interest issues on campuses.

### *Actions Taken at HMS Regarding Academic–Industrial Partnerships*

In 1998, a year after I'd arrived as dean, I asked Eugene Braunwald, an eminent cardiologist who had recently retired from his role as physician-in-chief at the BWH, to chair a distinguished panel of senior faculty from the basic science and clinical departments of HMS, including, of course, representatives from each of Harvard's major teaching hospitals.

The committee's work was nearly complete in the spring of 1999. The committee recommended permitting faculty to participate in industrial support of clinical trials with levels of personal financial involvement that exceeded those recommended by the federal government. The recommendations included new rules of disclosure and the use of committees to adjudicate in complex issues when they emerged.

The death of eighteen-year-old Jesse Gelsinger in September 1999 at the University of Pennsylvania, and the events that unfolded soon thereafter, changed everything. Gelsinger died while part of a clinical trial using a technique called gene therapy, apparently due to a severe immune response to the viral carrier that was used to transport the gene into his cells. It became apparent to me that the circumstances leading to his death raised ethical issues of the type not appreciated before: the relationships of the clinical investigators to industrial concerns; the role of the institution in endorsing the development of a new research entity focused on gene therapy with pressure to demonstrate success that overruled good judgment about when to introduce new trial therapies; failure to gain adequate and informed consent; failure to stay within the approved guidelines of the IRB; and worst, perhaps, failure to follow the clinical research protocol that led to the administration of an excessive dose of the viral carrier—a dose that earlier work in monkeys had shown to be potentially dangerous.

My response to this national crisis was that Harvard should not be seen as relaxing its rules in the face of such a disaster and that we would be better served by taking additional steps to assure that our investigators would not be caught in similar infringements of the rights of our patients and of the public entities that support their research. I met with the faculty committee and received their unanimous agreement to postpone a scheduled faculty-wide meeting and to reconsider our next steps, since the earlier recommendations had not been put in place. The final set of recommendations were agreed on in May 2001 and resulted in a few changes to the conflict of interest policy—fewer than some faculty expected. In addition, there were new rules aimed at protecting students and trainees: if their participation was being contemplated in a research project, the investigator was obliged to provide them with a full disclosure of the project.

The new policy guidelines passed without faculty dissent. In the meantime, largely as a result of the Gelsinger tragedy, conflict of interest issues had become a national concern. In 2000, with the sponsorship of the Josiah Macy Foundation, based in New York, I convened a group of medical school deans and academic leaders to consider the matter at a meeting in Washington, DC. We prepared a summary of our recommendations that was circulated to academic health center leaders.

A year later, I served on a committee formed by the Association of American Medical Colleges to review and develop guidelines for conflict of interest policies for academic health centers. The deliberations lasted over eighteen months and resulted in two separate but linked documents. The first dealt with individual faculty conflicts of interest and the second with guidelines for institutional conflicts. A key element in the first document was the concept that if the faculty member had any financial links to a company, relations that involved clinical trials or other patient engagement should be presumptively prohibited. However, this was a "rebuttable" presumption of prohibition. The guidelines supposed scenarios where faculty would be permitted to persuade their institutions that their circumstances were so exceptional that the prohibition should not apply. A number of medical schools, but not Harvard, subsequently adopted this model.

Returning to matters at Harvard Medical School, in 2004, I appointed two new committees to consider relevant revisions to the existing guidelines: one, chaired by Christopher T. Walsh, was to deal with basic sciences issues in academic–industrial relationships, and the second, chaired again by Barbara McNeil, with clinical matters. The effort led to revised guidelines and recommendations and emphasized the importance of full disclosure on an annual basis of any academic–industrial relationship exceeding the federal guidelines of $10,000; clearer definitions of terms; enhanced levels of protection for students and trainees; and new guidelines placing limitations on faculty serving as executive officers or board members of for-profit companies.

*Scandal at the NIH*

Incidents at the NIH between 2004 and 2005, where full-time federal employees failed to report outside consulting income from for-profit entities, triggered widespread concern by the NIH leadership, the US Congress and the research community at large. Reactions from congressional representatives were strong, to say the least. They were concerned that "federal employees" at the NIH were being allowed to get rich from extracurricular activities while serving full time in federally paid positions. Harold Varmus had vigorously promulgated the notion of such permission when he was director of the NIH, but it became clear to all of us that there were now different sensitivities about the issues, with growing attention from the congress and the public media about financial conflicts of interest, as well as conflicts regarding time commitments to their work at NIH.

The "extracurricular" events at the NIH triggered congressional investigations and an extensive internal review of NIH activities. The result, under the leadership of NIH Director Elias Zerhouni, was the drastic curtailment of interactions between federal employees and the industrial sector, perceived by many as an overreaction that almost certainly would inhibit productive interactions between government researchers and the pharmaceutical industry. Zerhouni's early tenure at the NIH, just as he was proposing a new emphasis on the importance of translational research, was considerably damaged, although he continued to provide strong leadership and selfless commitment to the strategic plan of fostering translational research he called the "Road Map."

The NIH inquiries regarding academic–industrial relations now extend beyond the federal laboratories to include academic investigators funded by the NIH. For reasons that are not entirely clear, many of the criticisms around the supervision of clinical trials have centered on the departments of psychiatry. The outcome has been the resignation of several academic leaders from their university positions and their withdrawal from ongoing clinical trials. The growing public perception generated by widespread reporting of these events in the *New York Times*, the *Wall Street Journal* and USA *Today* is that the time-honored physician commitment to do what is best for the patient has been replaced instead by doing what is best for the investigator.[11] The amounts of money involved in these misadventures are indeed large, in some cases reaching several million dollars.

*Reflections on Problematic Academic–Industrial Relationships and Accepting the Need for Reform: Five Practical Matters*

I fear, as I have watched the developments of the academic–industrial interface since 1990, that we are on a slippery slope that may well result in federal regulations that could in the end impair our efforts to develop effective relationships between our academic colleagues and industrial interests. The outcome of these events will ultimately hamper our search for better treatments for our patients.

Many of the perverse events, such as the NIH discrepancies described above, arise from a failure of full disclosure. Troublesome is the public perspective that clinical investigators have given tacit support to company claims of patient benefit from drugs and devices that lack the type of scrutiny the investigator employs in his or her own research efforts.

Given the challenges and opportunities of translational research available at biomedical research enterprises, what direction should academic institutions take? What type of faculty involvement in the pharmaceutical industry's marketing and business development plans should be deemed responsible? Should faculty serve on boards of directors of companies? What should be the rules of engagement for faculty in start-up companies that are often based on discoveries made in the faculty member's own laboratory? Should institutions accept equity in privately held, nonpublic companies? How will institutions manage their company portfolios when the services and products of these companies are purchased by the hospital or academic laboratory?

The matters under consideration are broad, complex and multifactorial, and they impact on most aspects of the academic mission. In seeking guidance for best practices, the perspectives of several constituencies require consideration. Universities play an important role in societies oriented toward a democratic marketplace. Beyond the "pure" academic mission of teaching and the provision of research guidance to undergraduates, graduates and professional students, universities serve significant advisory roles in broader economic and governmental arenas. The separation of the academic mission from the broader responsibilities of society, where government, business and community-based interests intersect, is arbitrary at best. And, inevitably, perspectives on the governing principles that connect these entities are always open to criticism from individual components of the complex matrices that emerge. An effort to understand these intersections and the interplay of these elements is an important first step in developing effective regulatory components. With these in mind, I would like to review five practical matters that confront us in current discussions on academic–industrial relations.

First are the pros and cons of industrial concerns marketing to professionals and academic hospitals, and to professional organizations. The sentiment currently expressed by a preponderance of observers in academic settings is that there ought to be a complete cessation of gifts to students, trainees, staff and faculty from commercial interests. It seems inescapable that these free items—in the form of pens, lunches or special rates for holiday travel—are designed to influence the prescribing behavior of professionals. In that sense, it constitutes marketing; we ought to acknowledge it and stop the practice.

Second is the provision of professional services to industry through speakers' bureaus and other company-sponsored marketing events. Criticism has been leveled at the practice of physicians participating in speakers' bureaus, where one is paid to accept speaking roles at company events. Companies wish to take advantage of faculty prestige and pay well to encourage participation.

The management of this problem is an extraordinarily complex task. Academic leaders cannot and should not impose rules on the activities the faculty undertake after work hours when it is unrelated to their faculty roles and responsibilities. But it does seem reasonable and wise to require faculty to disclose if they accept speaking roles at industry events. In the interests of transparency, many institutions are now disclosing all payments made to faculty on the school website. This seems a responsible way to manage this issue.

Third concerns the contributions industry makes to continuing medical education (CME). What are the current practices in this regard? Medical schools, hospital departments, medical societies and medical journals all depend on industrial advertising in one form or another to carry out their individual missions. Many of these activities use the awarding of CME credits to improve attendance. All states and provinces mandate a certain number of CME credits each year for maintaining medical licensure.

Fourth is the nature of academic–industrial collaborations in research contracting and support. Relations between academic institutions and industrial interests have changed over the years. As noted, the old notion of contracting for scientific expertise through payments to hospitals or universities is rarely undertaken these days. Open-ended agreements with academic investigators, even with milestones of discovery, have not usually been beneficial to industrial partners. As well, other relationships have certainly benefited the academy but not necessarily served the financial interests of the company, among them scholarships or fellowships to encourage trainees to enter industrial positions.

Finally, and fifth, is the relationship of academic investigators to companies they may have founded or with whom they have worked closely. This can be illustrated by some recent "success" stories that involve faculty at HMS (see the educational opportunities described in the next section). Controversy over relationships between HMS and drug companies provides an opportunity for educators to review their connections to industry and to consider improvements in what we currently do. But for that to happen, all sides must suspend the habitual assumptions that these relationships are either inherently unethical or are unassailable. Such hyperbole can fracture effective interactions that may, in the long run, endanger the progress that we all want: better treatments for the afflictions that cause human suffering.



### *The Education Opportunity*



Transactions between academic institutions and commercial enterprises in biomedical research provide an avenue for the education of future doctors. The goal of the educator in these matters is twofold. The first goal is to illustrate to our students, some of whom will seek careers in the commercial sector, the processes by which basic science discovery results in important, lifesaving, new therapies. Having observed the mechanisms that promote the development of new treatments for more than three decades, I can point to several examples of bias-free, industry-supported research that has led to important progress in health care. In each case, the drugs developed were compared by clinical trials with current best treatments.

One example is the lifesaving use of Gleevec in treating chronic myelogenous leukemia (CML). Ten years ago, the treatment of CML was marginally successful. Through frank discussions and cooperation between scientists at the Dana-Farber Cancer Institute and leaders of the pharmaceutical company Novartis, a compound that had been languishing on a laboratory shelf was evaluated in clinical trials. It progressed through the regulatory demands of the FDA in record time. The drug was brought to market, and now CML patients show a greater than 90 per cent response to treatment and are living productive lives.

The second example is the development of Velcade to treat multiple myeloma. A basic scientist in the Harvard Medical School Department of Cell Biology uncovered a new mechanism of cellular metabolism, which, when left unchecked, caused uncontrolled growth of plasma cells in bone marrow, often with fatal outcomes. This discovery was also at risk of remaining in the confines of the lab until collaboration with Boston-based Millennium Pharmaceuticals leveraged the finding to produce the drug Velcade, which is now being used to treat patients with multiple myeloma.

A third instance is the discovery of Enbrel, which is an entirely new class of drug. Research support to the Massachusetts General Hospital from Hoechst led to the creation of an entirely new Department of Molecular Biology, and to a scientist's discovery of how an antibody can fight the body's reaction to itself in rheumatoid arthritis. But it wasn't until the California-based biotechnology company Amgen intervened that the drug Enbrel moved to the fore and with it an entirely new biochemical pathway that now shows promise for the development of other drugs in this new class.

A goal of the educator is to convey the cultural differences between the academic and commercial worlds to students, and to make explicit every association that faculty have in these collaborations. If we are to fully educate our students about discovery in science and its application to medicine, we must detail every aspect of these discoveries. At the same time, we must describe and disclose the commercial relationships that have driven the success of these stories. We must also ensure that any faculty member who speaks of his or her work also describes, explicitly, his or her relationship with a commercial entity to avoid any perception of bias.

As educators, we have not done well on either count. Our students have not been told the true stories of how discovery occurs, and we have not been transparent in our explicit descriptions of the financial relationships involved. With the advances available through the websites of our institutions, we all need to provide this information, as some have already begun to do.

Recent news stories point out that even when academic–industrial relationships are transparent, they raise some complex questions. How should the leaders at the corporate levels of these enterprises appropriately interact? Should a dean sit on the board of a company? And why would the CEO of a for-profit entity want to serve on the boards of not-for-profit hospitals and research institutes?

As we explore the answers to these questions and work together to make these relationships more transparent, we must keep in mind the enormous benefits that these relationships have brought to our nation's patients, to our institutions and to our economy as a whole. At a time when both our economy and our health care system faces great challenges, we must remember that science and technology have brought us to the forefront of groundbreaking medical discovery, and that the collaborations between academia and industry have, in so many instances, led the way.

Faculty are often invited to serve on scientific advisory boards or even to function as corporate board members. But the rules remain unclear on whether or not it should be permissible to allow direct company investment in a faculty member's research laboratory if the faculty member has equity or other substantial financial investments in the company. The attitude of "let's keep it purely academic and not practical" or "such support contaminates the training of graduate students or post-doctoral fellows" trivializes the potential benefits of the research undertaken.

*Guidelines for Academic–Industrial Relationships*

I would offer the following guidelines as we continue to explore and develop principles for academic–industrial relations:

First, foremost and without exception, each institution, academic or commercial, needs to develop clear policy guidelines for their faculty, students and employees. Included in these recommendations ought to be rules of transparency in disclosure and monitoring to protect faculty and the institution from the surprises that have recently been so damaging. In the case of faculty, this may have to include random auditing to assure compliance.

Second, disclosure of all payments made by industry to faculty members ought to be publicly available, preferably on the institution's website. This is already the case at several leading institutions, such as the University of Pennsylvania and Stanford. The information ought to include faculty service on scientific advisory boards of companies, board memberships, consulting fees, speakers' bureau payments and the like.

Third, there ought to be greater transparency of "institutional" relationships to industry. These might include information on the institution's investment portfolio, stock equity in companies created by faculty, service contracts that conflict board of director members and so on.

Fourth, we have not done enough to assure that educational materials for students and CME updates are clear of any bias created by company involvement. New scrutiny ought to be directed at the relationships of faculty to commercial endeavors, to assure that perceptions of guilt by association are not in fact occurring.

Fifth, full disclosure to trainees must be made about the sources of money that support their work and the relationship of projects they undertake, if any, to industrial interests.

Disclosure, with attention to potential deleterious impacts, may provide an opportunity to construct the relationship with industry in a way that advances the interests of the company while providing experience that will enlighten the trainee regarding the differences in the two cultures. Let us not forget that many of our trainees will work in the commercial sector.

Sixth, the institution ought to form a visible faculty advisory committee with rotating terms of service to examine any relationship that appears questionable or that may be an exception to policy. Such exceptions may be important to some projects, including early-stage clinical testing of surgical methods or devices. To exclude the possibility of faculty involvement in these instances may delay the assessment of safety and efficacy and may not be in the best interests of the public.

Seventh, there is a critical need for every institution to establish an ombudsman's office to deal with issues that require complete confidentiality to protect individuals who come forward with evidence of misconduct or failure to adhere to recognized institutional policy.

Eighth, we, in the academic world need to step back from our shouting at one another and avoid the caterwaul of loud accusatory intonations that yield no positive results and only alienate us from the real challenges that lie ahead, namely, how to achieve better methods for advancing discoveries that will improve health care.[12]

The fundamental issue arising from these conflicts and controversies and the goal of all efforts of academic–industrial relationships ought to be the improvement of health care for our patients. Such advances are less optimal than they might be. It is here that we need to direct our focus and efforts. New modes and models of interaction urgently demand our consideration and evaluation. "At the heart of any failure to resolve conflicts, be they political, policy, or personal, is a deaf ear to the claims of legitimately competing priorities. Medicine's institutions must be willing to recognize and confront legitimate conflicts, not look to others to do it for them."[13]

## Health Care Reform

I feel a sense of sadness and betrayal as we enter the second decade of the twenty-first century. We were promised so much by a new administration; we relished the opportunity to support the new values and the sense of a bipartisan, more collaborative approach to national and international affairs.

Much of that has dissipated, and polarization has grown across the political spectrum. Hopefully, it is still too early to appreciate fully what may be accomplished in health care reform during the Obama presidency, but the signs are not encouraging. President Obama has led an effort to implement substantial changes in health care availability, including the requirement, modeled on what has been done in Massachusetts, of mandating that everyone obtain health insurance. This effort is designed to lead the US to near total coverage but currently with an intolerable delayed implementation—the target for implementation is 2014! The legislation has many additional flaws.

Let's begin with a fundamental moral issue. The US has never upheld the social values and societal responsibility to provide health care for all. It is the *only* industrialized society to fail in this regard. And, as the debate raged during the fall and winter of 2009, social values took a back seat to every argument from the supporters and opponents of reform.

In tracing the sequence of events that have led to so much dissent over the issue of health care for all—universal coverage—I am reminded of an episode that occurred years ago, having to do with the attempted sale of McLean Hospital in Belmont, Massachusetts. It is but one illustration of the path the country has taken, which has put us where we find ourselves today.

### *The Profit Center: An Attempt to Buy McLean Hospital*

In 1983 I chaired an HMS committee to review the proposal to sell Harvard's McLean Hospital, dedicated to psychiatric care, to the Hospital Corporation of America (HCA). It would be my first introduction to the dramatic transformations that were underway in the culture of medicine in America: namely, the emergence of widespread for-profit ownership of hospitals. I had arrived from Montreal a few years earlier, where we had been blessed with the introduction of the Canadian single payer system, which, according to many south of the border, smacked of "socialized medicine."

This is how it worked. Each resident had a health care card and flexible access to any physician of one's choice. The medical charges were codified, and payments to doctors and hospitals were made within thirty days. Each doctor had one of those now old-fashioned machines, much like the ones we used at gasoline service stations at the time. Place the card on the machine, run it back and forth to imprint the charges and mail one copy to the government, filing the other one in the office until payment arrived. It was efficient, there was no massive paperwork, administrative costs were negligible, everyone seemed satisfied and I never had to think about the "insurance status" of the patients I saw. But now I was in Boston, some would say the leading academic center for health care in the world, and here was the HCA, making the bet that psychiatric hospitals would be a potential profit center. As a flagship, McLean would help them get the effort off the ground.

The Harvard faculty committee deliberated for more than six months. We took testimony from numerous faculty and hospital administrators. We met with executives from HCA and listened to their assurances that all the components of the academic mission would be honored and supported financially. Passions ran high in the medical school over the potential dangers of a sale, and in the end, the committee ruled unanimously to reject the idea.

The matter died quietly, but the experience clarified how dramatically events were moving toward a new wave of medical care—the industrial-medical complex, which Arnold Relman, former editor of the *New England Journal of Medicine*, had written about in that publication a couple years earlier.[14] The McLean saga, now largely forgotten, amounted to nothing less than an emerging historic clash between a "not-for-profit" and a "for-profit" health care system. The huge lobbying network that emerged after this event, led by powerful business interests, has repeatedly defeated any serious efforts to "reform" the basic infrastructure of health care, where access to care is considered a right and not a privilege.

In 1982 Paul Starr published his treatise on the emerging character of the US health care system in a book entitled *The Social Transformation of American Medicine*.[15] No book since has so accurately captured the change that was overtaking the American medical scene at that time. More recently, the account of Kenneth Ludmerer in *Time to Heal* adds a more current perspective.[16]

We soon came to recognize new terms like "medical cost ratio," which describes the methods used to measure the percentage of dollars paid from insurance payments that actually go to the patient's benefit. The lower the "medical cost ration," the better and the more profitable the company becomes, with higher returns for investors. In the wake of such terms followed a series of pernicious ideas, such as the denial of insurance for "pre-existing conditions," lifetime limits on payments made, lack of portability from one job to another and so on.

The drama of failure of health care reform under President Clinton in 1994 led to a fifteen-year delay in legislative consideration. The issues in 2011 were well publicized and could be summarized in nine points:

1. The United States spends 16 per cent of the Gross Domestic Product on health care;
2. This amounts to approximately $8,000 per person per year, nearly twice that of Canada, the UK and Japan;
3. There are presently 50 million people without insurance, another 30 to 40 million who are uninsured for part of each year through lapses in coverage between jobs or during periods of growing unemployment, and many more whose insurance is inadequate to meet the expenses of a major illness;
4. Estimates indicate that up to 50 per cent of personal bankruptcies are triggered by excessive health care costs or catastrophic illnesses;
5. Many leading institutions, including major university hospitals, have grown enormously in size in terms of clinical care and research but have become unable or unwilling to provide equal growing capacity for primary care services;

6. An aging population with chronic diseases often have no "medical home" to coordinate care, which results in fragmented episodic care given mostly by specialists who communicate little or not at all with each other;
7. A new model for minor medical care is developing in pharmacies and in stores like Wal-Mart, with ineffective linkage to physicians for follow-up treatment. This business model is generally challenged by the deliverers of status quo medicine without adequate exploration of the possibilities this model represents;
8. Fewer and fewer medical school graduates are going into primary care; and
9. The dearth of primary care doctors has resulted in a proposed solution to increase the physician workforce by admitting more students, a solution that has already been implemented by many medical schools, based on an AAMC directive.

In 2011 we faced the dismal prospect of vested interests successfully overruling the interests of the public, as we watched the outcome of health care legislation that was introduced into law. The connection between this debate and the president's decision to increase spending for war by about $30 billion a year in Afghanistan was largely unnoticed. The total outlay will be about $100 billion per year, about the estimated cost of providing health care for all.

### *The Limitations of Recent Legislation*

I submit that the deliberations in Congress and the compromises made to pass the *Patient Protection and Affordable Care Act* fail to address any significant reform of the health care delivery system and have not succeeded in forging a path for control over the escalating costs of health care. The legislation provides a degree of "insurance reform," which should not be underappreciated for its importance, but "health care" reform has not been achieved.

I want to address three issues here that illustrate the limitations of the law passed by Congress: administrative costs, primary care networks and public health, and unsustainable medical care costs.

### *Administrative Costs*

The first has to do with the unnecessary administrative costs brought about by inefficiencies in the current system due to excessive paperwork. In 2000, at the beginning of my fourth year as dean at HMS, I made a pitch for a modest reform effort that remains valid today and aired my concerns in an op-ed piece in the *Boston Globe*. I called it "Health Care 101: Single Form, Single Plan, Multiple Payers":

*The financing of health care in the United States is a mess. As the leading democratic contenders for president spar with each other over tinkering with a broken system, I propose two simplifying steps to add to the debate as we approach the election in November 2000 [the result of which, as you will recall, saw Bush outlasting the challenges of the Florida election via a Supreme Court Ruling favoring him over Gore].*

*First, we could reduce the substantial proportion of health care expenditures that go to administrative costs (approximately 15 per cent to 20 per cent) by adopting a single, simple health insurance claim form. One of our faculty members recently stated that her office juggles thirty-eight different insurance forms. A typical office practice with two physicians hires six assistants. But 4.5 of them spend all of their time handling paper, not dealing with patients.*

*Using a single form and coding system to make claims for private insurance, like Medicare and Medicaid, would be enormously efficient. Ideally, in a computer-literate world, claims would be submitted electronically and payments made in a short turnaround of a few days or weeks. (After all, Quebec showed this could be done forty years ago).*

*The new form could also be used for tracking treatment for the uninsured, currently estimated to be forty to forty-four million, or approximately 16 per cent of the population. Submitting claims for the uninsured would help identify the sites they visit and the treatments they receive. These data would prove invaluable in assessing the true costs of caring for this often disadvantaged segment of our society and of determining the best way to bring them gradually into a health care insurance system.*

*The second step would follow. All currently insured Americans could be offered over time a single basic health insurance plan (like base-rate cable television) to be paid by multiple payers: the federal government through Medicare and Medicaid, private insurers, self-insurance, or a combination of employer and employee contributions. This could evolve as a single basic benefits plan with multiple payers rather than the controversial single payer option. To this base rate could be added a surcharge for more costly, complete or convenient services, such as open access to specialists, broader drug coverage, more frequent checkups, more comprehensive preventive measures and coverage for long-term care.*

*These initiatives would enhance access to care and provide vehicles to improve the general health of the nation. Lowered infant mortality rates, decreased morbidity from chronic unattended illness and higher rates of compliance with preventive measures and immunization might result.*[17]

As we all know, these changes never occurred; recent estimates suggest a range of 15–30 per cent of health care costs are linked to administrative inefficiencies. Various analyses give a wide range of estimates. According to a report from the American Medical Association in June 2010, one in five medical claims is processed inaccurately by commercial health insurers. The result is time wasted by physicians and their patients in attempts to adjudicate these clerical errors.

*Primary Care Networks and the Health of the Public*

The second issue is this nation's failure to develop an adequate primary care network or infrastructure. As an educator, I am fascinated by the current employment trends of medical school graduates and the failure to organize appropriate primary care systems. These were the concerns behind the question I raised in a commencement address to the graduating class at the University of Rochester School of Medicine in 2008. The title I chose was: "Where have all the Doctors Gone?" I first focused on the extraordinary opportunities that a career in medicine offers. What other career, I posited, offers so many opportunities? I suggested that a career in medicine affords one the opportunity to:

- Spend time in medicine or pediatrics or in surgery or neurosurgery;
- Work with pipettes, oscilloscopes, a PCR machine or move into whole genome mapping for your favorite disease;

- Live and work in Rochester, or Costa Rica, or Haiti, or Rwanda;
- Work on MRSA (methicillin-resistant *Staphylococcus aureus*) or a vaccine for malaria;
- Work on a Native American reservation or open an office on Fifth Avenue in New York;
- Work an eight-hour day as a dermatologist or anesthesiologist or settle for a sixteen-hour day in primary care; or
- Take care of live people or look after dead ones—the field of pathology has grown in interest among medical students.[18]

Or, I suggested, you might get an MBA and start a new Internet or biotech company. No other field offers so much: so where do all the doctors go?

Today, most graduates of medical schools, including Harvard, show little interest in primary care. Most specialize and only a few will go into rural areas, although I have observed that students from minority backgrounds are more likely to return to their communities to serve the underprivileged. Many recent graduates are hitting the ROAD, an acronym for the specialties that offer the best lifestyle conditions: Radiology, Ophthalmology, Anesthesiology and Dermatology.

Under urgent consideration today is whether or not we have enough doctors to care for our patients, particularly if we move toward a new scheme for universal health coverage. Fifteen to twenty years ago there were concerns that there were too many doctors, particularly in some specialties. Now, the Association of American Medical Colleges is asking medical schools to increase enrollments by 30 per cent over the next seven to ten years. There are fields like general surgery where serious shortages are expected, particularly in smaller urban centers and rural districts, and, in view of an aging population, there will be an increasing demand for geriatric medicine.

There is grave concern about the lack of primary care doctors to work in settings where the patient load is high and the pay is lower. Every year, US medical schools graduate about 18,000 students. We welcome another 7,500 foreign medical graduates (FMGS) each year into first-year residency slots, 80 per cent of whom will remain in the US. The impact of these graduates entering the US workforce is twofold. Unfortunately, some would say, their remaining in the US deprives their home countries of the workforce required to deliver adequate medical care there. On the other hand, while the majority of these FMGs also specialize, many of them seem willing to work in rural and underserved parts of the country.

There is an international issue at work here, with doctors from Canada and abroad too often eager to immigrate to the United States. As a Canadian colleague said recently, "I only wish the high salaries offered in the US did not drain away so many of our doctors..." I have often joked that when I graduated from medical school in Canada, the medical class differentiated along three academic lines. The top third of the class specialized, the middle third went into family practice or primary care and the bottom third went to the US. Doubtless an overstatement, but it usually resonates with audiences both in the US and Canada.

So what will we do to deliver the quality of care expected, and deserved, by our patients? How will we increase our focus on the importance of prevention and public health measures—encouraging parents to vaccinate their children, supporting major initiatives to stop smoking and developing regimens for weight control that actually work? I strongly believe that the answer is not to train too many more doctors but to give those we train the right jobs with pay commensurate with the contributions made. Perhaps we need to address the disparity in reimbursement wherein doing procedures pays well but thinking deeply about a patient's problems has financial limitations. Clearly, the role of primary care has not been a high priority; neither have the new requirements in medical care that will demand new models of health care delivery. For a priority shift to take place, there will need to be a new focus on teamwork, where, for example, doctors, nurses, pharmacists and social workers form efficient groupings to consider patient-centered care. And what of our responsibility to work with our governments, our cities and our health departments to accomplish this?

These issues deserve urgent attention. We must reorganize the hierarchy of care to include a larger role for nurse practitioners and physician assistants. We need to allow the physicians to do the work they were trained to do and want to do: namely, taking care of ill patients who need their attention, with less paperwork and more pay. Unless we address each of these issues, we will continue to see a decline in the numbers of our students willing to enter primary care medicine. These issues were highlighted at a Josiah Macy Conference that I was privileged to help organize in 2010.[19]

The debate about how to encourage more medical students to enter primary care will certainly continue for some time to come, but one suggestion for a course of action comes to mind: why not marry certain aspects of preventative care to primary care in our public schools, providing health care alongside education in a setting that could transform our efforts. As I drive around suburban America and visit schools in the inner cities, the facilities are often first-rate and could become centers for both education and health care.

### *Unsustainable Medical Care Costs*

The third issue illustrating the limitations of the law brought in by Congress has to do with our inability to sustain escalating costs within a payment system that rewards excess utilization by doctors and health care institutions and is driven by fee-for-service reimbursement. Anyone or entity involved in care—individual doctors, departments of academic health centers and hospitals—is a volume driver. Salaries and successful capital campaigns for new construction depend on doing more work, particularly the expensive type that generates the most profit. The opportunities for fraud in such a system are unlimited. The payment system can be gamed for financial advantage at any level, from patient to doctor to hospital to health care network. All incentives are focused on making more money for the enterprise rather than improving access (except through increasing volume) or quality of care (except as a marketing trick, too often based on unreliable data).

Atul Gawande, professor of surgery at HMS, brilliantly outlined these issues in a *New Yorker* article on health care costs in McAllen, Texas.[20] The doctors who run health care systems and order excessive testing can elevate costs twofold over those systems in more carefully managed environments close by. And, according to Arnold Relman, writing in the *New England Journal of Medicine*:

> *Most doctors are paid on a fee-for-service basis, which is a strong financial incentive for them to maximize the elective services they provide. There is little evidence that lawmakers are aware of, or understand the significance of, these facts or that—even if they did—they would have the stomach for the major reforms needed to solve this problem.*
>
> *...We are not likely to control medical inflation unless the incentives in the traditional fee-for-service payment of doctors are eliminated.*[21]

There are solutions out there to each of these problems, many of them successfully implemented in other countries. Leaders in Massachusetts concerned with the problems related to excessive provision of elective services are proposing what are called accountable care organizations (ACOs). Such an organization of health care aims to deliver care not just to the sick but also to the healthy, with an emphasis on health maintenance and not just disease treatment. Under such a system there would be financial rewards for keeping us healthy.

I have been particularly pleased in this regard by the superb efforts of the Massachusetts Medical Society, which, among other contributions, provides the world with one of the most respected of all medical journals, the *New England Journal of Medicine*.

## Conclusion

I cannot avoid the conclusion that the health care reform debate points again to a fundamental flaw in the social values of the US. The "exceptionalism" argument, that the United States is "different," can no longer be justified when considering the burden of responsibility for the people of this land who suffer most from the failure of our leaders to address their needs. As Nobel Prize–winning economist Paul Krugman wrote in December 2009 in the *New York Times*:

*Health care reform hangs in the balance. Its fate rests with a handful of "centrist" senators—senators who claim to be mainly worried about whether the proposed legislation is fiscally responsible.*

*But if they're really concerned with fiscal responsibility, they shouldn't be worried about what would happen if health care reform passes. They should, instead, be worried about what would happen if it doesn't pass. For America can't get control of its budget without controlling health care costs—and this is our last, best chance to deal with these costs in a rational way.*[22]

I agree with Krugman: what is being proposed here is better than nothing, and fixes can be made in later legislation.

I urge, as the process of reform implementation moves ahead toward an effective health care system, that legislation be anchored in some fundamental tenets. I have called these the Five Attributes (5 As) of Health Care Reform. They are:

*Accessibility*: Development of adequate primary and secondary care networks to provide the health care deserved by all Americans. Currently there are not enough primary care venues to deliver that care.

*Accuracy*: This depends upon providing the best evidence-based medicine, in accordance with recognized guidelines and tailored to the patient's phenotype, as it will emerge from genetic screening and pharmacogenomics.

*Advice*: What patients want most is sound advice and good judgment provided in a communication style and manner that evinces empathy and seeks to encourage compliance—true professionalism. Emphasis must include a focus on prevention and a healthy lifestyle

*Affability*: Our patients deserve health care that is caring and patient centered, with full recognition and acknowledgment of the patient's rights.

*Affordability*: Development of equitable sources of funding to lower the costs of coverage to match ability to pay. This will require new approaches to assess options for coverage among employer, employee, government and charitable organizations.

Throughout this debate, I have been reassured by how often recognition and affirmation has been given to the Canadian health care system, which, despite problems of access and escalating costs, remains capable of administering effective health care with statistical measures that outstrip the US data by a significant margin at approximately half the cost.

TWELVE

# *Maxims, Proverbs and Aphorisms: A Humble Guide to Successful (Enjoyable) Leadership*

AN INTERVIEW WITH CANADA'S LEADER of the Opposition, Liberal Leader Michael Ignatieff, in the September 2009 issue of *The New Yorker* provides brilliant insight into the political wisdom required of an academic leader.[1] Ignatieff excelled as a professor at the University of Cambridge and at Harvard, where he was revered as the author of treatises on political science. In 2006 he made the transition to the political scene, as a candidate for leader of the Liberal Party of Canada, which he achieved in 2008.

Ignatieff found the transition a transcending learning experience. He was refashioning the style he had honed as a professorial expert on political-philosophical positions to fit that of a politician who must sense the emotions of an audience for clues to their sentiments. This required a new social awareness of personal and group dynamics: What did they want? What did they expect of a leader? What were they really transmitting in the questions they asked? His transition from the academy to the House of Commons required relearning skills of communication from expert to advocate, of public recognition for intellectual prowess to appearing to appreciate the needs and sentiments of others—a form of emotional intelligence to be sure.

The role of the dean at Harvard Medical School is not unlike that of the head of a political party. To get appointed (elected) you need to tell a story enlivened by prior experiences and then balance the act by remaining "true to thine own self," demonstrating "trustworthiness with integrity" while morphing with the currents around you to accomplish the outcomes the institution requires. As my friend Holly Smith puts it, "Diplomacy is the art of getting others to see your way of doing it."

As I look back on four decades of academic experience in a number of different leadership roles and now frequently encounter younger colleagues who seek advice and counseling on their academic opportunities, I have been encouraged to summarize some of the lessons I've learned. The following closing comments in this book, therefore, are a humble offering of my insight into these matters, which I put forward in the hope that they will provide some useful guidance to those taking on administrative service in the academy. Many of the examples that follow come from stories already recounted, repeated here in summary form.

### 1. Be transparent: openness and honest disclosure spawn integrity

In the fall of 1981, after being appointed interim general director of the Massachusetts General Hospital, I received a call from Representative Al Gore Jr. of Tennessee. Gore was to the point. He said that the agreement with the Hoechst Corporation, headquartered in Germany, was "taking the cream off the top" of our research support and giving it away to a foreign country. I argued, apparently persuasively, that the hospital maintained fundamental rights to any discovery resulting from the collaboration and that development of promising new therapies would happen in the United States and not in a foreign country. I doubt I fully appreciated how impossible it would be to assure such an outcome. But I also pointed out a distinguishing feature of the agreement with Hoechst, which Howard Goodman had insisted upon, namely, that the research laboratories were to be open and accessible to members of the MGH and HMS communities.

Representative Gore listened, said I might expect to be called to congressional hearings and hung up. The conversation lasted about thirty minutes.

I read the Hoechst agreement again after our conversation. The arrangements were explicit, and there were no secret agreements that could not see the light of day. So I made the full document public for everyone to scrutinize. It subsequently came to be admired as a precedent for large contractual arrangements between academic and commercial entities.

I never heard from Gore again. My advice for faculty meetings, state of the school updates and town hall gatherings became: "Tell 'em what you've been up to, tell 'em what didn't work and then tell 'em what you plan to do next." And remember what Louis Brandeis once said, "Sunlight is the best disinfectant."

A word of caution clearly is needed. There are confidential matters that will always require wise judgment in how they are portrayed. The balance you strike between candor and circumspection can be critical.

## 2. Honor past agreements

I learned the importance of symbolic messages to the community outside the academy during my first year as chancellor at the University of California, San Francisco. A group of disgruntled medical faculty confronted me, as dean, with the urgent request of finding new research space. Many of the senior faculty and my own associate deans urged a resolution by expanding the tightly packed Parnassus site. This was challenging, if not impossible. To get the community's permission to allow modest new construction, the regents of the University of California had agreed in 1976 to a space ceiling on the development of the Parnassus site. We had already exceeded the limit agreed upon. Suits were pending, the faculty was restless and as new chancellor I felt trapped. I stepped back and decided to honor the past agreement, and we moved on to other options. The result today is a successful new campus at Mission Bay, the envy of academics everywhere.

It is always tempting for new administrations to make their mark by scuttling the work of previous leaders—the N.I.H. (not invented here) syndrome. Before doing so, make sure you understand all the ramifications that led to prior decisions and actions taken before your time. I don't recall ever observing that denigration of leaders who have gone before, or abrogating commitments that they may have made resulted in a positive outcome.

### 3. "Never attribute to malice what can be explained by incompetence"

The announcement that I would be moving to San Francisco as dean elicited a number of responses. One was a wonderful gift from Ken Tyler, a bibliophile and a former resident on my service at the MGH. It was, not surprisingly,.a book, entitled *To Rise Above Principle: The Memoirs of an Unreconstructed Dean*, by Josef Martin![2] Inside the back cover was the annotation: "Josef Martin is the pseudonym of a longtime dean at a major American university." To this day I been unable to determine the identity of the real author, but I would have been proud to pen it.

Among the maxims is the injunction: "Never attribute to malice what can be explained by incompetence." I have often taken the author's advice: "Incompetence really is so much more common than deliberate malice." I have found it wise to give individuals the benefit of the doubt, often withholding judgment on motivations resulting in behavior until some time has passed from the event. I have more often than not found that my initial suspicions about malicious behavior are either completely wrong or become tempered by consideration of other matters specific to the context of the problem.

### 4. "If a thing is not worth doing, then it is not worth doing well"



Once again, this is borrowed from my unknown namesake, Josef Martin. This important precept I have followed with fealty during my eighteen years of administrative service at UCSF and Harvard. Simply put, most of the activities demanded of deans are a waste of time. "Strategic planning," says the author, "was one of the activities of which much was made but which I could not take very seriously. It is carried on at a level of abstraction and ignores the nuts and bolts of the activity being planned for."

Most meetings with faculty are gripe sessions. One can usually decide quite quickly when an initiative is worth following up on. If not, you should then kill it before it assumes undeserved importance.

### 5. Never tell a lie so you won't need to remember what you said

The average tenure for a dean of US medical schools is less than four years, a statistic that has been surprisingly constant for the past several decades. I have found that a principal reason for the failure of deans to serve out their terms or to fail at reappointments is the perfectly understandable tendency to promise too much when pressed with demands from faculty and department chairs. It is tempting to acquiesce at once when approached by a request in order to make the encounter a positive one, but resources are always limited, and choices, often painful, need to be made. Try to remember that as dean you serve as "shepherd of the flock and department chairs are the crooks on which you lean."

Faculty and chairs rarely visit except to ask for something. I cannot recall a time when an appointment was made to tell me I was doing a good job. Deferral of response is the key: "I'll see what I can do," and "I'll get back to you on that," or "I need to check with finance and with space commitments we've already made." Here, the use of the first-person plural pronoun is important. Even as the dean, you have obligations to your team to be certain that they can deliver on what you promise.

### 6. Know when you need to pounce

Timing. The ability to sum up a set of circumstances and know when to act, to know when the vectors are aligned to take the next step toward the end game. To be an effective leader, you need to have the ability to know when enough information is in hand to come to a decision. This is the 80/20 rule: to act with 80 per cent of the information in hand, without worrying about the other 20 per cent. If you have gained this skill, you will be able to define and know when to apply Machiavellian principles to reach a good end for the circumstances.

On three occasions, at different institutions, the need to assert decisive action compelled planning that reshaped the future. In 1987, at the MGH, John Potts, chair of the Department of Medicine, and I spearheaded the bold move to lease space at the old Charlestown Navy Yard to develop research programs to stave off a decline in the institution's competitive posture. The move placed the hospital in a position to take advantage of expansion of the NIH budget, which doubled between the years 1996 and 2003.

In 1994–95, at UCSF, tensions within the faculty over lack of research space led, after a careful delineation of possible short-term and more substantial long-term opportunities, to the identification of the site now known as Mission Bay, once again giving the institution the means to capitalize upon expanding federal research support.

And in 1998, after my return to HMS, I knew we were greatly handicapped by lack of research space. I explored the options with the full support of President Rudenstine, whose friendship I had come to appreciate. He understood the dilemma facing the medical school with respect to alarmingly little expansion opportunities to support the growing research programs of younger investigators, more of whom were moving successfully up the tenure track. There was little opportunity to successfully recruit new department chairs or to expand the school's research into new areas of inquiry. Having learned that a site was possible, and knowing through early contacts with the mayor and with the Boston Redevelopment Authority of their keen interest to expand biomedical research in the city (having observed the enormous growth in Cambridge on the other side of the Charles River), we decided to test the waters. Compared to the experience in San Francisco, the approvals came with lightning speed, financing on favorable terms was available with Harvard's triple-A bond rating, and I had a team with Paul Levy and Eric Beurhens, who had experience in getting things done. We concluded the project in mid-2003 with construction of a 550,000-gross-square-foot research building ahead of schedule and below budget.

### 7. Know when to quit

I have always felt that academic leaders are most effective during the early years of their tenure, and individuals in positions of executive power are most effective in their first decade of work. "Hanging on" too long becomes a disservice not only to the community but to the incumbent as well. It is no accident that the US has adopted term limits for governors and presidents. Eight years of service, in two terms of four years each, is a good system. Some might argue that the politics of the president's re-election race every four years limits focus on effective outcomes, but no one argues that a president should serve more than eight years.

Successful academic warriors I have known almost always show great reluctance to step aside from the duties that carried them to the pinnacles of their careers. In every senior academic position that I have held, there have been forerunners who linger on, often with great reluctance to move aside from the limelight to make way for a fresh leader. The outcome is often resentment on the parts of both parties in the power exchange.

The trappings of an academic leadership position are hard to give up. There is the devoted office staff who shepherd one through the busy academic schedule, arrange talking points for speeches (of which several are often required in a day) and organize meetings with faculty and department chairs and with donors and alumni. Then, overnight, the power of the bully pulpit is transferred to a new incumbent. One's own views and opinions suddenly become less relevant. Free tickets to hockey and baseball games stop coming in, and the contacts and formalities of a daily routine dissipate almost overnight. Most of us choose to "be gone," to take a "sabbatical" to adjust to the dimming of the image, worrying all the while that we will soon be forgotten. In my own case, the appointment as the Edward R. and Anne G. Lefler Professor of Neurobiology provided a secure base to carry out my continuing efforts in teaching and clinical research. I did not find the transition difficult.

But knowing when to quit also involves knowing how to step aside from a strategic plan that has gone awry or from a plan for implementation that requires a different approach and another level of scrutiny to accomplish the most effective outcomes.

I recall a vivid example. Soon after returning to Harvard as dean, I assembled the hospital leaders and representatives of their management boards to discuss the possibility of greater collaboration, and to even consider mergers of selected aspects of their activities. I was troubled, for example, that there were four competing heart transplant programs in Boston, two of them at Harvard hospitals. This duplication of expertise was justified by the assertion that programs were excellent, when, in fact, there was little data to justify the small number of patients treated at each of the centers.

An example was the competition between Children's Hospital and the small pediatric service at the MGH, where, in the case of the MGH, transplants of various organs were so few in number that the outcomes for patients were worrisome. Despite conversations among the surgeons-in-chief, no accommodation was ever reached. I realized how impotent common sense is in the battles over turf that epitomize too much of the US health care system. I must admit I often thought of Schiller's famous saying: "Against stupidity the gods themselves struggle in vain" (*Mit der Dummheit kaempfen Goetter selbst vergebens*). I recognized that it was futile to waste further effort on grand schemes and instead focused on programmatic relationships among the hospitals, such as that which emerged in the nascent Harvard Clinical Research Initiative, the Harvard NeuroDiscovery Center and the Dana-Farber/Harvard Cancer Center.

## 8. "Rejoice with those who rejoice and weep with those who weep"

At my first meeting with the corporation members of Harvard University, hosted by President Rudenstine, one member asked, rather abruptly, about my views on the contentious mergers of the Harvard hospitals and what I intended to do to smooth the waters.[3] I began with a Biblical quotation, which I'd often used but had to later look up because I was uncertain of its origin.

I suggested that I would enter the fray with the attitude that "I would rejoice with those who rejoice, and I would weep with those who weep."[4]

Looking back, I'm not certain, even now, exactly what I meant, but I expanded on the extraordinary qualities and international reputations of each of the hospitals and said that I looked forward to learning about what each considered their strengths and weaknesses and where the challenges lay. Furthermore, I anticipated learning more about their perspectives on the role the medical school might play in their plans going forward.

As time passed during my time as dean at HMS, I came to appreciate a subtlety I'd perhaps overlooked at the beginning. Each time a hospital-based faculty member was responsible for a great act of public service, a clinical advance or a research discovery, they were from the MGH, from Children's or from the Dana-Farber. When things went amiss and required consideration of rebuke or discipline, they were always referred to in the press as "Harvard" faculty. Oh, well!

## 9. Learn to be generous

A singularity of leadership success is epitomized in the term "vicarious living." Simply put, a leader must relish the joy and satisfaction that accompanies watching the success of others. In an organizational setting, this type of generosity must be extended to freely giving credit where credit is due, to staff or faculty and department chairs. I met regularly with newly appointed department chairs to gauge their evolving leadership and to enable open discussions about any concerns or problems they might be experiencing. My hope for such meetings was to show that I could be a friend as well as a boss.

There is another aspect to generosity, which is the ability to forgive and forget. Holding a grudge is a powerful disincentive to forward progress. It is impossible to hold a position of leadership without being the recipient of bad news, or news that may reflect unfavorably on your performance or on you as a leader. The source of the derogatory comments may come from important individuals whose roles in subsequent actions are critical. Make an effort to understand the context of the criticism when it is first presented. Harboring negative feelings that surface from the inability to accept the comments for their potential value can lead to persistent counterproductive relationships in future interactions with naysayers.

I recall several contentious meetings with one basic science department chair at HMS whom I felt I could no longer work with until another more senior chair urgently demanded to meet with me to caution against alienating a powerful community leader. I called the individual, invited him to a nearby restaurant for lunch and we agreed to work together, becoming over time compatible colleagues. Not always easy to work with, Marc Kirschner went on to become the first chair of the new Department of Systems Biology and in 2009 was appointed University Professor by President Drew Faust.

### 10. Get out and about

One key to effective leadership is to get out and about. Leave the office and be visible to the community in ordinary ways. No executive ought to spend more than 60 per cent of his or her time in the office. The experiences there are too confining and the opportunities to check the pulse and blood pressure of the organization too limited.

Getting out for meetings with department chairs in their offices where you learn about the dynamics of their departments and see the inner sanctum of their operations can be very revealing. At the same time, the shift of the power base from the dean's office to the chair's office can lead to new insights and to greater comfort in relationships. I found it useful to schedule meetings formally with department faculty in their conference rooms, which would be led by department chairs and where any topic could be placed on the table. These meetings were tremendous opportunities for transparency and a chance to show that no discussion was out of bounds.

The complex setting of a medical school, with its relationships to the hospitals and other schools of the university, requires reciprocal interactions to achieve improved relationships. I met regularly with hospital CEOs, rotating between their offices and mine, with Dean Barry Bloom of the Harvard School of Public Health and with Dean Jeremy Knowles of the Faculty of Arts and Sciences. But getting away from the office can serve other purposes, as well. Attending lectures given by faculty to the students in a drop-in fashion provides evidence of the dean's interest in the educational mission. Attending seminars given by faculty, without always needing to sit in the "front row," sends a message of interest in the topic of presentation in which the dean is a faculty member and not a power figure.

Informal meetings are very important. Lunch in the cafeteria with students, faculty and staff allows down time spent on "ordinary" matters, where conversations turn to the avocations and outside interests not only of the dean but also of other members of the community. I also had regular open-door meetings with students. An approach I found particularly valuable both at UCSF and Harvard were luncheon meetings with eight to ten students, where the introductions included: "Where are you from and where did you go to college?" "What led to your decision to be a doctor?" and, "What do you expect to be doing in ten years?" The conversation was enlivened with each successive response, and the hour quickly passed with good feelings all around. I always shared my own experience when my turn came, trying to be honest about the events that had led to my assuming a full-time administrative position.

### 11. IQ and emotional quotient (EQ)

Efforts to define intelligence fill the pages of psychology and neurobiological journals and books. I find Harvard Professor Howard Gardner's description of what he labels "multiple intelligences" very useful.[5] By way of practical definition, I take intelligence to encompass the ability to learn, to remember, to synthesize, to create, to analyze, to differentiate, to classify according to type and condition, to construct new paradigms and to problem solve. IQ implies the ability to innovate, to think outside the box and to construct new scenarios. But intelligence alone is not sufficient. Individual brilliance may result in earth-shaking concepts, discoveries and Nobel prizes, but we expect more of academic leaders; we expect what is commonly called emotional intelligence or EQ.

EQ is the ability to understand another's position, to put oneself in the place and context of the whole, to empathize, to understand the impact of group dynamics on the outcome of a situation, to be able to reflect on one's own reactions, to feel and share another's disappointment and pain, to commiserate, and to initiate planning—bearing in mind the effect your actions will have on others. Simply put, EQ is the ability to listen and to recognize what the other person is *really* saying.

Daniel Goleman, a popular writer, defines the competencies of EQ as: self-awareness, self-management, empathy and relationship skills.[6] A person demonstrating a high EQ also has sufficient temerity and curiosity to want to understand another's perspective, to want to learn from another in order to "put right" one's own views and impressions.

When I think about EQ, I am reminded of the attributes of my colleague Bruce Spaulding, as we charted a course to solve the lack of research space at UCSF. Bruce was vice-chancellor for long-range planning and development and a consummate politician. He attended meetings I organized with other vice-chancellors, deans and faculty, showing constant vigilance to the words, facial expressions and body language he encountered. I would often notice, as I listened to a committee participant describing a view, that Bruce was watching me for my reaction even before I expressed it. He was an experienced observer of human behavior, and he used his observations to gain a sense of what was really taking place in discussions.

## 12. Don't forget the humor quotient!

IQ and EQ are important, but don't forget HQ, the humor quotient. This is the capacity to see the humor, folly, foible and absurdity in a situation. It encompasses the ability to use self-deprecation to accomplish an end, to exude a sense of lightness of being, of good cheer and hope. It is the ability to detoxify a situation by humor or self-effacement, to know how to relax the tension with a comment, a story or a well-told joke. It is the ability to bounce back after an untoward event.

George Valiant, a well-known Harvard professor of psychiatry, said, "Humor, like hope, permits one to focus upon and to bear what is too terrible to be borne." Quoting another unnamed source, Valiant states, "Humor can be marvelously therapeutic. It can deflate without destroying; it can instruct while it entertains; it saves us from our pretensions; and it provides an outlet for feeling that expressed another way would be corrosive." Which reminds me of my favorite neurology joke. Two men in a balloon drift over Boston. Upon entering a dense fog, they become lost. As a clearing appears below they notice a man standing in a field. Shouting to him they ask, "Where are we?" to which the man replies, "In a balloon." One of the riders comments to the other, "Just our luck we should run into a neurologist." The other counters, "How do you know he's a neurologist?" To which the first replies, "Easy, his information is accurate but totally useless."

### 13. Be ambitious: few things happen without ambition

Successful leadership emerges from the ambition to accomplish something. Self-confidence grows from knowing that a course of action is likely to succeed, if implemented openly, promptly and efficiently.

Anyone aspiring to success enjoys the recognition that comes from wealth, power, prestige and honor. Fear of failure is a powerful, nearly universal, motivating force, and when applied appropriately it can direct and guide ambition. Ambition overcomes procrastination, the bane of success, and collects, organizes and analyzes the available data and allows you to take action, in most cases without remorse. It allows you to press toward doing things well for their own sake, not just for compliments or kudos, but because self-satisfaction in doing the "right" thing is sufficient.

Second-guessing a decision is a destructive adventure. Remember that if a decision you made seems to have been wrong, you can adjust it with your next action. Ambition-driven self-confidence ought not to stave off saying sorry when things go wrong, or when a decision is shown to have been wrong. Apologies should be sincere and brief.

### 14. Learn to delegate

It is tempting to try and keep a finger on the pulse of everything that is going on in the orbit of the school, its affiliated hospitals and the university. Tempting, but impossible! It is impractical to personally try to do everything, so my advice is to stick to important issues.

Critical to success is a team of trusted, loyal, institutionally minded people. Here are two useful rules. The first is delegate and trust. It is empowering both to the chief and to the "Indians" (but inquire from time to time what progress is being made). Second, delegate and encourage. Empower with positive reinforcement for work going well and when it is completed. Give credit when and where credit is due. As Ronald Reagan once supposedly said, "There is no limit to what you can accomplish if you don't care who gets the credit."

### 15. Learn to manage up

It is common in management leadership reviews to ask for a 360 assessment—how does the dean or department chair relate to those above him or her, to peers and to employees who report to the individual? None of these matter as much how you deal with your boss. Effective relationships with the boss emerge from frequent contacts, both those scheduled regularly in a working day and one-on-one discussions.

The one-on-one connections are the most important. I always go with an agenda, even if the meeting is called by the boss. Try to find out what the topic of the meeting will be and plan on sharing or introducing some of your own points along the way. The meeting should begin with a cheery note of the things that are going well and with expression of appreciation for the help given. Point out a few successes and offer to help with any issues the boss deems important enough to ask about. Bosses love compliments, even if a bit of a stretch of the truth.

At the end of meetings, express thanks for the opportunity to work together (hopefully a sincere expression).

## 16. Lead by listening

Thousands of pages have been filled—from antiquity to the present era—about successful leadership and the set of attributes an ideal leader should possess. One of the oldest of these attributes, one that I especially like, comes from Plato's *Statesman*, where an analogy is drawn between leaders and weavers: a good leader weaves people of divergent and sometimes conflicting interests—including those who do not necessarily care for each other or for the leader—around a common mission.[7] For the successful leader to "weave" well in our world, he or she must have the ability and commitment to lead by listening, hence the final aphorism of this humble "guide." Everyone has a story to tell and most of us enjoy telling our story. But much of leadership is about listening to the stories others want to tell you; that's the only way you'll be able to assimilate the conversation and make an informed judgment. And informed judgment requires reflection before any action is taken. As Mike Brownstein, my colleague from NIH, puts it, "My dad's greatest gift was his ability to listen to all sides in a meeting, synthesize what had been said and then make a decision that was well informed and reasonably impartial."

Listen, reflect and respond.

## In Conclusion, a Word about Optimism

I sometimes joke that I suffer from terminal optimism; a fatal case. It is a valuable attribute when you have to fire someone. Leading them from the office, it's important to encourage them and convince them that something good is bound to happen.

Optimism helps when facing trying moments. The worst experiences I've had were when a brilliant faculty member, a successful department chair or an irreplaceable secretary met with me to tell me they were leaving. You want to cry, but you know that would be inappropriate. Quick rebound is critical. Allow yourself only one or two sleepless nights. Then move forward.

# EPILOGUE

## *Return to Duchess*

IN MAY 2009 I VISIT DUCHESS for my mother's ninety-fourth birthday. I approach the town by traveling north ten miles from the Trans-Canada Highway, which skirts the northern suburbs of Brooks, Alberta, a town of about 15,000 residents made rich by the booming oil and gas businesses that speckle the industrial areas of the town. When there is a westerly wind, the stink and airborne fumes from the local meat-packing plant are nearly unbearable. It is one of the largest beef-producing venues in Canada and serves as an employment locale for a Sudanese immigrant community.

The road to Duchess is now paved. This was the original "Alaska Highway" during the war and traverses the settlements of my grandparents, the Ramers, and passes by the tiny new house we built and moved into in 1945. The house still stands, looking quite chipper and owned by Gary Porter, a classmate of mine from high school, and his wife, Helen. The spruce trees we planted so many years ago appear healthy but show respect for their advancing ages. The house is a mere postage stamp on the corner of the original Ramer homestead, a piece of property that was willed to my mother.

Across the road to the west is the farm my father owned when he died, now placed in trust and owned by my two sisters and me. It is rented out for a nice profit (after paying the real estate and water taxes), which we give to Mother for her living expenses. The farm is a half section (320 acres) of irrigated, enriched, prairie soil. It now provides purchase for three disfiguring gas wells that bring in additional rent. In Alberta, the oil, gas and mineral rights belong to the government, which leases land for exploration to large national or international corporations, the owners receiving modest rents for the access to their lands.

Opposite and down the side road to the east is the original Martin homestead site, where the buildings have long been demolished and the land is now subsumed as a part of the half-mile-long field that grows grains and alfalfa. The farmland was sold to my sister Linda's son, Randy, who has built a huge house with a veranda at the most extreme end of the property.

It's a very dry spring, reminding me of the critical role of irrigation in this arid land. Giant sprinklers are spread out across the fields, rotating in grand arcs, sending out pulsed streams of water. The sprinklers are attached by pivots where pumps, connected to underground pipes, bring water from the nearby canal. Caught in the sunlight they appear like magnificent rural fountains blessed by the sun gods who provide sunshine almost nonstop from June through September, hence the designation "Sunny Alberta," promising warmth and long hiking days in the mountain parks and dinosaur valleys.

Just off the main road, continuing on toward Duchess, is the Ramer homestead. Grandmother's house is gone but the barn remains, repaired and moved across the highway to function as a storage facility. A mile farther on, the road takes an abrupt left turn into the Village of Duchess, now a quiet, tidy, bedroom community, with a paved main street and a population of close to eight hundred. My mother lives alone in the center of town, in the split-level, three-bedroom house with a full basement she and my father built in 1963. The garden, once my parents' delight, shows signs of neglect. The roses that my father used to carefully nurture don't look tended to. I sense that Mother just

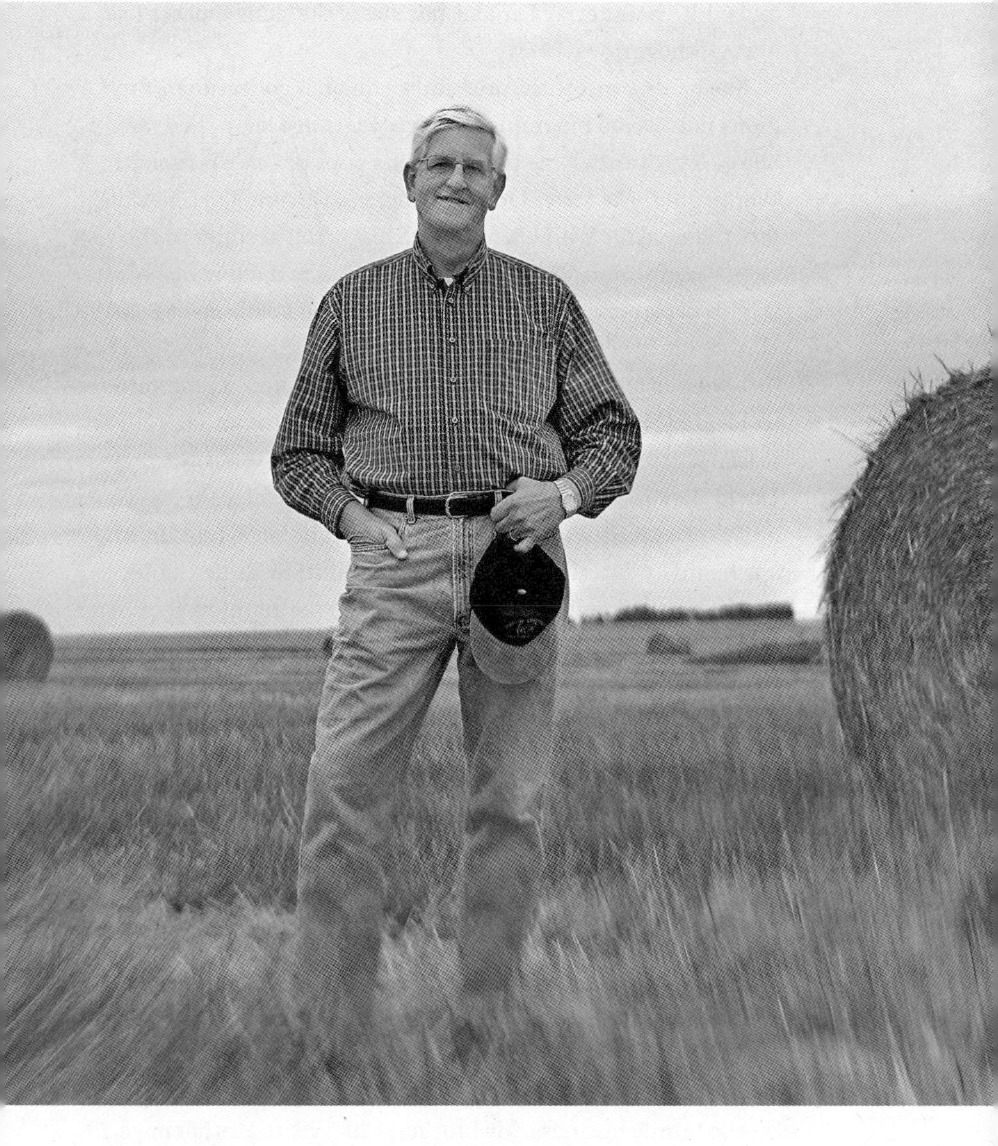

On the Martin family farm, Duchess Alberta.

can't look after it the way she used to. Dad died in 2005, but he had not been out there actively caring for the yard for a couple of years before that.

I arrive at my mother's home. She greets me affably from her chair in the living room, rising effortlessly to cross the room to my embrace. She is prim, poised and prepared to offer me a mid-morning coffee and raspberries, my favorite fruit. Her mind is clear, and she speaks effortlessly with normal cadence. Her face and white hair betray her age, but she is the same mother I've always known.

She reads constantly, preferably from her collections of religious novels and biographies. A few years ago she called me before a visit to ask me to bring her a copy of *One Christmas in Washington: The Secret Meeting Between Roosevelt and Churchill that Changed the World*, a narrative historical account of the visit to the White House by Winston Churchill just a few weeks after the US declared war on Japan following the bombing of Pearl Harbor on December 7, 1941.

I ordered the book online and came to appreciate her interest as I leafed through it on my flight west from Toronto to Calgary. It was written by a history professor at the University of Calgary, David Bercuson, director of the university's Centre for Military and Strategic Studies. The book had caught her attention when she heard an interview with the author on a local TV channel. The book's subject matter, she said, was an interest of hers because she so vividly remembered the war and the events scaling it up into a world war. The book was a difficult read. It was fully annotated and had a dense bibliographic listing at the end along with a detailed index. A few weeks later, I asked whether she had been able to find time to read it. "Oh," she said, "I finished it right away."

My sisters, Marian and Linda, raised their families in Duchess, and both live only a couple of blocks from my mother's house. Linda's sons, Jamie and Randy, took over the Martin Chrysler business straight out of high school after it moved from Duchess to Brooks. The business has thrived during the oil boom, mostly through truck sales and a few minivans. Mother worries constantly about the impact of Chrysler's bankruptcy on the family business. My brother, Dale, visits Mother once a month or so from his home in Red Deer, north of Calgary.

The highway through the village meets Main Street in a third of a mile, and then it continues on west to rejoin the Trans-Canada Highway in Bassano, my birthplace, thirty miles away. The portion of the highway through the village is the main business strip with a new post office, an automobile repair shop, a meat preparation store, a small general store and an expanding mobile home park along the old railroad, where the two grain elevators once stood. A left turn puts me on Main Street, which shows little evidence of activity; old buildings have been torn down and a new motel with fourteen rooms has just opened. The old pool hall is still there, looking forlorn and apparently unoccupied. But the Duchess Hotel sits on one corner, and the bar seems active in the evenings. Across the street on the opposite corner is the famous Duchess Café, where my father and his retinue broke for coffee each morning and afternoon. It is now one of the ubiquitous Chinese restaurants that dot the small towns and villages across the province. The old Duchess Garage building has been replaced by a new warehouse, looking tidy and well appointed.

Off to the west are the elementary and high schools, bracketed by the modern skating and hockey rink on one side and the curling club and indoor soccer field on the other. During the fall and winter, the ice in the hockey arena is kept frozen by pipes beneath the surface and the curling rink shimmers with a majestic smooth surface. The season has ended for both winter sports by May, and the area seems desolate. A large community center sits across from the curling rink; it is the site used for any gathering requiring room for a crowd of a couple hundred or more. A Martin family reunion was held there in 2007.

The Duchess Mennonite Church is a thriving community church. It was constructed in the 1980s to replace the original one that first opened in 1928. The old church building was transported carefully to a farm site south of Brooks, where it still serves admirably as a well-kept private dwelling. The church now has regular attendance of one hundred to 150 people on Sunday mornings. The services are modernized, with springy gospel ditties appearing as PowerPoint projections on one of the bare walls. The minister is a Mennonite with seminary education. The audience and attendees are almost entirely unfamiliar, although my uncle Sam and aunt Beulah Martin still attend regularly, as do my sisters and my mother, when she feels up to it. I have a handful of first cousins who remain in the area.

The Village of Duchess is home primarily to young families and retired local farmers. The housing market is booming, with four or five houses being built each year. My sister's husband, Dale Shantz, served as mayor of the village for over twenty years. The town has a modern water supply from a reservoir kept brim full with irrigation water, as well as a septic system with a modern treatment plant. The taxes are modest and the town receives an ample provincial budget. Duchess now has a successful high school; the school system expanded to twelve grades a few years after I graduated from Rosemary High School, ten miles away. Many graduates go on to university.

That afternoon, I visit the cemetery. In the first row, left side, facing the road is the oldest tombstone in the graveyard. It identifies the site where my great-grandfather, Jacob S. Ramer, lays buried next to Hettie, his wife. It is marked 1925. The other tombstones and ground-level plaque markings cover about an acre squared off from the road, each separated by a carefully tended and manicured lawn.

In the cemetery there is a single rather majestic spruce tree about twenty-five feet tall. Next to it is my father's grave. My father's granite marker has a blue hue, to recall and honor his preferred color for clothes—light-blue, button-down, long-sleeved cotton or polyester shirt and blue jeans. The gravestone marks his time here: November 2, 1913, to February 9, 2005. Half of the face of the block of granite is empty, reserved for my mother's name.

Many of my aunts and uncles, as well as my two closest cousins, Charles Ramer and Evangeline Martin, lay buried here. The other names are from the community, most of them familiar from childhood and youth. I search out the modest marking for my sister, Betty, born premature and stillborn. I recall, with little residual emotion, my father taking the body in a shoebox with me and my brother, Dale, to bury it. For years, we were uncertain where the location was, but my mother insisted later that a remembrance be placed; so a spot was selected and marked.

The cemetery abuts the old railroad, the Royal Line, now gone and all the steel rails, wooden supports and spikes sold or given away. The grain elevators, which stood forty to fifty feet tall, lined the tracks to facilitate loading for transport to the east or west for loading onto ships at Thunder Bay or Vancouver, respectively. They, too, are gone, replaced by the faceless mobile home park.

As I leave the small cemetery, I turn right, traveling for half a mile outside the village, where a green nine-hole golf course beckons the local duffers. It is now tree lined with spruce and pine, most planted by my father over the years. A favorite fall gardening adventure for him consisted of visits to the local nurseries in Brooks as the growing season wound down to purchase at great discounts the small fragile trees, six to twelve inches high. He planted them in his own garden behind the house in Duchess until they were substantial enough to be transplanted to the golf course. This effort he carried out with great joy, and over the years as I watched them grow, I was reminded again of his passion for the good earth and what it could "bring forth."

The regional health care system is focused on private practitioners in Brooks who work in competing offices and staff the twenty-bed hospital. Serious health problems are dealt with in Medicine Hat, sixty-two miles to the east on the Trans-Canada Highway or in Calgary to the west, just one hundred miles away, where a full array of high-quality specialty care is available, although elective surgery requires a wait of a few months. My niece, Stephanie, Linda's daughter, works as a nurse in the usually quiet emergency ward in Brooks. She finds her experience there quite different from that of nurses in the Wichita General Hospital in Kansas, where she and her American husband lived for more than a decade before returning to her roots.

The next morning, I travel the familiar route from Duchess to Brooks, now a wide, two-lane, paved road, to visit Uncle Sam and Aunt Beulah. His health has been failing in recent years, and I want to garner some of his recollections about the "old days." He is eighty-six years old, in good spirits and with an excellent recall of details, so I ask him about Grandpa Martin. "What was he like?" Sam reflects, "He was a generous man. I remember when I was fifteen or sixteen years old, I went with him to peddle vegetables and fresh meat and eggs from our farm to neighbors and ranchers across the river. One lady came out and said she had no money. 'Give her what she wants,' Dad said." Sam thinks for a second and then adds, "I sometimes thought that he was enjoying the Depression just so he could help others."

Sam goes on with his recollections: "I went with him and Mom on one of their trips back east to visit relatives. We stopped to see Uncle Jason in Wisconsin, who asked Dad for $650. He reached for his wallet and without a word spoken gave it to him. I don't know if Jason ever paid it back."

Sam recalls another event. One day in Slatter's Meat Shop, there was a visit from Mrs. Hole (pronounced Holy), wanting to buy a pound of hamburger. When she protested the price, Grandpa said, "Well, go ahead and take it." Mrs. Hole protested that it wouldn't be right. "Then pay for it and shut up," was Grandfather's answer.

"What about Grandma?" I ask.

"She was always depressed. She seemed to be unhappy most of the time. She missed her sisters who had never left Pennsylvania." He recalls a vivid memory. "I overheard Mother complaining to Dad that she was having trouble sleeping. He replied that was not the case with him, and concluded, 'Something must be on your conscience.'"

My conversation with Sam turns, as it so often has, to his prison experience. The details are fresh in his mind. Tears well up as he begins talking about it. I ask about the details of the arrest and how he felt about it, living now in the same town where sixty-five years ago he had been handcuffed and trundled off to the train station for the ride to Calgary. He remains baffled, he says, about how it had happened, but there was a sensitivity, he thinks, to his having left the farm to work for Uncle Fred, when they had failed to immediately notify the Mobilization Board.

The visit ends with recollections of their son, Murray, the brilliant family doctor who died suddenly just eighteen months before. "He always complained that he was working too hard. Here I am going on at eighty-seven, and two of the kids are gone. [Glenda was killed at age eight.] I wonder why they had their lives shortened and I have lived this long."

He looks tired after an hour of chatting. The oxygen tank is nearby; his cardiac condition has threatened his survival on numerous occasions over the past decade. I am glad to see him again and promise to let him read what I am writing. Little do I know that this will be the last time I will have a chance to chat with him.

Uncle Sam passed away on April 8, 2010, after a brain hemorrhage that resulted from a fall.

I HAVE BEEN BACK TO ALBERTA often over the years, not only to visit family or to attend the triennial Martin family get-togethers in the Canadian Rockies but also to visit and consult with the two medical schools, one in Calgary and the other, my alma mater, in Edmonton. The place has been bred in my bones, and I shall never be able to entirely escape it.

Looking back, I wonder how elements of character and personality develop from the template we are born with? How does experience imprint later characteristics that come to define us? How do sensory perceptions early in life affect who we think we are? How do these play out with the genes we inherit from our parents and grandparents? Nature versus nurture—likely not either, but rather both.

Three elements of my "roots" influenced my life.

The first was early awareness of my family origins. This arose from family stories of generational migrations and movements of the Mennonites that brought my parents to the expansive plains of Alberta, Canada.

As a child, I heard of the tragic consequences of radical belief and of the persecution of Anabaptist revolutionaries (precursors of the Mennonites) who fled Europe for the freedom of William Penn's Pennsylvania. The *Martyrs Mirror* and the Bible were fixtures in our house. Translated into English with numerous reprintings, the *Martyrs Mirror* revealed in words and graphic illustrations the brave stubborn folks whose beliefs led to death and persecution well into the eighteenth century. The tales of their persecutions were hardly imaginable in my young mind.

The second formative element was the realization that the happenstance of one's placement on the planet is a matter of extraordinary luck. As Wendell Berry, the American poet put it, "The world is full of places; why is it that I am here?" Perceptions from everyday experiences embed biases about the cultural, societal, religious and economic realities of that placement. These affect one's goals and aspirations. Mine were indelibly linked to my early religious experience and the symbolism it provided. Ideas about equality and diversity emerged. I was taught that God had created all of us equal—despite obvious differences in fortune in life. But we were to help with the inequities through acts of kindness to benefit those less well off than we were. These notions, taught through Bible stories read to me by my mother, led to my aspirations to become a doctor.

The third element that shaped my perspective relates, in a different way, to my origins in Canada, where values and sociological underpinnings had a powerful effect on my views of a citizen's rights and expectations, particularly as they relate to health care and the responsibility of government and society to work to serve the common good, with interests for the whole, without bias toward the wealthy. Starting early on in my academic career, this "socialist" perspective—now ensconced in the United States as a fundamental "evil"—gave me a desire to give back to my native country.

I am grateful for my Canadian medical education. Not inconsequential in this regard were the low tuition expenses I incurred, which allowed me freedom to undertake prolonged post-graduate training in the US without accruing large indebtedness, such a common issue now for graduates in the US.

When I returned to Canada in 1970, I witnessed the implementation of Medicare, with universal health care coverage, financed by joint agreements between federal and provincial governments. In Quebec, the government insurance scheme worked brilliantly. There was no concern about whether a patient had insurance, and the billing procedure was so simple and straightforward that an office clerk could manage every detail.

I have no doubt that these experiences frame my present bias toward a universal health care system in the US, based upon a single-payer system. However, I recognize this is presently a political impossibility. The current system in the US is broken, not only because of the uninsured but also because health care costs of the traditional fee-for-service reimbursement mechanism are unsustainable, and primary care networks essential for proper delivery of health care and for prevention are simply not in place. I have a sense of outrage at the social injustices that derive from the big business model of insurance and health care administration now extant in the US.

In this volume, I have reflected on four decades of academic experience, time spent in various leadership positions. In the first two, I served as chair of two very different clinical departments: neurology and neurosurgery at McGill University and then neurology at the Massachusetts General Hospital. The third big job was as dean and then chancellor at the University of California, San Francisco; the fourth as dean of Harvard Medical School.

My academic experience has spanned two countries, both public and private institutions, and health care systems organized with disparate philosophical backdrops. The most complex of these experiences was my service at Harvard where intense intra-institutional rivalries and cross-faculty debates, during a time of presidential precariousness, shook the institution to its roots.

Each step of my life has been heralded by unexpected opportunities where serendipity played a major role. I have often said that I never looked at a job I didn't take—each of these adventures came along by way of circumstances that were unpredictable and unanticipated. Today, looking back, I feel enormous gratitude for these experiences, resulting in a compelling drive to reflect on lessons learned along the voyage.

# POSTSCRIPT

*Dr. Ed Benz*
*President and CEO of the*
*Dana-Farber Cancer Institute*

THERE ARE CERTAIN THINGS WE CAN TAKE for granted about colleagues we encounter during our careers in academic medicine. First, everyone in the business is smart—exceedingly smart. Second, virtually everyone is intense and admirably hardworking. Third, while our community may seem disproportionately endowed with large egos, almost everyone is, in his or her own way, highly dedicated to improving the state of human health. Far less commonly encountered, however, are highly successful academic physicians who are also low-key, disarmingly charming and able to take themselves less seriously than they take their work and their responsibilities.

Joe Martin falls squarely in that category of low-key, affable and self-transcendent individuals. There is no question that he is exceedingly smart, hardworking, intense and dedicated, yet, he is also remarkably accessible, likeable and warm. I think these qualities, even more than his brilliance, enabled him to thrive as a leader in highly competitive organizations such as Massachusetts General Hospital, University of California in San Francisco and Harvard Medical School. It is this side of Joe that makes it a particular honor to write this postscript and to share my observations about the very pleasurable decade we shared at Harvard Medical School.

Although he was well known to me by reputation, I did not meet Joe personally until I was the Osler Professor at Johns Hopkins in 1997. At the time, Johns Hopkins was in a period of crisis. The pressures of the "managed care era" of the 1990s had fractured the relationships between a renowned hospital and an esteemed school of medicine. The faculty was caught in the middle. The trustees recognized the need for united leadership and for a single leader, a dean/CEO. I was serving on that search committee. Even though he was in the midst of his efforts to forge a UCSF–Stanford merger, Joe agreed to visit as a consultant. Hopkins, of course, was hoping that he might become attracted to the position. I remember arriving early for the introductory dinner and finding Joe waiting politely for all of us. We had a chance to chat one-on-one for a few minutes, and I was immediately taken by his sociability, grace and warmth. This was not the hard-charging, aggressive neuroscientist/chancellor that I had anticipated on the basis of his resume and accomplishments. The memory of that dinner still lingers as one of the more pleasant encounters that I have had in academics.

> Amphitheater of the Joseph B. Martin Conference Center in the New Research Building, dedicated September 23, 2003.

Joe provided us with good insights and strong advice. He also let us know, very politely, that the charms of San Francisco Bay were a bit more suitable for Rachel and him than those of Chesapeake Bay. Though disappointed that he would not be coming to Hopkins, I was pleased to have made a new friendship. Hopkins did manage to integrate its components, and I settled in, expecting to finish my career in Baltimore.

In late 1999 the University of Pennsylvania convened an external committee to recommend future directions in its gene therapy programs. Joe and I were appointed to that panel. After our first meeting, he called to invite me to have breakfast with him before the start of our second meeting, in order to "get my thoughts about the leadership of the Dana-Farber Cancer Institute (DFCI) at Harvard."

Having trained at Harvard, I was familiar with its culture of fiercely independent hospitals. I assumed that he might be interested in comparisons and contrasts with the integration

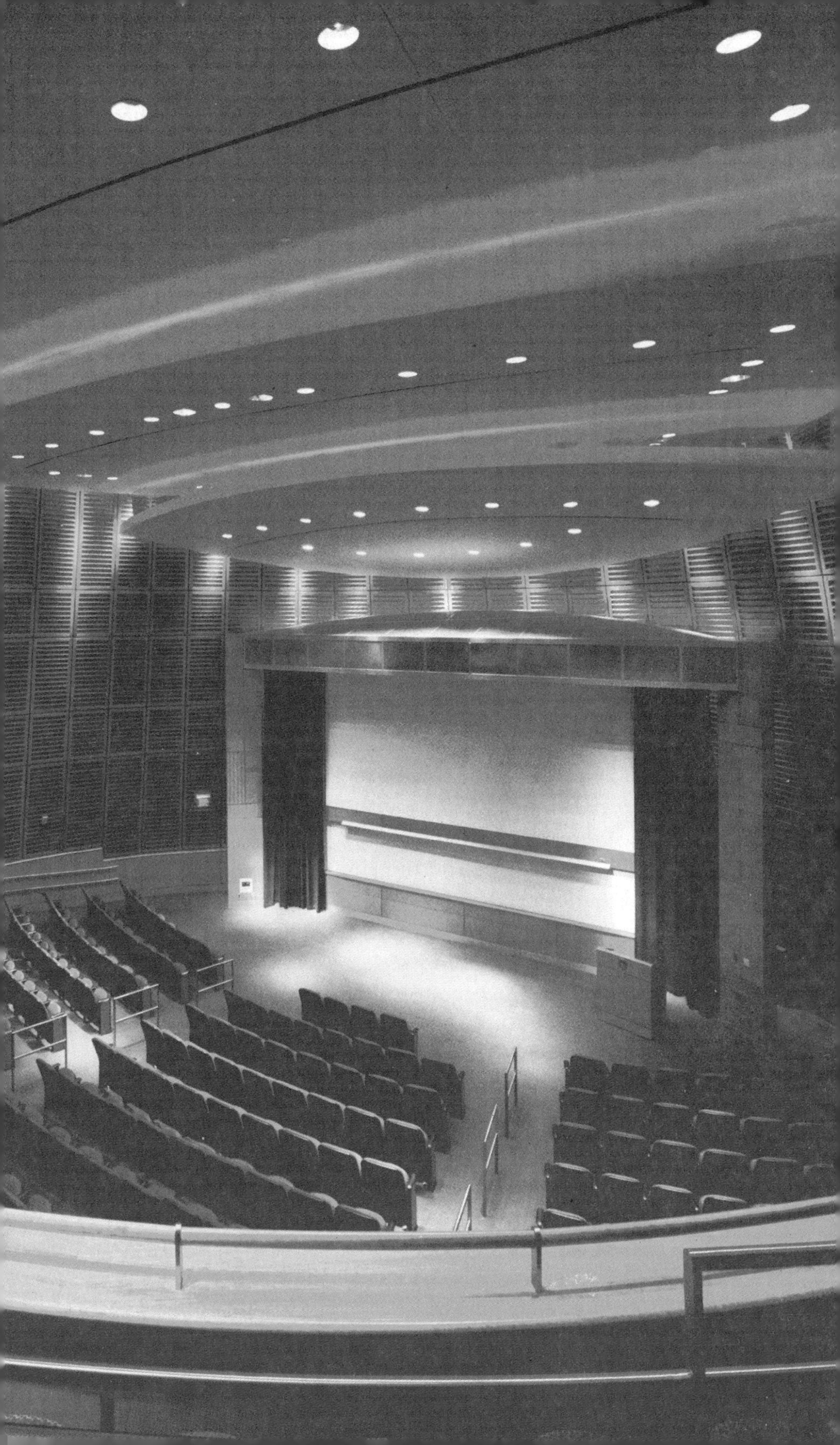

that we had achieved at Hopkins. At that breakfast, he outlined the ambitious initiative that he and the retiring president of the DFCI, David Nathan (my med school mentor) had launched. DFCI had been, for fifty years, a pre-eminent cancer hospital and research institute. It functioned like all Harvard hospitals, that is, as a silo within Harvard's federation of teaching hospitals and health schools. Joe and David had created the Dana-Farber/Harvard Cancer Center, a consortium of the five principal teaching hospitals, HMS and HSPH. All seven institutions would share the designation of "Comprehensive Cancer Center" from the National Cancer Institute, and share in the governance and resources of the core grant that supported it. In this way, Joe and David hoped to turn an intensely competitive and sometimes cannibalistic set of relationships around cancer research into something collaborative and synergistic. The president of DFCI would also serve as the director and principal investigator of the DF/HCC.

Joe's charm and low-key negotiating power were fully in evidence. He told me that he and the DFCI board chair were co-chairs of the search for David Nathan's successor and described in very compelling terms what a superlative opportunity this position constituted. The new president would be not merely be the CEO of a premier cancer institute but also have the major leadership role in galvanizing all of Harvard's research power in the cancer field. I started thinking of names to suggest to him. However, before the second cup of coffee was poured, he looked at me and said,"might *you* have some interest in exploring this extraordinary opportunity?"

At the time, I was quite happily ensconced in a position at Johns Hopkins that one was not supposed to leave until one retires or dies. I had never worked in a cancer center. Even though I had cared for patients with hematologic malignancies as a clinical hematologist, I was not a "cancer doctor" by any stretch of the imagination. Nonetheless, I found myself agreeing to bring Peggy to Boston for a visit in the early spring. During that visit, Joe and Rachel took Peggy and me to a quiet dinner, after which Peggy said, "You will not be able to say no to him." She was right. We moved to Boston in the autumn of 2000, beginning what has been by far the most challenging,

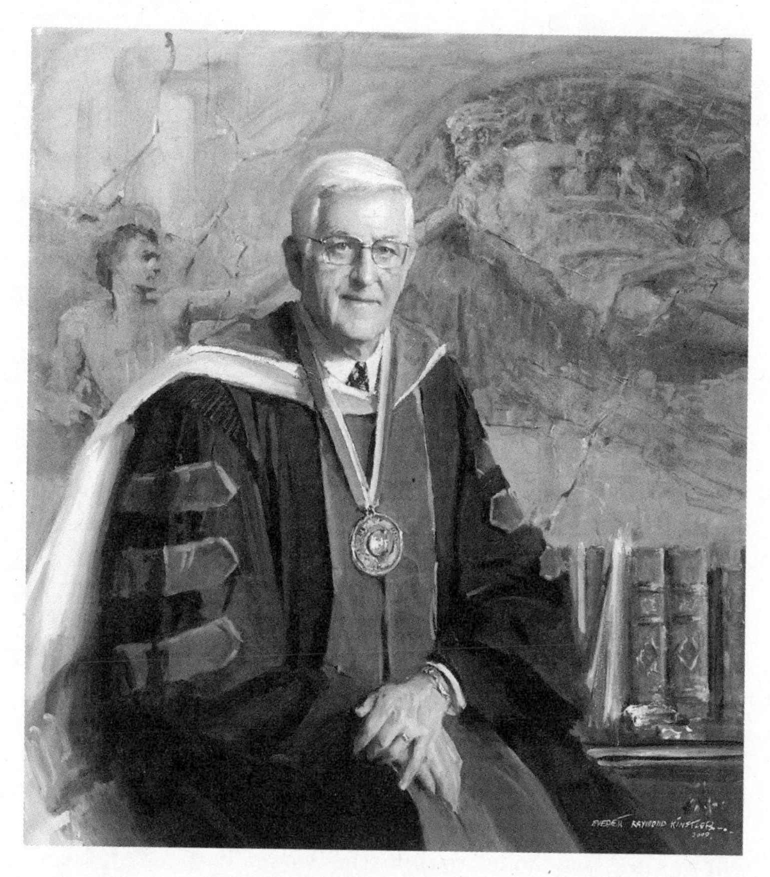

Portrait of the author, presented to faculty June 27, 2009. The portrait hangs in the Benjamin Waterhouse Faculty Room of Gordon Hall at Harvard Medical School. (Portrait by E. Raymond Kinstler of New York City)

exhilarating and fulfilling decade of my career. In a very real way, I am indebted to him for these years in Boston.

The same characteristics that I found so engaging in our early encounters with Joe have been consistent threads throughout his life and career. Joe's brilliance, vision and drive do not wash over you when you meet him. Rather, they seep in over time in a series of pleasant and enjoyable interactions. First, you enjoy being with him. Next, you are impressed with his vision and what he wants to accomplish with you. Then you do what he is asking of you.

Among the many highlights in Joe's life and career, I have first-hand knowledge only of those occurring during the last decade before his retirement, when he was serving as dean of Harvard Medical School. This decade embraced the transition to a new century, the exuberance of the late nineties, the devastation of September 11 and the twin revolutions of the Internet and the human genome project. Joe worked tirelessly to foster a local revolution at HMS. Under his tutelage, we began to feel our way toward being a more unified and interactive network of institutions rather than a loose and often counterproductive federation of competing hospitals and schools. Joe spent much of his deanship working tirelessly to achieving this greater cooperation and synergy among Harvard's many moving parts. He, perhaps more than any dean before him, tried to actuate the vision of the Harvard enterprise being all it could be.

The DF/HCC was a centerpiece of these efforts. It is the context within which I interacted most frequently and intensely with Joe. At the time of my arrival, the entire concept of a trans-Harvard collaboration around cancer research was in a very fragile state. The initial parties had been brought to the table somewhat reluctantly, and centrifugal forces were already high, even though the effort was only two years old. Without Joe's calm and even-handed use of the prestige of the dean's office, the DF/HCC would have unraveled while I was still getting my sea legs in a new institution. As chair of the governance committee of DF/HCC, Joe constantly stood up for the need to cooperate and collaborate. He did not pretend that the tensions did not exist, nor was he naïve enough to think they would disappear. Rather, he insisted that we achieve the vision despite these obstacles. By the time of his departure, while tensions still flared on a recurring basis, the DF/HCC was firmly established as Harvard's signature effort in cancer research.

Harvard should be indebted to Joe for his unflagging dedication to pulling the many pieces of the Harvard medical community together. While this unity still very much a work in progress, it has become much more widely accepted as the most desirable vision for all of us, even while we stumble over institutional needs and priorities. Other deans will probably reap the rewards of the early successes that he engendered, but his galvanizing role must be remembered.

I hope that Joe will think of his role in founding DF/HCC as one of the brightest areas of his legacy. I regard it as one of the major contributions he has made during his entire career. By any measure, DF/HCC has been an enormous success and a proof of the principle that Harvard hospitals do much better working together, collaborating and sharing, than they do by trying out-compete colleague institutions. Prior to the creation of DF/HCC, the Dana-Farber Cancer Institute represented the predominant institutional force nationally and internationally in cancer. Now, each of the five hospitals is clearly respected in the field individually, as well as in the context of DF/HCC. Prior to the formation of DF/HCC, there were no SPORE grants at Harvard. (SPORE grants are special awards given by the NCI for collaborative projects focused on translating discoveries into improved clinical outcomes. They are highly prestigious and one of the "marks" of a successful comprehensive cancer center.) Since it was formed, DF/HCC has received eight, among the highest in the country. Prior to the formation of DF/HCC, there was only one program project grant that involved investigators from more than one institution. There are now over forty. Major national awards for team science, two of the five trans-institutional Stand Up to Cancer awards, and innumerable individual and team science awards recognizing seminal research breakthrough have resulted from the formation of interactive programs and initiatives in DF/HCC. All institutions are well represented in these recognitions. Most important, major new advances that improve care have resulted from these projects in ways that would not have occurred had the individual institutions continued to flail at the problem on their own. DF/HCC has established itself as a clear world leader in cancer genomics, as a pioneer in the identification of molecular targets, the development of targeted therapies for diseases such as chronic myelogenous leukemia, multiple myeloma and lung cancer, outcomes and comparative effectiveness research, and numerous other areas.

When the new consortium was first reviewed for its core grant in 1999, the academic world was highly skeptical and cynical about the likelihood that the Harvard institutions could work together. To everyone's surprise, DF/HCC not only made it through the review process but got the highest priority score in the country. When renewal of the core grant was conducted in 2005, skepticism in the outside world was again high that the institutions could stay together and actually accomplish anything that "added value" to what the individual entities could do. Once again, a review of accomplishments and the working relationships in DF/HCC surprised everyone and the center once again received the highest priority score. Now as DF/HCC approaches its third competing renewal, in its eleventh year of existence, the center is considered a national model for trans-institutional collaboration. It has inspired formation of other consortia at major medical centers in the Midwest and West Coast. Research funding, the numbers of cancer-oriented research faculty, and cancer philanthropy have increased dramatically at every participating institution. The DF/HCC annually brings in over $600 million in extramural research support to the Harvard institutions and to Boston. Nearly five thousand cancer patients a year now enroll in clinical trials. At any given time nearly 15,000 patients within the Harvard hospitals participate in one of over seven hundred clinical trials, several of which, such as recent vaccine and immunotherapy trials for prostate cancer and melanoma and those introducing targeted therapy for lung cancer, melanoma and sarcoma, have been groundbreaking.

The state-of-the-art conference center in the New Research Building at Harvard is named for Joe Martin. At its dedication, many expressed their admiration for the contributions he had made and the person that he is. However, having a space named after him, even one as magnificent as that conference center, is not a wholly adequate reflection on Joe's legacy. DF/HCC, the Harvard NeuroDiscovery Center and other trans-Harvard consortia that will follow will be his lasting and living legacy as dean of Harvard Medical School.

Joe Martin led major academic institutions through times that were both evolutionary and revolutionary. He maintained a strong profile of the health science schools that he led when we were experiencing tumultuous changes in leadership, public support and finances. He finished his career at a place all good leaders should aspire to: having made the organizations he led both better than they were and doing many good things that they were not before he arrived. For that, we all owe Joe our deepest appreciation.

DR. ED BENZ is president and CEO of Dana-Farber Cancer Institute, HMS, director of Dana-Farber/Harvard Cancer Center, HMS, the Richard and Susan Smith Professor of Medicine, HMS, as well as professor of pediatrics, HMS, and professor of genetics, HMS.

# NOTES

## ONE
### *The Journey from Bern to Duchess*

1. Primary sources and documents at the State Archives in Bern, the Dutch Mennonite Archives in Amsterdam, as well as legal documents, such as tax records, deeds and wills at Lancaster, Pennsylvania, are listed in Jason Martin's "Christian and Ells Martin: Immigrant Patriarch and Matriarch," *Pennsylvania Mennonite Heritage*, Volume x, No. 3 (Lancaster, PA: Lancaster Mennonite Historical Society, July 1987), 13f., and in his "Immigrant Christian Martin and the European Background of the Martin Family," *Lancaster Mennonite Historical Society*, Quarterly Meeting (Lancaster, PA: Lancaster Mennonite Historical Society, September 18, 1989) 2ff. The Martin family origins and background are also discussed by John L. Ruth, *The Earth is the Lord's* (Scottsdale, PA, and Waterloo, ON: Herald Press, 2001), 228–30, and in the online *Global Anabaptist Mennonite Encyclopedia*, accessed January 12, 2011, www.gameo.org/encyclopedia/contents/M3784ME.html.
2. See the sixth edition of the *Martin Genealogy Project*, with a listing of 34,285 individuals, accessed January 12, 2011, www.genealogygoldmine.com/martin.
3. Their names appear in Daniel Rupp's *Names of Immigrants in Pennsylvania, 1727–1776* (Philadelphia: Leary, Stuart, Co., Publishers, 1898), 50–54. Rupp's book, along with Carl Boyer's *Ship Passenger Lists, Pennsylvania and Delaware, 1641–1825* (Newhall, CA: Carl Boyer, 1992), includes numerous ship passenger lists.
4. *Martyrs Mirror* was first published in Dutch (Nederlandish) by author Tieleman Jansz van Braght in two parts, the first recounting martyrdom from the time of Jesus to 1500 CE and the second those dying of the Anabaptist-Mennonite faith. The first German edition was published at the Ephrata Cloister in Pennsylvania in 1748–49. The first English edition appeared in 1837, also published in Pennsylvania.

5. From their origins in the German-speaking regions of Switzerland, Alsace and the Rhineland, Mennonite descendants followed two main routes as they fled persecution. The first path was followed by my ancestors, who began immigrating to the US in 1683 with subsequent waves of newcomers over the next century. This group of Mennonites became known as the Pennsylvania Dutch Mennonites. Another wave of Mennonites took up the second route and migrated to Prussia, and at the invitation of Czar Catherine the Great, in 1768, they moved on to the region north of the Black Sea, later part of the Ukraine. These German Mennonites came to North America in the nineteenth and early twentieth centuries, settling in many parts of the US and Canada and in South America (Paraguay and Uruguay). Today the major Mennonite groups in North America usually worship separately, but they work together in support of the Mennonite relief agencies: Mennonite Central Committee (MCC) and Mennonite Disaster Service (MDS).
6. Mennonite Archives, Amsterdam, *Inventaris* no. 2281.
7. The online essay by Kraig Ruckel, "Palatine Emigrants: Emigration from the Rhineland to America—Eighteenth Century," accessed March 14, 2011, www.cc.utah.edu/~pdp7277/palatine.html, summarizes the palatine immigration to the New World. For a full discussion see Walter Knittle, *Early Eighteenth Century Palatine Emigration: A British Government Redemptioner Project to Manufacture Naval Stores* (Westminster, MD: Heritage Books, reprinted 2006 from 1937 original).
8. The Berwangen Lutheran Church records, discussed by Jason Martin, "Immigrant Christian Martin," 7f., are in the Evangelische Pfarramt in Berwangen.
9. See The Palatine Project, Reconstructed Passenger Lists for a listing of the Wengers, accessed January 12, 2011, www.progenealogists.com/palproject/pa/1727molly.htm, and the Martin Genealogy Project, accessed January 12, 2011, www.genealogygoldmine.com/martin/shiplists/Molly.html.
10. Accessed January 12, 2011, http://files.usgwarchives.org/pa/1pa/ships/britann.txt (File contributed for use in USGenWeb Archives by Faye Moran).
11. *Global Anabaptist Mennonite Encyclopedia*, accessed January 12, 2011, www.gameo.org/encyclopedia/contents/M3784ME.html, and Ruth, *The Earth is the Lord's*, 228–30.
12. The Anabaptist movement included three principle lineages: the Mennonites, founded by Menno Simons in 1536; the Amish, named for a secession movement led by Jakob Ammann in 1693; and the Hutterites, named after Jakob Hutter in 1536. Today there are about 1.5 million Mennonites worldwide distributed in over forty

countries, with the largest memberships in Canada, the US and the Democratic Republic of Congo. The Amish number about 250,000 and are scattered throughout the middle states and Canada. The Hutterites, who live together in colonies and share all economic resources equally among members, number about 45,000 and are mostly located in the western Canadian provinces and the adjacent states in the US.

13. George Hantsch's journal—discussed by Jason Martin, "Immigrant Christian Martin," 7—is located at the Moravian Archives in Bethlehem, Pennsylvania.
14. Pierre Berton, *The Last Spike: The Great Railway, 1881–1885* (Toronto: McClelland and Stewart, 1971), 394. "On July 28, 1874, near Calgary, the workers set a record never surpassed for manual labor on a railroad: 6.38 miles finished in a single day."
15. Wallace Stegner, *Wolf Willow: A History, a Story, and a Memory of the Last Plains Frontier* (New York: Penguin, 2000).
16. R. Gross and N. Kramer, *Tapping the Bow* (Brooks, AB: Eastern Irrigation District, 1985), 6–7.

## TWO
## *Emerging as a Family in the New Land*

1. Uncle Clarence married Ethel, my father's older sister. The Ramer children were my "double-first cousins."
2. Uncle Sam Martin's audio interview, accessed January 12, 2011, www.alternativeservice.ca/sacrifice/prison/prison3.htm. See also William Janzen and Frances Greaser, *"Sam Martin went to Prison" a story of conscientious objection and Canadian Military Service* (Winnipeg, MB, and Hillsboro, KS: Kindred Press, 1990).
3. Two of Uncle Sam's six children became medical doctors. Rodney, a John W. Scott Award winner from the University of Alberta, is a radiologist who works in Lethbridge, not far from where Sam had been imprisoned, and Murray, the oldest brother, practiced family medicine after graduating from the University of Calgary until he died unexpectedly of a cardiac arrest at age sixty in 2007.
4. My hunting escapades left more than memories. After one hunting experience in August, lying among the swaths of grain with my 12-gauge shotgun, shooting at wave after wave of ducks descending for an afternoon feast of wheat, I returned home with severe tinnitus (ringing in my ears) that lasted for three days. Years later in a laboratory of our first-year medical school physiology class we performed audiograms on each other that revealed a significant high-frequency hearing loss in my left ear. "Oh, were you left-handed?" I've been asked. No, with the right cheek resting on the

stock, sighting down the barrel with the right eye (dominant), the left ear is most exposed to the blast from the gun's muzzle. My dad had the same problem.

## THREE
## *Transitions*

1. Dr. Lionel McLeod was appointed a Markle Scholar, which included a research grant and was a rare award for a Canadian. His friendship with William Drucker, another Markle Scholar, who was a surgeon at Case Western Reserve University, would be a key to my introduction to that academic community and my eventual decision to train in neurology there. Lionel would later be appointed dean of the University of Calgary's Faculty of Medicine and would be the principal academic leader in the formation of the Alberta Heritage Foundation for Medical Research, in which capacity he invited me to serve on the scientific advisory committee during the 1980s.
2. We visit Ben and Carol Ruether now whenever our travels take us to Calgary, where Ben is now retired from his position as professor of medicine (hematology/oncology) at the University of Calgary.
3. J.B. Martin and H.E. Bell, "Association of splenic atrophy and intestinal malabsorption: report of a case and review of the literature," *Canadian Medical Association Journal* 92 (1965): 875–78.
4. Herman Bleibtreu went on to the Department of Anthropology at the University of Arizona, where he is currently listed as an emeritus faculty member.
5. Victor McKusick together with John Hostetler and investigators from Johns Hopkins and the University of Pennsylvania went to on to characterize many of the autosomal recessive genetic disorders resulting for consanguinity among the Amish and Old Order (horse and buggy) Mennonites. Today that work goes on in the Clinic for Special Children in Strasburg, Pennsylvania, led by D. Holmes Morton, an HMS graduate and pediatrician. I visited the clinic founded in 1989 on the occasion of its twentieth anniversary in 2009. I was amazed at the cooperation the clinic doctors are given by the grateful families, who raise money to support the effort through quilt sales and auctions.
6. In addition to Cleveland, I considered training programs at Queen Square, London, the Montreal Neurological Institute, the University of Minnesota , the University of Michigan, New York Presbyterian Neurological Institute and, of course, the Massachusetts General Hospital. The latter never replied to my

queries for an application until pressed some months later when they responded bluntly with a rejection. I was delighted to arrive there fifteen years later as the chief!

7. Vilnis Ciemins entered private practice in neurology in the western part of Cleveland after his Case Western Reserve University internship.
8. Ingo Weiderholt returned from Case Western Reserve University to Germany and became a forensic psychiatrist. On a visit to San Francisco in 1996, we learned of his unfortunate illness that had led to a liver transplant, after infection with hepatitis C.
9. Michael Swash returned to England from Cleveland as an advanced registrar (a senior resident in training), obtained his qualifications as a neurological consultant and eventually became the chief of the service at London Hospital.
10. Michael Cohen returned to Buffalo and became chief of neurology at the Buffalo Children's Hospital and later chair of the department.
11. John Conomy, a talented junior resident at Case Western Reserve University, one year behind my group, went on to be chief at the Cleveland Clinic.
12. Michael Genco returned to Buffalo for a lifetime of clinical practice associated with the university there.
13. Berch Griggs would later be appointed chief of the Department of Neurology at the University of Rochester in New York.
14. J.B. Martin, R.H. Travis, and S. van den Noort, "Centrally mediated orthostatic hypotension," *Archives of Neurology* 19 (1968): 163–73.
15. J.B. Martin, R. Boshans, and S. Reichlin, "Feedback regulation of TSH secretion in rats with hypothalamic lesions," *Endocrinology* 87 (1970): 1032–40.
    S. Reichlin, J.B.Martin, R.I. Boshans, D.S. Schalch, J.G. Pierce, and J. Bollinger, "Measurement of TSH in plasma and pituitary of the rat by radioimmunoassay utilizing bovine TSH: effect of thyroidectomy or thyroxine administration on plasma TSH levels," *Endocrinology* 87 (1970): 1022–31.
16. J.B. Martin and S. Reichlin, "Thyrotropin secretion in rats after hypothalamic electrical stimulation or administration of synthetic TSH-releasing factor," *Science* 168 (1970): 1366–68.
17. J.B. Martin, G.M. Brown, and S. Reichlin, eds, *Clinical Neuroendocrinology* (Philadelphia, PA: F.A. Davis Company, 1977). A second edition was published in 1987 by the same publisher.

## FOUR
*Montreal*

1. Garth M. Bray and Donald W. Baxter, "Neurology at the Montreal General Hospital," in Joseph Hanaway and John Burgess, eds, *The General: A History of the Montreal General Hospital 1819–1996* (Montreal: McGill-Queens University Press, Forthcoming).
2. Ibid.
3. J.B. Martin, "Plasma growth hormone (GH) response to hypothalamic or extra-hypothalamic electrical stimulation," *Endocrinology* 91 (1972): 107–15.
4. L.P. Renaud, J.B. Martin, and P. Brazeau, "Depressant action of TRH, LHRH and somatostatin on activity of central neurons," *Nature* 255 (1975): 233–35.
5. J.B. Martin, L.P. Renaud, and P. Brazeau, "Hypothalamic peptides: new evidence for 'peptidergic' pathways in the CNS," *The Lancet* 2 (1975): 393–95.
6. G.S. Tannenbaum and J.B. Martin, "Evidence for an endogenous ultradian rhythm governing growth hormone secretion in the rat," *Endocrinology* 98 (1976): 562–70.
7. J.O. Willoughby, J.B. Martin, L.P. Renaud, and P. Brazeau, "Pulsatile growth hormone release in the rat: failure to demonstrate a correlation with sleep phases," *Endocrinology* 98 (1976): 991–96.
8. J.B. Martin, "Neural regulation of growth hormone secretion, Medical Progress Report," *New England Journal of Medicine* 288 (1973): 1384–93.
9. K.W. Cheng, H.G. Friesen, and J.B. Martin, "Neurophysin in rats with hereditary hypothalamic diabetes insipidus (Brattleboro strain)," *Endocrinology* 90 (1972): 1055–63.
   K.W. Cheng, J.B. Martin, and H.G. Friesen, "Studies of neurophysin release," *Endocrinology* 91 (1972): 177–84.
   J.B. Martin, S. Lal, G. Tolis, H.G. Friesen, "Inhibition by apomorphine of prolactin secretion in patients with elevated serum prolactin," *Journal of Clinical Endocrinology and Metabolism* 39 (1974): 180–82.
10. For more information on the House of Friendship, see www.maisondelamitie.ca/html/indexe.html.
11. W. Penfield, *No Man Alone: A Surgeon's Life* (New York: Little, Brown and Company, 1977).
12. Preston Robb, *The Development of Neurology at McGill* (Montreal: self-published, 1989).

13. During the 1980s and 1990s some of the most forward-looking academic developments in neurology at McGill University occurred at the MGH North. Under the skillful guidance of Albert Aguayo, a McGill Centre for Research in Neuroscience was created, with a focus on developmental neurobiology and nervous system regeneration. Aguayo was awarded the prestigious Gairdner Prize for Medical Research in 1988 for his work on regeneration in the central nervous system.

## FIVE

### *Boston: The MGH Years*

1. Webster Bull and Martha Bull, *Something in the Ether: A Bicentennial History of the Massachusetts General Hospital, 1811–2011* (Beverly, MA: Memoirs Unlimited, 2011).
2. Susan Leeman and I re-established contact and renewed our friendship through three meetings I invited her to attend over breakfast and in my office. I was grateful when reconciliation was achieved. Leeman remains active in research and teaching at Boston University in 2011.
3. Charlie did leave on September 1. Over time, he ascended quite remarkably in the pharmaceutical industry to become chairman and CEO of Glaxo Inc. from 1989 to 1995, a position he held until his planned retirement. He later ran as a democratic candidate for the United States Senate for North Carolina, losing in the primary by a narrow margin to Harvey Gantt, who subsequently lost to Jesse Helms in the Senate race that fall. Our close friendship, always tremendously valuable to me, was maintained over the twenty-five years following his departure from the MGH. I was thrilled when Charlie and his wife, Ann, provided funding for a chair in cardiovascular research at the MGH in 201, a position held in 2011 by Dr. Kenneth Chien, director of the Cardiovascular Research Center, who works on stem cell biology relevant to heart disease.
4. The Kennedy family had developed close personal interactions with my MGH predecessor, Raymond D. Adams. Eunice devoted her effort in both time and money to the study of neurological developmental disabilities and went on to establish the extraordinary Special Olympics to encourage active participation of these individuals in athletics events. Members of the Kennedy family later came forward with the resources to establish the Joseph and Rose Kennedy Professorship in Child Neurology at the MGH and the Shriver Center.

5. By 1997 there were over thirty faculty members in the two units of the department, one at HMS and one at MGH, the vast majority of whom went forward to tenure appointments at HMS. Two professors, Jack Szostak and Gary Ruvkin, were awarded the esteemed Lasker Prize for their work, and Szostak was a 2009 co-recipient of the Nobel Prize in Physiology or Medicine. In 2003 Howard retired from the chair and was succeeded by Robert Kingston, whom Howard had recruited as a junior investigator. Phil continued as chair of the HMS department until 2005, when Cliff Tabin, whom Phil had recruited to HMS over a decade earlier, succeeded him.
6. O.P. Rorstad, A. Schonbrunn, and J.B. Martin, "Somatostatin radioreceptor assay: development and application to the measurement of somatostatin-like activity in the rat central nervous system," *Canadian Journal of Biochemistry and Cell Biology* 61 (1983): 532–37.
7. W.J. Millard, S.M. Reppert, S.M. Sagar, and J.B. Martin, "Light-dark entrainment of the growth hormone ultradian rhythm in the rat is mediated by the arcuate nucleus," *Endocrinology* 108 (1981): 2394–96.
8. P.E. Cooper, M.H. Fernstrom, O.P. Rorstad, S.E. Leeman, and J.B. Martin, "The regional distribution of somatostatin, substance P and neurostensin in the human brain," *Brain Research* 218 (1981): 219–32.
9. N.H. Kowall, M.F. Beal, R.J. Ferrante, and J.B. Martin, "Topography of nicotinamide adenine dinucleotide phosphate-diaphorase staining neurons in rat striatum," *Neuroscience Letters* 599 (1985): 61–6; R.J. Ferrant, N.W Kowall, E.P. Richardson Jr., E.D. Bird, and J.B. Martin, "Topography of enkephalin, substance P and acetylcholinesterase staining in Huntington's disease striatum," *Neuroscience Letters* 71 (1986): 283–88; N.W. Kowall, R.J. Ferrant, and J.B. Martin, "Patterns of cell loss in Huntington's disease," *Trends in Neuroscience* 10 (1987): 24–29.
10. The opportunities that came with the revolution in molecular genetics has offered new approaches to these conditions that I described in some detail in my lecture upon receiving the first Henry G. Friesen International Prize in Health Research, given in Ottawa in September 2006. It was an enormous privilege to see Henry again. He has now retired to his alma mater, the University of Manitoba.
11. J.B. Martin, "Molecular basis of the neurodegenerative disorders," *New England Journal of Medicine* 340 (1999): 1970–80. See also J.B. Martin, ed., *Scientific American Molecular Neurology* (New York: Scientific American Inc., 1998).

12. M.F. Beal, M.F. Mazurek, C.N. Svendsen, E.D. Bird, and J.B. Martin, "Widespread reduction of somatostatin-like immunoreactivity in the cerebral cortex in Alzheimer's Disease," *Annals of Neurology* 20 (1986): 489–95; M.F. Beal and J.B. Martin, "Neuropeptides in neurological disease," *Annals of Neurology* 20 (1986): 547–65.
13. Flint remained at the MGH in his own independent laboratory after my exit to San Francisco in 1989 and was later recruited to chair the Department of Neurology at Weill Cornell Medical College in New York.
14. John's own family would face the extraordinary challenge of ALS when his wife, Elvira, became ill in 2007, a few months after John stepped down as AD Center director, with rapid deterioration in motor function. She passed away in January 2009.
15. David and I remain close friends. Rachel and I have visited their family compound in Bradford, Pennsylvania, near the original oil well that led to the founding of Forest Oil, as well as at their home in Denver. David, now in his mid-eighties, visits Boston for regular annual meetings as a member of Anne Young's external advisory committee, giving us the opportunity to spend time with him and his wife, Catherine, in Boston.

**SIX**

## *A Science Saga: The Search for the Huntington's Disease Gene*

1. Michael Hayden, *Huntington's Chorea* (New York: Springer, 1981).
2. G. Huntington, "On Chorea," *Medical and Surgical Reporter* 26 (1872): 317–21.
3. J.B. Martin and J.F. Gusella, "Huntington's disease: pathogenesis and management," *New England Journal of Medicine* 315 (1986): 1267–276.
4. Alice Wexler, *Mapping Fate: A Memoir of Family, Risk and Genetic Research* (Berkeley, CA: University of California Press, 1996).
5. H.F. Judson, *The Eighth Day of Creation: Makers of the Revolution in Biology, 25th Anniversary Edition* (Cold Spring Harbor, NY: Cold Spring Harbor Laboratory Press, 1996).
6. J.D. Watson, F.H. Crick, "Molecular structure of nucleic acids: a structure for deoxyribose nucleic acid," *Nature* 171, no. 4356 (1953): 737–38.
7. D. Cook-Deegan, *The Gene Wars: Science, Politics, and the Human Genome* (New York: W.W. Norton, 1994).

8. D. Botstein, R.L. White, M. Skolnick, and R.W. Davis, "Construction of a genetic linkage map in man using restriction fragment length polymorphisms," *American Journal of Human Genetics* 32, no. 3 (1980): 314–31.
9. Y.W. Kan and A.M. Dozy, "Polymorphism of DNA sequence adjacent to human beta-globin structural gene: relationship to sickle mutation," *Proceedings of the National Academy of Sciences* 75, no. 11 (1978): 5631–35.
10. J.F. Gusella, N.S. Wexler, P.M. Conneally, S.L. Naylor, M.A. Anderson, R.E. Tanzi, P.C. Watkins, K. Ottina, M.R. Wallace, A.Y. Sakaguchi, A.B. Young, I. Shoulson, E. Bonella, and J.B. Martin, "A polymorphic DNA marker genetically linked to Huntington's disease," *Nature* 306 (1983): 234–38.
11. Huntington's Disease Collaborative Research Group, "A novel gene containing a trinucleotide repeat that is expanded and unstable on Huntington's disease chromosomes," *Cell* 72 (1993): 971.
12. G.J. Meissen, R.H. Myers, C.A. Mastromauro, W.J. Koroshetz, K.W. Klinger, L.A. Farrer, P.A. Watkins, J.F. Gusella, E.D. Bird, and J.B. Martin, "Predictive testing for Huntington's disease with use of a linked DNA marker," *New England Journal of Medicine* 318 (1988): 535–42.

**SEVEN**

## *From Bethesda to San Francisco*

1. D.T. Krieger and J.B. Martin, "Brain peptides," *New England Journal of Medicine* 304 (1981): 876–85, 944–51.
2. Bob Martuza would later leave to chair neurosurgery at the Georgetown University School of Medicine, and a decade later would return as chief of neurosurgery at the MGH.
3. Steve Hyman later headed the National Institute of Mental Health and served as provost of Harvard University from 2001 to 2011.
4. Steve Fink went on to chair the Department of Neurology at Boston University before succumbing to a rapidly progressive course of malignant glioma.
5. Mike Comb later went into industry as a research scientist.
6. Holly Smith, *My Life and Hard Times: The Autobiography of Dr. Holly Smith*, conveyed in personal communication with the author.
7. Kate Volkman, "UC: Under Construction," UCSF *Medical Alumni Bulletin* (Fall 2008), 8.
8. W. Francis Ganong Jr. was a Harvard Medical School educated physiologist, one of the first neuroendocrinologists to elucidate the functions of the nervous system in homeostasis. He was born in Northampton, Massachusetts, the son of the distinguished

Canadian botanist, William Francis Ganong. He was renowned, in addition, for his book, *Review of Medical Physiology*, first published in 1963, which by the time of his death in 2007 was in the 23rd edition and had been translated into eighteen languages.

9. Prior to his decline in effectiveness at UCSF, Richard had been invited to join the ranks of editors of *Harrison's Principles of Internal Medicine*. I liked Dick a great deal and offered him a position in the dean's office to head clinical affairs to help him through the professional rough patch he was in. He functioned adequately in that role for two years before returning to the University of Washington, where he thrived as chief of the medical service at Harbor Bay Hospital until his retirement seven years later. Unfortunately, Dick had a double dollop of tragedy. Soon after returning to Seattle, his wife, Marilyn, developed amyotrophic lateral sclerosis (ALS) and died a few years later. Dick remarried and became involved in HIV-AIDS research work in West Africa. Tragically, however, while boating on a river there, he was attacked by a crocodile. His body was never found.
10. Both Bargmann and Tessier-Lavigne rapidly ascended the academic ladder at UCSF. Both were recruited away, Bargmann to Rockefeller University in New York and Tessier-Lavigne to Stanford. In the spring of 2011 they were reunited when Tessier-Lavigne became the newly appointed president of Rockefeller University.
11. J.A. Kastor, *Mergers of Teaching Hospitals in Boston, New York, and Northern California* (Ann Arbor, MI: University of Michigan Press, 2001).

## EIGHT
## *Return to Harvard Medical School*

1. Another member of the corporation who had close ties to the medical school was Richard Smith, whose family had been generous in donating to the Dana-Farber Cancer Institute.
2. Ray would eventually succeed Dennis in the role of academic dean when Dennis received institutional funding from the National Institute of Allergy and Infectious Diseases, part of the National Institutes of Health, to support the New England Regional Center of Excellence (NERCE) as one of the government's bioterrorism initiatives.
3. I would call upon Eric to succeed Paul when Paul was recruited to the position of CEO at the BIDMC in the fall of 2001. Eric's outstanding work led to the completion of the NRB in 2003 on time

and below budget, a unique experience, I've been assured, in the recent history of Harvard University projects. The total cost of the project came to $280 million.

4. The NRB has no other formal name, but hopefully it will be named in honor of a donor at some point in the future.
5. Larry Tye, "Harvard Medical Dean in the hot seat," *Boston Globe*, December 29, 1997.
6. Nora N. Nercessian, *A Legacy So Enduring: An Account of the Administration Building at Harvard Medical School from its Foundation to its Rededication as the Gordon Hall of Medicine* (Cambridge, MA: Harvard College, 2001).
7. Ibid.
8. D.C. Tosteson, "New Pathways in General Medical Education," *New England Journal of Medicine* 233 (1990): 234–38.
9. I was fortunate that Dan Federman was assisted in the annual fundraising efforts by Tenley Albright, a surgeon and HMS graduate, who was widely admired for her gold-medal performances in figure skating in the 1956 Olympics. She would continue to work with me as director of the annual fundraising effort for the remainder of my deanship.
10. L. Kowalczyk, "Busy Harvard doctors balk at teaching," *Boston Globe*, June 1, 2003.

## NINE
## *Working with Larry Summers*

1. R.E. Rubin, *In an Uncertain World* (New York: Random House, 2004).
2. W.C. Willett, *Eat, Drink and Be Healthy* (New York: Free Press, a division of Simon and Schuster, Inc., 2005).
3. The Harvard Institute for International Development (HIID) was dissolved in June 2000. From 1974 to 2000, HIID was Harvard University's multidisciplinary center for coordinating development assistance, training and research in Africa, Asia, Central and Eastern Europe, and Latin America. Events in Russia resulted in federal charges of money mismanagement that led to a fine of $25 million, which the university paid just as Larry Summers was beginning his term as president of Harvard. He was later criticized by faculty for his management of the issue after disclosure that several faculty members involved had been close colleagues.
4. C.P. Snow, *The Two Cultures*, first published in 1954. The talk was delivered May 7 in the Senate House, Cambridge, and subsequently published as *The Two Cultures and the Scientific Revolution*. The lecture and book expanded upon an article by Snow published

in the *New Statesman* on October 6, 1956, also entitled *The Two Cultures.* Published in book form, Snow's lecture was widely read and discussed on both sides of the Atlantic, leading him to write a 1964 follow-up, *The Two Cultures: And a Second Look: An Expanded Version of The Two Cultures and the Scientific Revolution.* In 2008, the *Times Literary Supplement* included *The Two Cultures and the Scientific Revolution* in its list of the one hundred books that most influenced Western public discourse since World War II.

5. Michael Lewis, *MoneyBall: The Art of Winning an Unfair Game* (New York: W.W. Norton, Inc., 2003).
6. L. Summers, The Seidman Lecture in Health Policy, delivered to faculty, sponsored by Department of Healthcare Policy, October 2004 (provided for the author's use by Barbara McNeil).
7. L. Summers, Fiftieth Anniversary Blackfan Lecture: "Science, Business, Medicine, and the University," delivered at the Children's Hospital of Boston, June 11, 2003 (provided for the author's use by Fred Lovejoy).
8. In "An Address on the hospital unit in university work," *The Lancet* 177, no. 4561 (January 28, 1911): 211–13.
9. J.B. Martin, "Summer's Bold Vision for the Life Sciences," *Boston Globe*, Op-Ed, February 24, 2006.
10. J.D. Watson, *Avoid Boring People: Lessons from a Life in Science* (New York: Random House, 2007).
11. S. Bagley, "Why Pundits get things wrong," *Newsweek* (February 23, 2009), 45.

## TEN

## *Harvard Medical School: 1997–2007*

1. Spencer Goldsmith, in an e-mail to the author, December 16, 2009.
2. Professor Paul Farmer was also elevated to this status in 2011.
3. R. Dolin in letter to D. Bok, May 11, 2007.
4. Joseph C. Rost, *Leadership for the Twenty-First Century* (New York: Praeger, 1991), 37ff.
5. For a full discussion, see Mary Louise Gill, "Method and Metaphysics in Plato's Sophist and Statesman," in Edward N. Zalta, ed., *The Stanford Encyclopedia of Philosophy* (Winter 2009 Edition), accessed February 17, 2011, http://plato.stanford.edu/archives/win2009/entries/plato-sophstate/. Of special interest is the section entitled "Weaving and Statecraft."
6. Gabriel García Márquez, *The Story of a Shipwrecked Sailor* (New York: Random House, 1986).

**ELEVEN**

## *Issues Facing Academic Medical Health Centers Today*

1. The name Mentor arises from Greek mythology. In *The Odyssey*, Odysseus sets out and leaves his son Telemachus to the tutelage of Mentor, who was actually the goddess Athena, disguised as a man. See Ann Shearer, *Athene: Image and Energy* (New York: Viking Arkana, the Penguin Group, 1996).
2. Neil L. Rudenstine, *Diversity and Learning at Harvard: A Historical View; Pointing our Thoughts: Reflections on Harvard and Higher Education: 1991–2001* (Cambridge, MA: Harvard University Press, 2001), 19–32.
3. Jeffrey Toobin, *The Nine: Inside the Secret World of the Supreme Court* (New York: Anchor Books, 2007), 256–57, 248–49.
4. Privileged communication by Jacob Yost, Harvard graduate student, April 2009.
5. H.T. Moses and J.B. Martin, "Biomedical Research and Health Advances" *New England Journal of Medicine*, 364 (2011): 567–71.
6. Drummond Rennie, "Thyroid Storm," *Journal of the American Medical Association* 277 (1997): 1238–43.
7. D.G. Nathan and D.J. Weatherall, "Academic Freedom in Clinical Research," *New England Journal of Medicine* 347 (2002): 1368–71.
8. Elizabeth Kagedan, "Mum's not the word," in the University of Toronto newspaper, *The Varsity*, accessed February 2010, www.thevarsity.ca, February 22, 2010.
9. Joyce Brinton, Personal communication to the author, June 9, 2009.
10. J.B. Martin, "The Pervasive Influence of Conflicts of Interest," *Neurology* 74 (2010): 2016–21.
11. Numerous reports appeared in these papers on these topics from 2008 to 2010. See Gardner Harris, "Academic researchers' conflicts of interest go unreported," *New York Times*, November 19, 2009; Rita Beamish, "HHS watchdog to recheck ethics," *USA Today*, March 30, 2007; "Feeling heat over financial conflicts, NIH mulls new rules for grantees," *Wall Street Journal*, December 8, 2008.
12. These eight points are included in J.B. Martin, "The Pervasive Influence of Conflicts of Interest," 2016–21. Also, many of these issues have been addressed in the most recent formulation of guidelines at Harvard Medical School under the leadership of Dean Jeffrey Flier. See http://hms.harvard.edu/public/coi/policy/integritypolicy.html.
13. Drummond Rennie, "Thyroid Storm," *Journal of the American Medical Association* 277 (1997): 1238–43.
14. Arnold S. Relman, "The New Medical-Industrial Complex," *New England Journal of Medicine* 303 (1980): 963–70.

15. Paul Starr, *The Social Transformation of American Medicine: The Rise of a Sovereign Profession and the Making of a Vast Industry* (New York: Basic Books, 1982).
16. Kenneth Ludmerer's *Time to Heal: American Medical Education from the Turn of the Century to the Era of Managed Care* (Oxford: Oxford University Press, 1999).
17. J.B. Martin, "Health Care 101: Single Form, Single Plan, Multiple Payers," *Boston Globe*, 2000, Op-Ed.
18. J.B. Martin, "Where have all the Doctors Gone?" Commencement Address, University of Rochester School of Medicine and Dentistry, May 2008.
19. Josiah Macy Foundation Report *"Preparing Health Professionals for a Changing Health Care System,"* 2010. See www.josiahmacyfoundation.org.
20. Atul Gawande, "McAllen, Texas, and the Cost of Medical Care," *The New Yorker*, June 1, 2009.
21. Arnold Relman, "Doctors as the key to health care reform," *New England Journal of Medicine* 36 (2009): 1225–27.
22. Paul Krugman, "Pass bill," *New York Times*, December 18, 2009.

**TWELVE**

## *Maxims, Proverbs and Aphorisms*

1. Adam Gopnik, "The Return of the Native," *The New Yorker*, September 7, 2009.
2. Josef Martin, *To Rise above Principle: The Memoirs of an Unreconstructed Dean* (Chicago: University of Illinois Press, 1987).
3. The corporation consisted of the president and six other internally appointed members. In 2010 this number was expanded to thirteen members in total.
4. Romans 2:15.
5. Howard Gardner, *Frames of the Mind: The Theory of Multiple Intelligence* (New York: Basic Books, 1993).
6. David Goleman, *Emotional Intelligence* (New York: Bantam Books, 1995).
7. For a full discussion, see Mary Louise Gill, "Method and Metaphysics in Plato's Sophist and Statesman," in Edward N. Zalta, ed., *The Stanford Encyclopedia of Philosophy* (Winter 2009 Edition), accessed February 17, 2011, http://plato.stanford.edu/archives/win2009/entries/plato-sophstate/. Of special interest is the section entitled "Weaving and Statecraft."

# PHOTO CREDITS

Page 71: Photo courtesy of Eastern Mennonite University.

Page 81: Photo courtesy of Case Western Reserve University School of Medicine.

Page 257: © 1998 President and Fellows of Harvard College on behalf of HMS Media Services (617) 432-0905. Photo by Liza Green. All rights reserved.

Page 265: Photo by Steve Gilbert, StudioFlex Productions, © 2001. All rights reserved.

Page 266: © 2002 President and Fellows of Harvard College on behalf of HMS Media Services (617) 432-0905. Photo by Liza Green. All rights reserved.

Pages 294 and 295: Aero Photo Inc., 801 Main Street, Wareham, MA 02571. All rights reserved.

Page 335: Photo by Graham G. Ramsay.

Page 389: Photo by Trudie Lee.

# INDEX

NOTE: The abbreviation "JBM" refers to the author, Joseph B. Martin. His father, of the same name, is abbreviated "JBM Sr."

# Other Books by The University of Alberta Press

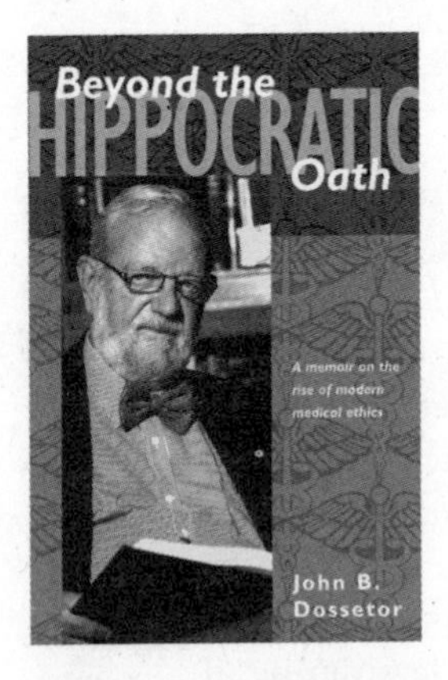


*Beyond the Hippocratic Oath*
*A Memoir on the Rise of Modern Medical Ethics*
John B. Dossetor

320 pages | B&W photographs, tables, figures, appendices, notes, bibliography, index
978-0-88864-453-4 | $39.95 (T) paper
Biography

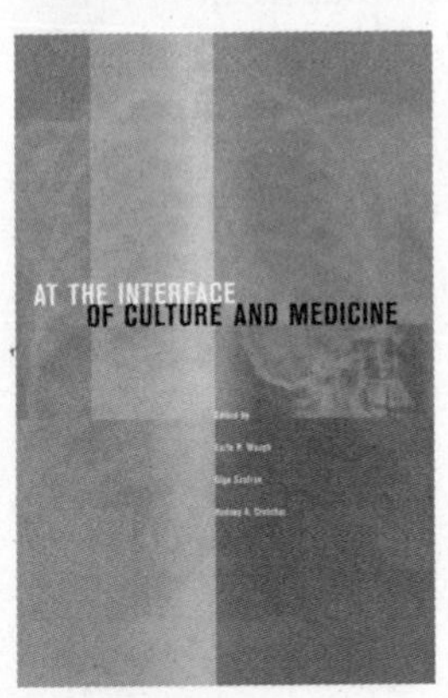


*At the Interface of Culture and Medicine*
Earle H. Waugh, Olga Szafran &
Rodney A. Crutcher, Editors

316 pages | Colour section, maps, figures, bibliography, index
978-0-88864-532-6 | $49.95 (S) paper
Medicine/Cultural Studies

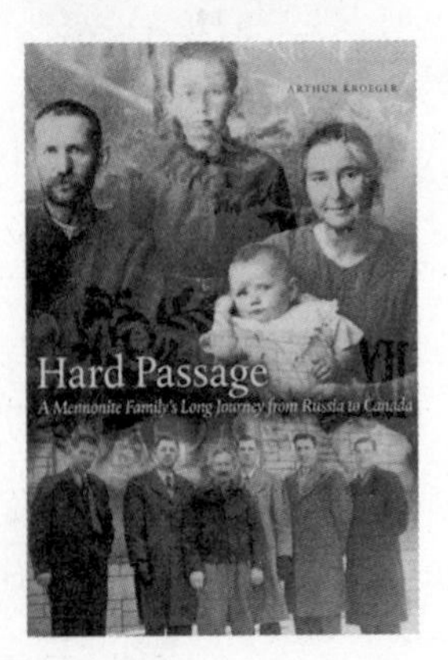


*Hard Passage*
*A Mennonite Family's Long Journey from Russia to Canada*
Arthur Kroeger

288 pages | B&W photographs, maps, notes, bibliography, index
978-0-88864-473-2 | $34.95 (T) paper
History/Immigration